ARTIFICIAL INSEMINATION IN FARM ANIMALS

Edited by **Milad Manafi**

Artificial Insemination in Farm Animals
Edited by Milad Manafi

Published by InTech

Janeza Trdine 9, 51000 Rijeka, Croatia

Publishing Process Manager Ana Pantar

Technical Editor Teodora Smiljanic

Cover Designer InTech Design Team

Additional hard copies can be obtained from orders@intechopen.com

Artificial Insemination in Farm Animals, Edited by Milad Manafi
p. cm.
ISBN 978-953-307-312-5

For EU product safety concerns:
IN TECH d.o.o., Prolaz Marije Krucifikse Kozulić 3, 51000 Rijeka, Croatia,
info@intechopen.com or visit our website at intechopen.com.

Meet the editor

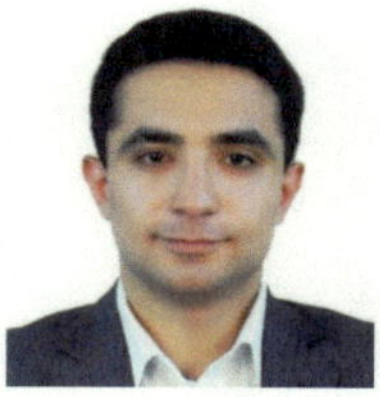

Dr. Milad Manafi has been Assistant Professor and Head of the Department of Animal Science at Malayer University (Iran) since 2009. Following his undergraduate studies at the Department of Animal Science, University of Applied Science, Damghan (Iran), he gained his Master degree and Ph.D. at the Department of Poultry Science, Bangalore Veterinary College, Bangalore (India) in 2009. After research appointments at various international companies, in 1999 he became the co-founder of the Animal Research Unit at the Simorgh Pvt., Ltd. (Iran), where he acted as its Scientific Coordinator until its transfer to India. His research interests are poultry nutrition, digestive physiology, poultry production and management, development of digestive function in poultry and other farm animals, as well as mycotoxins in poultry feed and mycotoxin resistant chickens. He has co-authored more than 60 scientific publications and presentations and holds 10 patents in Australia, France, China and India.

Contents

Preface

As we look back over the millennium, it is difficult to imagine man's evolution in the absence of domesticated livestock. Likewise, domesticated animals are so dependent upon man that in his absence their very existence would be jeopardized to the point where they would not thrive and some would fail to survive. Artificial insemination (AI) - one of the most important techniques ever devised for the genetic improvement of farm animals - is a widely used tool for livestock breeding and management programs and is a process by which sperm are collected from the male, processed, stored and artificially introduced into the female reproductive tract for the purpose of conception. A male animal produces millions of sperms daily. Theoretically, it can inseminate females regularly and produce several offsprings.

Artificial insemination is used instead of natural mating for reproduction purposes. This is when a male animal, for example, a bull, is kept with a herd of cows and 'covers' (copulates with) them when they are ready to mate (in oestrus) so the bull's semen fertilizes the cow's eggs to produce calves. Fertilization can take place away from the bull and the two animals do not even meet! Although AI (in the form of intrauterine insemination) is not frequently used in human patients, it is the most commonly used method of breeding food production animals in developed countries, with more than 90% pigs and almost the same proportion of dairy cattle bred by this method in the European Union and North America. In the actual procedure used, semen is obtained from a male animal and, after being diluted, is deep-frozen, after which it can be stored for long periods of time without losing its fertility. For use, the semen is thawed and then introduced into the genital tract of a female animal.

The first successful experiment with artificial insemination in animals was performed by an Italian physiologist *Lazzaro Spallanzani,* who in 1780, while investigating animal reproduction, developed a technique for artificial insemination in dogs. This approach was refined in the 1930s in Russia, and the subsequent development of methods for the cryopreservation (preservation through freezing) of semen led to the widespread use of AI in animals.

There are many advantages to artificial insemination (AI) in domesticated and zoo animals, such as smaller chance of injury to either partner during the mating process, less stress to the female, who is often the one that has to be transported to and from the home of the male, but one should keep in the mind that the system of reproduction is perfect, including artificial insemination. The chief priority of artificial insemination is that the desirable characteristics of a bull or other male livestock animal can be passed on more quickly and to more progeny than if that animal is mated with females in a natural fashion. Ten thousand or more calves are produced annually from a single bull through the use of artificial insemination.

Artificial insemination has been most widely used for breeding dairy cattle and pigs and has made bulls of high genetic merit available to all. It has been used to facilitate the reproductive success and conservation of threatened or endangered animals. Although AI (in the form of intrauterine insemination) is not frequently used in human patients, it is the most commonly used method of breeding food production animals in developed countries, with more than 90% pigs and almost the same proportion of dairy cattle bred by this method in the European Union and North America. Examples of wild animals that have been successfully impregnated through artificial insemination include big cats (e.g., the tiger, the puma, the cheetah, and the clouded leopard), the white rhinoceros (*Ceratotherium simum*) and the onager (*Equus onager*).

This book contains under one cover 16 chapters of concise, up-to-date information on artificial insemination. AI in buffalos, ewes, pigs, swine, sheep, goats, pigs and dogs will be detailed in different chapters. Cryopreservation effect on sperm quality and fertility, new method and diagnostic test in semen analysis, management factors affecting fertility after cervical insemination, factors of non-infectious nature affecting the fertility, fatty acids effects on reproductive performance of ruminants, particularities of bovine artificial insemination, sperm preparation techniques and reproductive endocrinology diseases will be described in these chapters.

The purpose of this book is to provide, as both a college text book and a reference source, a comprehensive text that contains current information on artificial insemination. This book is not a presentation of concepts of artificial insemination with an extensive list of references, but rather a consensus of important information with key references to allow the reader to further explore the artificial insemination field.

This book will deal with the use of artificial insemination (AI) in animals, currently and in the future, with particular emphasis on comparative aspects between species. This book will explain the advantages and disadvantages of using AI, the various methodologies used in different species, and how AI can be used to improve reproductive efficiency in farm animals.

I hope this book will be used worldwide as a college textbook and authoritative reference book for research and extension specialists, AI practitioners, teachers and students.

When preparing this book, I obtained numerous suggestions from eminent scientists in both Iran and other countries. I wish to express my sincere appreciation to them.

Milad Manafi
Assistant Professor and Head, Department of Animal Science,
Faculty of Agricultural Sciences, Malayer University, Malayer,
Iran

1

Artificial Insemination: Current and Future Trends

Jane M. Morrell
Swedish University of Agricultural Sciences, Uppsala, Sweden

1. Introduction

The chapter will deal with the use of artificial insemination (AI) in animals and humans, both currently and in the future, with particular emphasis on comparative aspects between species. Although AI (in the form of intrauterine insemination) is not frequently used in human patients, it is the most commonly used method of breeding food production animals in developed countries, with more than 90% pigs and almost the same proportion of dairy cattle bred by this method in the European Union and North America. This chapter will explain the advantages and disadvantages of using AI, the various methodologies used in different species, and how AI can be used to improve reproductive efficiency in farm animals, sport animals, and human patients. To finish, some speculation is made about future trends for this biotechnology.

1.1 What is artificial insemination (AI)?

Artificial insemination (AI) is the manual placement of semen in the reproductive tract of the female by a method other than natural mating. It is one of a group of technologies commonly known as "assisted reproduction technologies" (ART), whereby offspring are generated by facilitating the meeting of gametes (spermatozoa and oocytes). ART may also involve the transfer of the products of conception to a female, for instance if fertilization has taken place *in vitro* or in another female. Other techniques encompassed by ART include the following: *in vitro* fertilization (IVF) where fertilization takes place outside the body; intracytoplasmic sperm injection (ICSI) where a single spermatozoon is caught and injected into an oocyte; embryo transfer (ET) where embryos that have been derived either *in vivo* or *in vitro* are transferred to a recipient female to establish a pregnancy; gamete intrafallopian transfer (GIFT) where spermatozoa are injected into the oviduct to be close to the site of fertilization *in vivo*; and cryopreservation, where spermatozoa or embryos, or occasionally oocytes, are cryopreserved in liquid nitrogen for use at a later stage.
AI has been used in the majority of domestic species, including bees, and also in human beings. It is the most commonly used ART in livestock, revolutionising the animal breeding industry during the 20th century. In contrast to medical use, where intra-uterine insemination (IUI) is used only occasionally in human fertility treatment, AI is by far the most common method of breeding intensively kept domestic livestock, such as dairy cattle (approximately 80% in Europe and North America), pigs (more than 90% in Europe and North America) and turkeys (almost 100% in intensive production). AI is increasing in

horses, beef cattle and sheep, and has been reported in other domestic species such as dogs, goats, deer and buffalo. It has also been used occasionally in conservation breeding of rare or endangered species, for example, primates, elephants and wild felids. The other ARTs in animals are generally confined to specialist applications or for research purposes, since the cost would be prohibitive for normal livestock breeding. In contrast, IUI is used less often in human fertility treatments than IVF or ICSI.

1.2 Advantages and disadvantages of artificial insemination

AI in animals was originally developed to control the spread of disease, by avoiding the transport of animals with potential pathogens to other animal units for mating and by avoiding physical contact between individuals. The use of semen extenders containing antibiotics also helped to prevent the transmission of bacterial diseases. The advantages and disadvantages of AI are as follows:

Advantages:

- AI helps prevents the spread of infectious or contagious diseases, that can be passed on when animals are in close contact or share the same environment;
- The rate of genetic development and production gain can be increased, by using semen from males of high genetic merit for superior females;
- It enables breeding between animals in different geographic locations, or at different times (even after the male´s death);
- Breeding can occur in the event of physical, physiological or behavioural abnormalities;
- AI is a powerful tool when linked to other reproductive biotechnologies such as sperm cryopreservation, sperm sexing;
- AI can be used in conservation of rare breeds or endangered species.

Disadvantages:

- Some males shed virus in semen without clinical signs of disease ("shedders").
- Some bacterial pathogens are resistant to the antibiotics in semen extenders or can avoid their effects by forming bio-films;
- There has been a decline in fertility in dairy cattle and horses associated with an increase in AI;
- The focus on certain individuals may result in loss of genetic variation.

1.2.1 Viruses in semen

Cryopreserved semen doses can be "quarantined" until the male is shown to have been free of disease at the time of semen collection. In contrast, the short shelf-life of fresh semen doses means that they must be inseminated into the female before the disease-free status of the male has been established. Breeding sires used for semen collection are tested routinely for the presence of antibodies in serum as being indicative of past infection, but some viruses, e.g. equine arteritis virus, may be shed in semen for several weeks before there is evidence of sero-conversion. In other cases, usually of congenital infection, individuals may be permanent virus "shedders" without ever developing antibodies. Semen from these individuals represents a source of pathogens for disease transmission to naive females.

1.2.2 Bacteria in semen

Normally, in a healthy male, the ejaculate itself does not contain microorganisms, but contamination occurs at semen collection from the prepuce and foreskin, the male´s abdomen and the environment. Semen processing from livestock usually takes place without access to a laminar air flow hood, resulting in potential contamination from the laboratory environment. Antibiotics are added to semen extenders to limit the growth of these contaminants and prevent disease in the inseminated female. Although the female reproductive tract has well-developed physiological mechanisms for dealing with contamination introduced during mating, these can be overwhelmed by bacteria multiplying in semen extenders or where semen is deposited in a non-physiological location.

1.2.3 Antibiotics in semen extenders

The addition of antibiotics to semen extenders is controlled by government directives, both nationally and internationally, which state the types of antibiotic to be used and also their concentrations. In general, there is a tendency to use broad spectrum, highly potent antibiotics in various combinations to reduce sperm toxicity. However, these antibiotics may exacerbate the development of resistance, both for the people handling the semen extenders and in the environment during the disposal of unused extenders or semen doses. The scale of the problem becomes apparent if one considers that approximately **four million liters** of boar semen extender containing antibiotics are used in Europe alone per year.

2. Pre-requisites for AI

Pre-requisites for AI include a supply of semen, reliable methods for oestrus detection in the female and a means of inserting the semen into the female reproductive tract.

2.1 Collection of semen

In most domestic animals, semen is collected by means of an artificial vagina, for example, bull, ram, stallion, after allowing the male to mount either an oestrous female or a phantom. The artificial vagina consists of a lubricated liner inserted into an outer jacket, the space between the two being filled with warm water. The pressure can be increased by adding air. The ejaculate is deposited into an insulated collecting vessel attached to one end of the liner. Boar and dog semen is usually collected by manual stimulation.

In some species that are accustomed to being handled, it is possible to obtain semen by vaginal washing after natural mating, for example, dogs and marmoset monkeys. However, in this case the spermatozoa have already been exposed to vaginal secretions which may be detrimental to sperm survival. Human males can usually supply a sample by masturbation, except in the case of spinal injury when electroejaculation may be necessary. Some other primates can be trained to supply a semen sample on request in the same manner. For other species, for example, most non-domestic species, electroejaculation represents the only possibility for obtaining a semen sample. The problem with electroejaculation is that the secretions of the accessory glands may not be present in the usual proportions, which may have a detrimental effect on sperm survival.

2.1.1 Constituents of semen

Semen consists of spermatozoa contained in a watery fluid known as seminal plasma that represents the combined secretions of the different accessory glands, such as the seminal vesicles, bulbourethral gland and prostate. The relative contributions of these different glands vary between species. In some species, such a most primates, the semen coagulates immediately after ejaculation and then liquefies over a period of approximately 30 minutes. In most other species, the ejaculate remains liquid, the exception being in camelids where the seminal plasma is highly viscous and does not liquefy readily *in vitro*. The addition of enzymes has been suggested as a means of liquefying primate or camelid semen. However, all the enzymes tested thus far (collagenase, fibrinolysin, hyaluronidase and trypsin) have been seen to cause acrosomal damage in spermatozoa (Wani et al., 2007) and are contra-indicated if the spermatozoa are to be used for AI. Recent advances have shown that camelid semen, extended 1:1 volume to volume, will liquefy in 60-90 min at 37°C.

Seminal plasma contains an energy source (often fructose), proteins and various ions such as calcium, magnesium, zinc and bicarbonate. Seminal plasma not only activates the spermatozoa, which have been maintained in a quiescent state in the epididymis, but also functions as a transport medium to convey the spermatozoa into the female reproductive tract and to stimulate the latter to allow spermatozoa to swim to the site of fertilization. It has been suggested that seminal plasma, at least in horses, is also a modulator of sperm-induced inflammation, which is thought to play an important role in sperm elimination from the female reproductive tract (Troedsson et al., 2001). Various proteins in the seminal plasma, such as spermadhesins and the so-called CRISP proteins (CRISP = cysteine-rich secretory proteins) are thought to be associated with sperm fertility. It is likely that these proteins bind to spermatozoa immediately, setting in motion a sequence of intracellular events via a second-messenger pathway. In some species, small membrane-bound vesicles have also been identified in seminal plasma, apparently originating from different accessory glands in various species. These vesicles, variously named prostasomes, vesiculosomes, or epididysomes depending on their origin, fuse with the sperm outer membrane, increasing motility and possibly being involved in sperm capacitation and acquisition of fertilizing ability. However, their exact mechanism of action has yet to be elucidated.

Seminal factors promote sperm survival in the female reproductive tract, modulate the female immune response tolerate the conceptus, and to condition the uterine environment for embryo development and the endometrium for implantation (Robertson, 2005). The mechanism of action in the endometrium is via the recruitment and activation of macrophages and granulocytes, and also dendritic re-modelling, that improve endometrial receptivity to the implanting embryo. Cytokine release has embryotrophic properties and may also influence tissues outside the reproductive tract.

Exposure to semen induces cytokine activation into the uterine luminal fluid and epithelial glycocalyx lining the luminal space. These cytokines interact with the developing embryo as it traverses the oviduct and uterus prior to implantation. Several cytokines are thought to be involved, for example granulocyte-macrophage colony stimulating factor (GM-CSF), a principle cytokine in the post-mating inflammatory response, targets the pre-implantation embryo to promote blastocyst formation, increasing the number of viable blastomeres by inhibiting apoptosis and facilitating glucose uptake (Robertson et al., 2001). Interleukin-6 (IL-6) and leukocyte inhibitory factor (LIF) are similarly induced after exposure to semen (Gutsche et al., 2003; Robertson et al., 1992).

Clinical studies in humans showed acute and cumulative benefits of exposure to seminal fluid but also a partner-specific route of action. Live birth rates in couples undergoing fertility treatments are improved if women engage in intercourse close to embryo transfer (Bellinge et al., 1986; Tremellen et al., 2000). The use of seminal plasma pessaries by women suffering from recurrent spontaneous abortion is reported to improve pregnancy success

(Coulam and Stern, 1993, cited in Robertson, 2005). Partner-specificity of the response is suggested by increased rates of preeclampsia in pregnancies from donor oocytes or semen when prior exposure to the donor sperm or conceptus antigens has not occurred (Salha et al., 1999).

2.1.1.2 Semen processing

Although seminal plasma plays such an important role in activating spermatozoa and in the female reproductive tract, it is detrimental to long-term sperm survival outside the body. Under physiological conditions, spermatozoa are activated by seminal plasma at ejaculation and then swim away from the site of semen deposition in the female. It is only during *in vitro* storage that spermatozoa become exposed to seminal plasma long-term. Thus it is customary to add a semen extender to the semen, to dilute toxic elements in seminal plasma, to provide nutrients for the spermatozoa during *in vitro* storage and to buffer their metabolic by-products. The addition of extender also permits the semen to be divided into several semen doses, each containing a specific number of spermatozoa that has been determined to be optimal for good fertility in inseminated females.

2.1.2 Semen preservation

Semen is used either immediately after collection ("fresh") for example turkeys, human beings; after storage at a reduced temperature ("stored") for example horses, pigs, dogs; or after freezing and thawing ("cryopreservation") for example, bulls.

2.1.2.1 Fresh semen

In contrast to animal species, human semen is not extended prior to processing (see previous section) and is not usually kept for more than a few hours before use. Poultry semen cannot be extended as much as is customary for other species since the spermatozoa are adversely affected by increased dilution. Goat semen cannot be kept at 37°C because an enzymatic component of the bulbo-urethral gland secretion hydrolyses milk triglycerides into free fatty acids, which adversely affects the motility and membrane integrity of buck spermatozoa (Pellicer-Rubio and Combarnous, 1998). For liquid preservation, goat semen can be stored at 4°C although fertility is retained for only 12-24h. The rate of extension used for stallion semen varies between countries but rates of 1:2, 1:3 or even 1:4 (v/v) semen:extender are common. The standard practice in some countries is to have 500 million or one billion progressively motile stallion spermatozoa for fresh or cooled semen doses respectively. Boar semen doses contain three billion progressively motile spermatozoa.

2.1.2.2 Stored semen

Storing extended semen at reduced temperature helps to extend sperm life by slowing their metabolism as well as by inhibiting bacterial growth. Bacteria grow by utilizing the nutrients in semen extenders, thus competing with spermatozoa for these limited resources, and release metabolic byproducts, thus creating an environment that is not conducive to maintaining viable spermatozoa. Furthermore, as bacteria die, they may release endotoxins that are toxic to spermatozoa. However, cooled stored semen is the method of choice for breeding horses and pigs, enabling the semen dose to be transported to different locations for insemination. Stallion semen is stored at approximately 6°C while boar semen is stored between 16 and 18°C.

Most boar semen doses are sold as cooled doses. In contrast, some stallions produce spermatozoa that do not tolerate cooling, rapidly losing progressive motility. In such cases, the only option currently is to use fresh semen doses for AI immediately after semen collection, although a new method of processing, centrifugation through a single layer of colloid, has been shown to solve the problem, as discussed later.

2.1.2.3 Cryopreservation

Semen is most useful for AI if it can be cryopreserved, since this method of preservation ideally enables the semen to be stored for an unlimited period without loss of quality until needed for AI. Since the frozen semen does not deteriorate, it can be quarantined until the male has been shown to be free from disease at the time of semen collection. However, the spermatozoa of various species differ in their ability to withstand cryopreservation: ruminant spermatozoa survive well whereas poultry spermatozoa do not, with less than 2% retaining their fertilizing ability on thawing (Wishart, 1985). For farm animal breeding, the cost of cryopreservation and the likelihood of a successful outcome following AI must be considered when deciding whether to use fresh, cooled or frozen sperm doses.

The spermatozoa are mixed with a protective solution containing lipoproteins, sugars and a cryoprotectant such as glycerol. These constituents help to preserve membrane integrity during the processes of cooling and re-warming. However, sperm motility must also be maintained, so that the thawed spermatozoa can reach the oocytes after insemination and fertilize them. In most species, the seminal plasma is removed by centrifugation before mixing with the cryoextender, for example, stallion, boar, goat and human semen. The extended semen is packed in straws and frozen in liquid nitrogen vapour before plunging into liquid nitrogen for long-term storage. There is considerable variation in the success of sperm cryopreservation between different species, despite intensive research into the constituents of cryoextenders and the rates of cooling and re-warming. Human spermatozoa can be frozen relatively successfully using commercially available cryoextenders and programmable freezing machines.

2.2 Oestrus detection and ovulation

Successful AI also depends on depositing the semen in the female tract at around the time of ovulation. Like human beings, some domestic animals breed throughout the year, for example cattle and pigs, but others show a defined period of reproductive activity known as the breeding season, for example sheep and horses. The onset of the breeding season is controlled by photoperiod. Both of these patterns of reproductive behaviour are characterised by waves of ovarian activity, culminating in ovulation. However, in some other species ovulation occurs in response to the stimulus of mating, for example, cats, rabbits and camels. In spontaneously ovulating species, ovulation occurs at some time during, or shortly after, oestrus, which is the period of time when the female is receptive to the male. Since a successful outcome for AI depends on the deposition of spermatozoa at a suitable time relative to ovulation, oestrus detection is crucial if the female is to be inseminated at the correct time. Males of the same species are, of course, very good at detecting oestrus females, but since many livestock breeding units that practice AI do not have male animals in the vicinity, it is essential that husbandry personnel become good at recognising oestrous behaviour.

Although some domestic animals may show well-developed oestrous behaviour, e.g. dairy cows, others may not. Behavioural signs of oestrus in cows include restlessness or increased activity, vocalization, chin resting, swelling of the vulva, vaginal discharge and mounting other cows, although there are breed differences in the frequency and intensity of these signs. In sheep and goats, vulval swelling and vaginal discharge may be seen, and there is usually pronounced male-seeking behaviour. When AI is to be used in sheep, it is usual to synchronize oestrus with hormones: intravaginal sponges impregnated with progestagens are inserted to suppress the ewe´s natural ovarian cycle for 12 days. On sponge removal, pregnant mare serum gonadotrophin is administered, with AI taking place at a set time thereafter. Alternatively, a vasectomised ram wearing a marker can be run with the females. When the females are in oestrus, the vasectomised ram marks them as he mounts, thus enabling them to be identified for AI. Oestrous sows and mares can be identified by the behaviour exhibited towards teaser males.

2.2.1 Induced ovulation

When AI is performed in species that are normally induced ovulators, such as rabbits, cats and camels, it is necessary to stimulate ovulation. The easiest way to achieve this stimulation is to mate the female with a vasectomised male, but this practice is not desirable from the point of view of disease control and necessitates having vasectomized males available. The most acceptable alternative is to administer luteinising hormone , usually in the form of human chorionic gonadotrophin. However, the major disadvantage is that repeated injections of this foreign protein may cause the female to develop antibodies, thus inactivating subsequent doses.

2.2.2 Artificially induced ovulation

Hormones may be administered to spontaneous ovulators to ensure that ovulation occurs at the correct time relative to AI. However, since 2006, the use of hormones in food-producing animals has been forbidden in the European Union, and local regulations may also apply in other parts of the world. Previously most dairy goats in France were inseminated out of the breeding season with deep frozen semen, after induction of oestrus and ovulation by hormonal treatments. This protocol provided a kidding rate of approximately 65% (Leboeuf et al., 2008). As an alternative to administering artificial hormones, out-of season breeding may be induced by altering the photoperiod or by introducing a buck to the herd. This practice is also widespread in intensive sheep flocks.

2.3 Deposition of semen in the female

There are differences between species in the site of semen deposition during natural mating. In ruminants and primates, semen is deposited in the vagina whereas in pigs, dogs, camels and horses, semen deposition is intrauterine. In most species, it is possible to pass an insemination catheter through the cervix, thus enabling semen to be deposited in the uterus during AI. Exceptions are sheep and goats, where the tightly folded nature of the cervix does not permit easy passage of an insemination catheter. The advantages of depositing the semen in the uterus are that the spermatozoa have less far to travel to reach the oviducts and fewer spermatozoa are lost through back-flow. A smaller volume of semen can be used per insemination dose than for intravaginal deposition, thus permitting an ejaculate to be divided into several AI doses, and the cervix, which can act as a barrier to the passage of spermatozoa, is bypassed. A disadvantage, particularly for human IUI, is that seminal plasma is also introduced into the uterus, unless specific steps are taken to separate the spermatozoa from seminal plasma before IUI.

3. Species differences in the use of AI

Despite the fact that the basic principles of AI are the same in all species, there is wide variation in the uptake of this biotechnology in different species.

3.1 AI in cattle

In cattle, frozen semen doses are used most widely in Europe and North America, since there are well-established protocols for cryopreserving bull semen. Semen doses typically contain approximately 15 million motile spermatozoa. In New Zealand, however, fresh semen doses are used instead, with AI occurring within 24h of semen collection.

3.2 AI in pigs

The porcine AI industry uses liquid semen that has been stored for one to several days at 16-18°C. In contrast, AI with cryopreserved boar spermatozoa results in lower farrowing rates and litter sizes than with cooled, stored spermatozoa, making the use of frozen-thawed sperm doses unattractive for commercial pig breeders. Exceptions to this rule are when semen is transported over long distances, which creates problems in temperature regulation, and in instances where it is vital that the boars can be shown to be free of disease at the time of semen collection. The ability of boar spermatozoa to survive cool storage so well is attributed to low levels of reactive oxygen species (ROS) in semen or to the efficient scavenging of ROS by anti-oxidative components in seminal plasma.

3.3 AI in horses

AI has increased in horses in the last 25 years. Initially, fresh semen was used for AI shortly after semen collection, but nowadays the use of cooled semen has largely replaced fresh semen in Europe and North America. The extended semen is cooled to approximately 5°, and transported in insulated containers, together with a cold pack. The fertility of the cooled semen is maintained for approximately 24h. Frozen semen doses are used infrequently, although this trend may change with the development of better freezing protocols. However, with the increased use of cooled semen, a concomitant decrease in foaling rate has been observed in several countries, such as Finland and Sweden, although the reason for this apparent decline in fertility is unknown. Unlike bulls and boars, which are selected for their semen quality as well as for their potential "genetic merit" in production characteristics (body composition, weight gain, milk production etc), the choice of stallions as breeding sires is based solely on their performance in competition. Thus, considerable variation in semen quality exists between stallions. This variation, coupled with increased use of a wider range of stallions, may be contributing to the observed decline in foaling rate. Other important considerations are the lack of established standard methods for cooling and freezing of stallion spermatozoa, for the sperm concentration in the insemination dose, or for quality control of raw or frozen/thawed spermatozoa.

3.4 AI in sheep

Ram semen differs from stallion and boar semen in consisting of a small volume (a few mL) of seminal plasma containing a very high concentration of spermatozoa. In Europe, reproductive research in livestock has tended to focus on cattle and pigs rather than on small ruminants, with the result that sperm handling and cryopreservation for AI is less advanced in the latter species. In addition, the anatomy of the female reproductive tract in these species presents more of a barrier to successful insemination than in cattle, since the cervix is tightly folded, making insertion of the insemination catheter difficult. Productivity in sheep and goats could be increased, by improving the quality of the spermatozoa assigned for use in AI, and improving the AI techniques in these species. Recent innovations in sheep breeding include the development of a flexible catheter at the National Center for Genetic Resource Preservation, Fort Collins, Colorado, that can be inserted through the ovine cervix, thus overcoming the barrier to effective AI in this species.

AI in sheep and goats is traditionally performed with fresh or cooled spermatozoa, with acceptable fertility results. However, use of foreign breeds, genetic improvement and the use of "safe" semen from other countries requires the use of frozen semen, to enable analyses for contaminants or diseases in the "donor" male to be completed before the semen doses are used for AI. Although the post-thaw motility of frozen semen from goats and sheep is usually considered acceptable, low fertility has been associated with its use in AI, mainly owing to a shortened lifespan of the spermatozoa.

3.5 Intrauterine insemination in human fertility treatment

It is estimated that 10-20% of couples wanting to conceive are unable to do so without some assistance. In 40% of cases, sub-fertility is due to female factors, with a further 40% being due to male factors. The remaining cases may be multifactorial or idiopathic in origin. The use of IUI is generally contraindicated in male factor infertility, with IVF or ICSI being the treatments of choice. Since spermatozoa must be able to reach the site of fertilization and the products of conception must be able to reach the uterus for implantation, female factor infertility due to blockage of the oviducts is better treated by IVF or ICSI than by IUI. The patient´s own semen or donor semen may be utilized for these fertility treatments.

4. AI - State of the art

AI can help to improve reproductive efficiency in animals for food production or sport. We are living in a world of scarce resources where there is constant competition for water, food, land and energy. Since protein of animal origin continues to be one of the most important forms of nourishment for human beings, animals are an essential part of the ecosystem and must be husbanded in a sustainable fashion. Animal production not only "competes" with human beings for the aforementioned resources, but also produces large amounts of effluent and gaseous emissions which can affect the environment. Therefore, it is vital for the survival of the planet that all aspects of animal production are justified and optimized. Through grazing or browsing and the recycling of nutrients, animals also contribute to maintaining the landscape in a productive state.

The production of food of animal origin is based on breeding offspring to enter various husbandry systems. Therefore, one of the first points for optimization is in increasing reproductive efficiency, using an holistic approach. Females should be bred for the first time at an appropriate age to ensure the birth of healthy offspring and optimum lactation, without compromising the health of the female. Subsequent breeding attempts should also be timed appropriately to balance the metabolic requirements of lactation and early pregnancy. Females not conceiving or showing early embryonic loss should be identified at an early stage for re-breeding or culling. However, optimizing female reproduction demands a supply of spermatozoa. The spermatozoa must be readily available (i.e. can be stored), robust, and capable of fertilization, initiation of early embryonic development and regulation of placental formation, and there must be a means of delivery to an appropriate site in the female.

5. AI in other species

AI in non-domestic species presents several new challenges compared with domestic species. In many cases little is known about the reproductive biology of the species in question, and handling the animals may cause them stress, with the attendant risk of injury. The animals must be managed correctly for the establishment and maintenance of pregnancy. There are reports of successful AI in deer, buffalo and camelids.

6. Future trends in AI

It is highly probable that the use of AI in livestock will continue to increase. AI not only facilitates more effective and efficient livestock production, but can also be coupled to other developing biotechnologies, such as cryopreservation, selection of robust spermatozoa by single layer centrifugation, and sperm sex selection.

6.1 AI in increasing the efficiency of livestock production

Apart from some specialist sheep or goat units focussing on milk production for cheese and intensive meat production, farming of these species tends to be confined to marginal land that is unsuitable for crop production or grazing for dairy cattle. There has been limited selection for production traits. However, there is a resurgence of interest in them now in developed countries because of growing awareness that small ruminants could represent better utilization of scare resources than larger ones, such as cattle, while producing less methane and effluent. In many developing countries, sheep and goats are better suited to the climate than cattle, and it is culturally acceptable to eat their meat and milk products. Thus it is likely that there will be an upsurge in the use of AI in sheep and goats in the future, with an emphasis on improving production traits by the introduction of superior genes. However, it is essential that any A.I. scheme aimed at large scale improvement of the national herd must be supported by improved animal husbandry and animal health, otherwise the pregnancies resulting from AI will not go to term, and the offspring will either not survive or will fail to thrive. Many of the advanced ART are of little help in areas where basic husbandry skills are inadequate.

6.2 Biomimetic sperm selection

One potential disadvantage of AI is that the natural selection mechanisms within the female reproductive tract to select the best spermatozoa for fertilization may be bypassed when AI is utilized. Biomimetics is the use of technologies and/or processes that mimic a naturally occurring event. Several *in vitro* procedures have been suggested that could be used to mimic selection of good quality spermatozoa in the female reproductive tract and thus fit the definition of biomimetics in ART. These include sperm processing procedures such as swim-up, sperm migration, filtration and colloid centrifugation (reviewed by Morrell & Rodriguez-Martinez, 2009). Of these methods, the one that is most applicable to livestock and human spermatozoa is colloid centrifugation.

6.2.1 Density gradient centrifugation

Human spermatozoa for fertility treatment are usually processed to remove the seminal plasma and to select those of better quality. In most cases, this is achieved either by sperm migration, in which the more motile spermatozoa are separated from the rest of the ejaculate, or by density gradient centrifugation, where the most robust spermatozoa are selected. The benefits of density gradient centrifugation are as follows (Morrell, 2006):

i. Poorly motile and abnormal spermatozoa are removed,
ii. Sources of ROS (cell debris, leukocytes, epithelial cells and dead or dying spermatozoa) are removed;
iii. Sperm survival is improved during frozen and non-frozen storage;
iv. Bacterial contamination is controlled without antibiotics.

6.2.2 Single layer centrifugation

Density gradient centrifugation is seldom used when processing animal semen because of the limited volume of semen that can be processed at one time and the time taken to prepare the different layers. A novel sperm preparation technique, Single Layer Centrifugation (SLC) through a colloid, was developed at the Swedish University of Agricultural Sciences (SLU) to select the most robust spermatozoa from ejaculates. This method is similar to density gradient centrifugation (DGC), but is better suited for animal semen since it has been scaled-up to process whole ejaculates. The major applications for SLC-selection are similar to DGC end have been reviewed extensively by Morrell & Rodriguez-Martinez (2010)

6.3 Sex selection

For many centuries, animal breeders and researchers have endeavoured to control the sex of the offspring born, for various reasons. Initially male offspring were preferred for meat production, because of the better feed conversion efficiency and lean-to-fat ratio of males, whereas females were preferred for dairy purposes, except that some males of high genetic merit were still required as sires. Couples may want a child of a specific sex to avoid the expression of sex-linked disorders.

Many methods have been proposed for separating X- and Y-chromosome bearing spermatozoa, based on physical properties, e.g. size of the sperm head, or functional properties e.g. swimming speed. However, the only method which has been shown to work reliably is that of selection and separation of spermatozoa whose DNA is stained with a bis-benzimidazole dye, H33342, using the sorting capacity of a flow cytometer (Morrell et al., 1988; Johnson et al., 1989). This method functions because the X chromosome is larger than the Y, therefore taking up more of the DNA-specific stain and showing a higher fluorescence when the spermatozoa are passed through a laser beam. In bulls, for example, the difference in DNA content between the X and Y- chromosome is approximately 4.2%. However, the process of sorting sufficient numbers for an insemination dose in the flow cytometer takes too long, since the stained spermatozoa must pass one at a time through a laser beam for detection of their DNA content. Moreover, the pregnancy rate after insemination of sexed bull spermatozoa is lower than with unsexed spermatozoa, making the procedure inefficient and expensive. Experience has shown that the staining profiles are highly individual, with the result that it is not possible to separate the X- and Y-chromosome bearing spermatozoa efficiently from all males.

Alternative methods of sex selection are also being investigated. A company in Wales, Ovasort, has identified sex-specific proteins on the sperm surface and have raised antibodies to them. It is intended to use the antibodies to aggregate spermatozoa bearing a specific sex chromosome, thus enabling them to be removed from the general population.

A combination of ARTs would also be relevant for sperm sexing. Thus, the speed of flow sorting can be increased by first removing the dead and dying spermatozoa from the population, for example by density gradient centrifugation or single layer centrifugation. Such a combination may increase the "sortability" of sperm samples. Sufficient sexed spermatozoa may be obtained from flow sorting for IVF, thus generating embryos or blastocysts for subsequent transfer. However, methods of speeding up the selection process are needed if flow cytometry is to become useful for species other than the bovine.

6.4 Sperm cryopreservation

As previously mentioned, the ability of cryopreserved spermatozoa to retain their fertilizing ability varies widely between species. New cryoextenders and new protocols are being developed constantly in an effort to address this issue. One recent advance has been the introduction of dimethylsulphoxide and the amides formamide and dimethylformamide as cryoprotectants, in place of glycerol. These molecules seem to function better than glycerol for some individuals whose spermatozoa do not freeze well, for example, some stallions. One explanation for this observation is that these molecules are smaller than glycerol and therefore may cause less damage when they penetrate the sperm membrane. However, no method appears to be universally successful within one species. As far as turkey spermatozoa are concerned, it seems that the development of a successful freezing method will require more than new cryoprotectants and additives (Holt, 2000).

6.5 Removal of viruses from ejaculates

Viral infectivity can be removed from the semen of patients with viral infections such as HIV and hepatitis, by a sequential method of sperm preparation i.e. centrifugation on a density gradient followed by a "swim-up" (reviewed by Englert et al., 2004). Spermatozoa from virally infected men prepared by this method have been used in assisted reproduction attempts, apparently without sero-conversion of mothers or children. However, some studies with HIV report that density gradient centrifugation alone will not remove all viral infectivity (Politch *et al.,* 2004). Since spermatozoa may function as vectors for viruses (Chan *et al.,* 2004), further work is required to investigate how closely different viral particles are associated with the sperm membrane with putative carry-over during processing. The double method of processing has also been successful in removing equine arteritis virus from an infected stallion ejaculate in a preliminary study (Morrell & Geraghty, 2006). SLC together with swim-up was used to reduce viral infectivity from boar semen spiked with porcine circo virus 2 (Blomqvist et al., 2011).

6.5 AI in conservation biology

It has been suggested that AI and other forms of ART could be useful for genetic conservation and preservation of rare breeds. Many of these technologies have been successful to some degree in a research setting, but none have produced results sufficient to effect population-wide improvements in genetic management (Morrow et al., 2009). Cryopreservation of semen has been the most widely applied ART in this respect, but much of the frozen semen in so-called gene banks has never been tested for fertility. A lack of suitable females or dearth of knowledge about the reproductive biology of the species involved may contribute to this deficit. However, long-term storage of frozen gametes of unknown fertility is not a sustainable policy for the conservation of rare breeds and endangered species. The development of *in vitro* methods of testing sperm fertility would contribute considerably to conservation efforts. Since the semen quality in these animals may be poor (Gamboa et al., 2009), techniques such as SLC of samples prior to AI could be of considerable benefit in conservation breeding.

7. Conclusion

AI revolutionized animal breeding in the 20th century, particularly in combination with sperm cryopreservation. The AI industry has developed dramatically in most domestic species in the last few decades and its use is now widespread in intensive animal production. The development of other associated technologies, such as sperm selection and sex selection, are predicted to create powerful tools for the future, both for domestic livestock breeding and for the purposes of conservation. AI will continue to play a role in fertility treatment for human patients, although it may be superseded by IVF or ICSI. It has been suggested that AI (in animals) is entering a new era where it will be used for the efficient application of current and new sperm technologies (Roca, 2006). Exciting possibilities are offered by emerging techniques, such as Single Layer Centrifugation, for improving sperm quality in AI doses as well as for increasing sperm survival during cryopreservation.

8. References

Bellinge, B.S., Copeland, C.M., Thomas, T.D., Mazzucchelli, R.E., O'Neil, G., Cohen M.J. (1986). The influence of patient insemination on the implantation rate in an in vitro fertilization and embryo transfer program. *Fertil Steril,*, Vol. 46, 2523–2526.

Chan, P.J., Su, BC., Kalugdan, T., Seraj, J.M., Tredway, D.R., King, A. (1994). Human papillomavirus gene sequences in washed human sperm deoxyribonucelic acid. *Fertil Steril.*, Vol. 61, pp. 982-985.

Englert, Y., Lesage, B., van Vooren, J.P, Liesnard, C., Place, I., Vannin, A.S., Emiliani, S., Delbaere, A. (2004). Medically assisted reproduction in the presence of chronic viral disease. *Hum. Reprod. Update,* Vol. 10, pp. 149-162.

Gamboa, S., Machado-Faria M,, Ramalho-Santos J. (2009). Seminal traits, suitability for semen preservation and fertility in the native Portuguese horse breeds Puro Sangue Lusitano and Sorraia: Implications for stallion classification and assisted reproduction. *Anim Reprod Sci.*Vol.113, pp.102-113.

Gutsche, S., Wolff, M., von Strowitzki, T., Thaler CJ. (2003). Seminal plasma induces mRNA expression of IL-1β, IL-6 and LIF in endometrial epithelial cells in vitro. *Mol Hum Reprod,* Vol. 9, pp. 785–791.

Holt, WV. (2000). Basic aspects of frozen storage of semen. *Anim. Reprod. Sci.*, Vol. 62, 3–22.

Leboeuf, B., Delgadillo, JA., Manfredi, E., Piacere, A., Clement, V., Martin, P., Pellicer, M., Boue, P., de Cremoux, R. (2008) Management of Goat Reproduction and Insemination for Genetic Improvement in France *Reprod Dom Anim,* Vol. 43 (Suppl. 2), pp. 379–385

Johnson, L.A., Flook, J.P. and Hawk, H.W. (1989). Sex preselection in rabbits: live births from X and Y sperm separated by DNA and cell sorting. *Biol Reprod.* Vol. 41, pp.199-203.

Morrell, J.M., Keeler, K.D., Noakes, D.E., MacKenzie, N.M. & Dresser, D.W. (1988). Sexing of sperm by flow cytometry. *Veterinary Record,* Vol. 122, pp. 322-324.

Morrell, J.M. (2006). Update on semen technologies for animal breeding. *Reproduction in Domestic Animals,* Vol. 41, pp. 63-67.

Morrell, J.M. & Geraghty, R.J. (2006). Effective removal of equine arteritis virus from stallion semen. *Equine Veterinary Journal.* Vol.38, pp. 224-229.

Morrell, J.M., Rodriguez-Martinez, H. (2009). Biomimetic techniques for improving sperm quality in animal breeding: a review. The Open Andrology Journal, Vol. 1, pp. 1-9.

Morrell, J.M., Rodriguez-Martinez, H. (2010). Practical applications of sperm selection techniques as a tool for improving reproductive efficiency. *Veterinary Medicine International,* doi:10.4061/2011/2984767

Morrow, C.J., Penfold, L.M,, Wolfe, B.A.(2009). Artificial insemination in deer and non-domestic bovids. Theriogenology. Vol. 71, pp. 149-65

Pellicer-Rubio, M., Combarnous, Y. (1998). Deterioration of goat spermatozoa in skimmed milk-based extenders as a result of oleic acid released by the bulbourethral lipase BUSgp60. *J Reprod Fertil,* Vol. 112, pp. 95–105.

Politch, J.A., Xu, C., Tucker, L., Anderson, D.J. (2004). Separation of human immunodeficiency virus type 1 from motile sperm by the double tube gradeint method versus other methods. *Fertil. Steril.,* Vol. 81, pp. 440-447.

Robertson, S.A., Mayerhofer, G., Seamark, R.F. (1992). Uterine epithelial cells synthesize granulocyte-macrophage colony-stimulating factor and interleukin-6 in pregnant and nonpregnant mice. *Biol Reprod,* Vol. 46, pp. 1069–1079

Robertson, S.A., Sjoblom, C., Jasper, M.J., Norman, R.J., Seamark, R.F. (2001). Granulocyte-macrophage colony-stimulating factor promotes glucose transport and blastomere viability in murine preimplantation embryos. *Biol Reprod* Vol. 64, pp. 1206–1215

Robertson, S.A. (2005). Seminal plasma and male factor signalling in the female reproductive tract. *Cell Tissue Res,* Vol. 322, pp. 43–52

Roca, J., Vazquez, J.M., Gil, M.A., Cuello, C., Parrilla, I., Martinez, E.A. (2006). Challenges in Pig Artificial Insemination. *Reprod Dom Anim,* Vol. 41 (Suppl. 2), pp. 43–53.

Salha, O., Sharma, V., Dada, T., Nugent, D., Rutherford, A.J., Tomlinson, A.J., Philips, S., Allgar, V., Walker, J.J. (1999). The influence of donated gametes on the incidence of hypertensive disorders of pregnancy. *Hum Reprod,* Vol. 14, pp. 2268–2273.

Tremellen, K.P., Valbuena, D., Landera, S. J., Ballesteros, A., Martinez, J., Mendoza, S., Norman, R.J., Robertson, S.A., Simon, C. (2000). The effect of intercourse on pregnancy rates during assisted human reproduction. *Hum Reprod,* Vol. 15, pp. 2653–2658.

Troedsson, M.H., Loset, K., Alghamdi, A.M., Dahms, B., Crabo, B.G. (2001). Interaction between equine semen and the endometrium: the inflammatory response to semen. *Anim Reprod Sci* , Vol. 68, pp. 273–278.

Wani, N.A., Billah, M., Skidmore, J.A. (2007). Studies on liquefaction and storage of ejaculated dromedary camel (*Camelus dromedarius*) semen. *Anim Reprod Sci,* Vol. 109, 309-318.

Wishart, G.J. (1985). Quantitation of the fertilising ability of fresh compared with frozen and thawed fowl spermatozoa. *British Poultry Science,* Vol. 26, pp. 375–380.

2

Artificial Insemination at Fixed Time in Bufalloes

Gustavo Ángel Crudeli[1] and Rodolfo Luzbel de la Sota[2]
[1]*Professor of Theriogenology, Faculty of Veterinary Sciences, Nor Eastern National University, Corrientes,*
[2]*Professor of Theriogenology, Faculty of Veterinary Sciences, National University of La Plata, La Plata, Argentina*

1. Introduction

To maintain a calving interval of 13-14 month in buffaloes, successful breeding must take place within 85-115 days (d) after calving. Complete uterine involution and resumption of ovarian activity and heat expression usually takes place around 20-50 d post partum (dpp); therefore, there is a window of 35-95 d to rebreed a cow and get her pregnant to maintain the desired calving interval. Although artificial insemination (AI) has the potential to make a significant contribution to genetic improvement in buffaloes, its practical application has been difficult because poor estrus expression by cows and poor estrus detection by humans, a variable duration of estrus and the difficulty to predict time of ovulation. More recently, the development of protocols for synchronization of ovulation and fixed timed insemination (TAI) in buffaloes have been used to overcome these constrains and be able to use more extensively AI in commercial herds. Nevertheless, resynchronization of ovulation and TAI still remains a problem herds managed under extensive conditions for similar reasons abovementioned.

Very recently, we did four field trials to study the efficacy of different protocols that combined use of GnRH, or estradiol benzoate (EB), prostaglandin (PGF) and intravaginal progesterone (P_4) releasing device (PIVD) or norgestomet ear implant (NOR) to resynchronize estrus and ovulation at day 18 post AI in buffalo cows under commercial conditions.

2. Materials and methods

2.1 First trial

In the first field trial, we assessed with ultrasonography the ovarian follicular dynamics to study the efficacy of a combined treatment of GnRH, PGF and NOR to synchronize and resynchronize ovulations in TAI programs. Eighteen Mediterranean buffalo cows with a body condition score (BCS) of 2.70±0.26 (scale 1-5) from a farm in northeastern Corrientes Argentina (27° 20′ 33″ S and 58° 08′ 27″ W) were used in the study. Cows were randomly assigned to one of 3 treatments (TRT, **Figure 1**): 1) TRT1 (n=6); synchronization: day (d) -10,

8 ug GnRH (buserelin, Receptal®, Intervet SA, Argentina); d -3, 150 ug PGF (cloprostenol, Preloban®, Intervet SA, Argentina); resynchronization: d18 8 ug GnRH; d 25, 150 ug PGF; 2) TRT2 (n=6); synchronization: d -10, 8 ug GnRH and ½ ear implant for 7 days (norgestomet, Crestar®, Intervet SA, Argentina); d -3, 150 ug PGF; d -1 8 ug GnRH; resynchronization: d 18, 8 ug GnRH and ½ NOR ear implant for 7 days; d 25, 150 ug PGF; d 27 8 ug GnRH; 3) TRT3 (n=6): same protocol as TRT2 but without ear implant during synchronization and resynchronization (Figure 1). Daily ultrasounds and blood samples were taken from day -3 to day 2 during synchronization and from day 18 to day 30 during resynchronization (Figure 1). Blood samples were stored at -20 C° until P4 concentrations were analyzed by RIA (Count-A-Count®, DPC, Los Angeles, USA; intra-assay CV, 3.78%; Inter-assay CV, 9.28%).

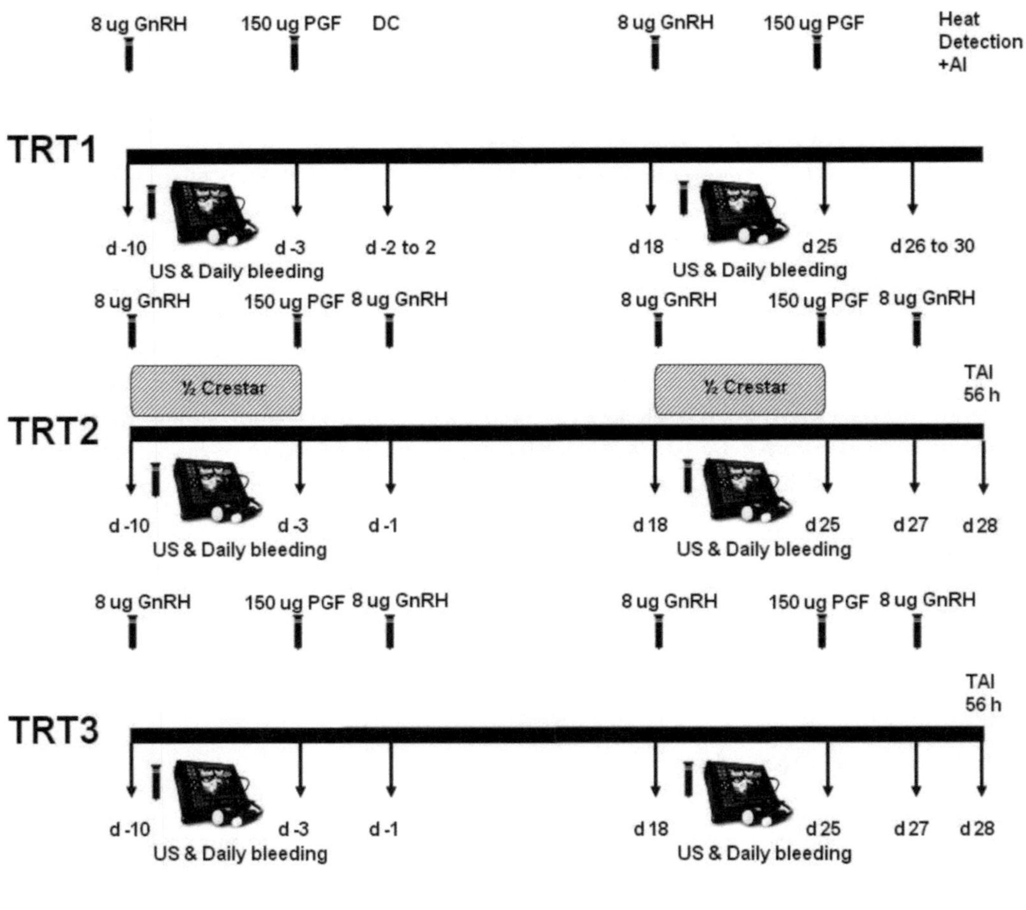

Fig. 1. Experimental design for studying follicular dynamics, time of ovulation, and fertility after synchronization and resynchronization of estrus and ovulation in buffaloes in field trials 1 and 2.

2.2 Results and discussion

Dominant follicle diameter prior to ovulation tended to be bigger in TRT1 compared to the TRT2 and TRT3 (12.58±0.67 vs. 10.97±0.74 mm; P<0.07), and it was bigger in resynchronization compared to synchronization (12.56±0.46 vs. 10.70±0.51 mm; P<0.02). On the contrary, even though the diameter of subordinate follicle was bigger with TRT3 compared to TRT1 and TRT2 (5.73±0.45 vs. 4.18±0.43 mm; P<0.02), the diameter of the subordinate follicle was of equal size during synchronization and resynchronization (4.70±0.35 mm). During synchronization, dominant follicle, subordinate follicle, and dominance daily growth rate was 0.55 mm/d, 0.25 mm/d and 0.75 mm/d respectively (**Figure 2**). During resynchronization, dominant follicle and dominance growth rate changed with a different pattern between treatments (**Figure 3**). Dominant follicle and dominance growth rate was bigger in TRT1 and TRT2 compared to TRT3 alone (0.87 mm/d and 0.81 mm/d vs. 0.68 mm/d; 0.65 and 0.68 mm/d vs. 0.40 mm/d; respectively; P<0.01; **Figure 3A and C**). In addition, during resynchronization, subordinate follicle diameter tended to increase continuously for the TRT3, whereas tended to increase and then to decrease with the other two treatments (P<0.09; **Figure 3B**). Even though the interval from PGF injection to ovulation was longer for TRT1 compared to the TRT2 and TRT3 groups (112.16±7.30 vs. 85.16±8.16 mm; P<0.03), the interval GnRH-ovulation was equal for TRT2 and TRT3 groups (36.54±5.36 vs. 37.83±5.73 mm; P>0.37). During resynchronization, a new wave started and divergence took place at day 19 and 22 for TRT1, at day 20 and 22 for TRT2, and at day 21 for TRT3. TRT2 treatment tended to be more effective in inducing follicle turnover compared to TRT1 and TRT3 alone (100% vs. 81%; P<0.07; (**Figure 3**). During resynchronization, more dominant follicles ovulated compared to synchronization (100% vs. 81%; P<0.04). Lastly, even though if all 3 treatments were equally efficacious to produce follicle turnover in 90 % of cows, that efficiency tended to be higher during synchronization compared to resynchronization (100% vs. 75%; P<0.07).

The diameter and growth rate of the DF reported in our study agree with those reported previously by Presicce et al., (2004). They reported that in pluriparous cows, DF diameter in the first wave was 13.3±0.5 mm and for the second wave was 13.8±0.6 mm and the growth rate was 1.6±0.1 and 1.3±0.1 mm respectively. Similar results were reported very recently by Barkawi et al., (2009). In their study DF diameter for cows with 2 waves was 13 and 15 mm and for cows with 3 waves was 11, 10, and 14 mm. In our study, the DF diameter during synchronization was similar to cows with 3 waves and during resynchronization with cows of 2 waves of their study. Furthermore, the DF growth rate reported in our study is quite similar to that reported by Awasthi et al., (2007). In their study, cows with normal estrus had similar diameter and growth rate compared to our cows during synchronization but was smaller compared to our cows during resynchronization.

Progesterone concentrations previous to PGF reported by us in this study are higher than those reported previously by Chauman et al., (1983) and by Kumar et al., (1991). Maybe these higher P_4 concentrations reported here are responsible for lower growth rate of DF prior to PGF administration when compared to growth rates reported previously by others (Presicce et al., 2003, 2004; Awasthi et al., 2006, 2007; Barkawi et al., 2009).

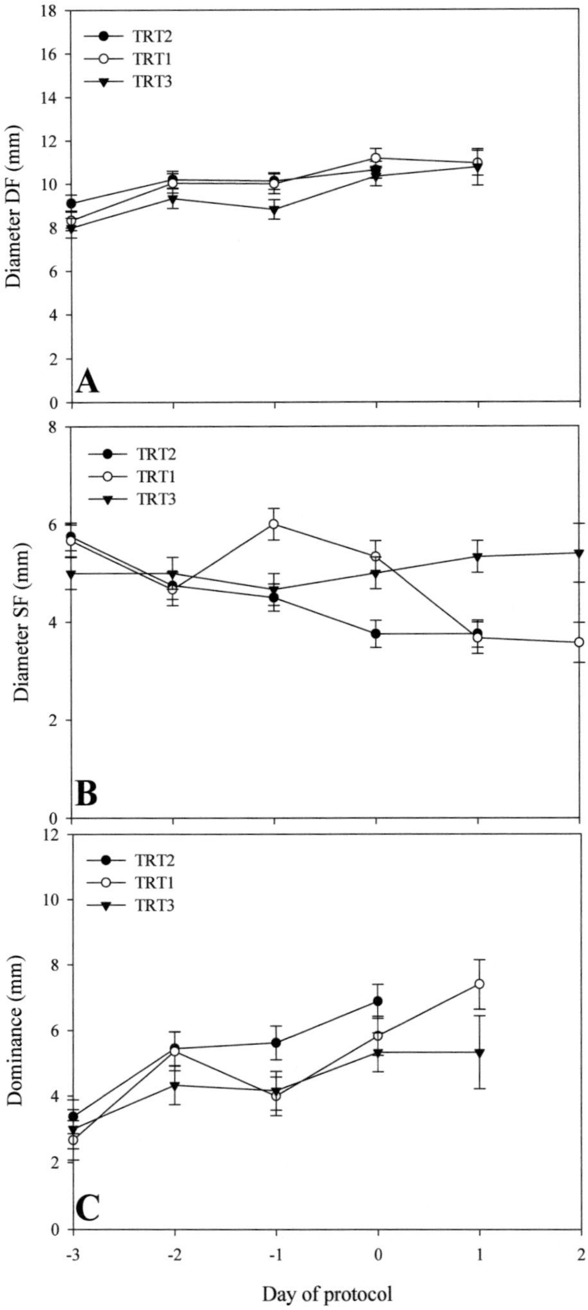

Fig. 2. Follicular dynamics by day of protocol during synchronization: diameter of the dominant follicle (A), diameter of the subordinate follicle (B), and dominance (C). TRT1: 8 ug GnRH (d-10), 150 ug PGF (d-3), heat detection every 12 h; TRT2: ½ Crestar ear implant (d-10 al -3), 8 ug de GnRH (d-10), 150 ug PGF (d-3), 8 ug GnRH (d -1); TRT3: 8 ug GnRH (d - 10), 150 ug PGF (d -3), 8 ug GnRH (d -1).

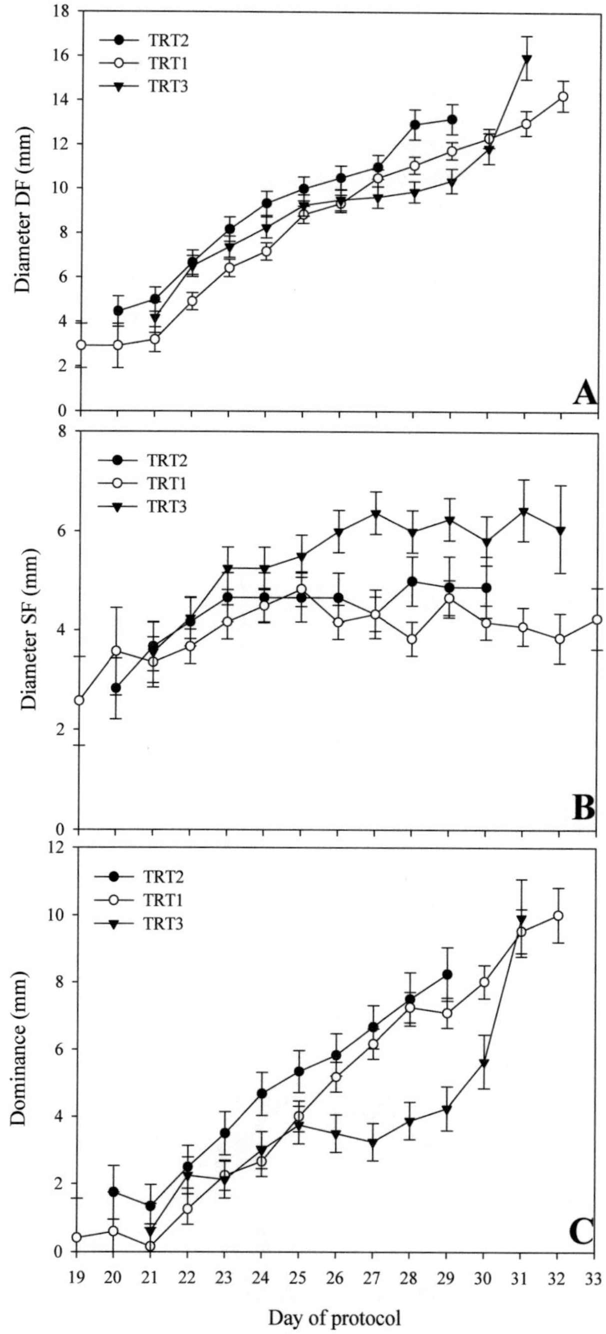

Fig. 3. Follicular dynamics by day of protocol during resynchronization: diameter of the dominant follicle (A), diameter of the subordinate follicle (B), and dominance (C). TRT1: 8 ug GnRH (d-10), 150 ug PGF (d-3), heat detection every 12 h; TRT2: ½ Crestar ear implant (d-10 al -3), 8 ug de GnRH (d-10), 150 ug PGF (d-3), 8 ug GnRH (d -1); TRT3: 8 ug GnRH (d -10), 150 ug PGF (d -3), 8 ug GnRH (d -1).

3. Material and methods

3.1 Second trial

In the second field trial, we assessed the fertility obtained with protocols used in the previous experiment in a commercial farm. We used 57 Mediterranean buffalo with a BCS of 4.41±0.12 (scale 1-5) from a farm in northeastern Corrientes Argentina (29° 42′ 20″ S and 59° 23′ 17″ W). Cows that were randomly assigned to one of three TRT (**Figure 4**): 1) TRT1 (n=20); 2) TRT2 (n=18); 3) TRT3 (n=19).

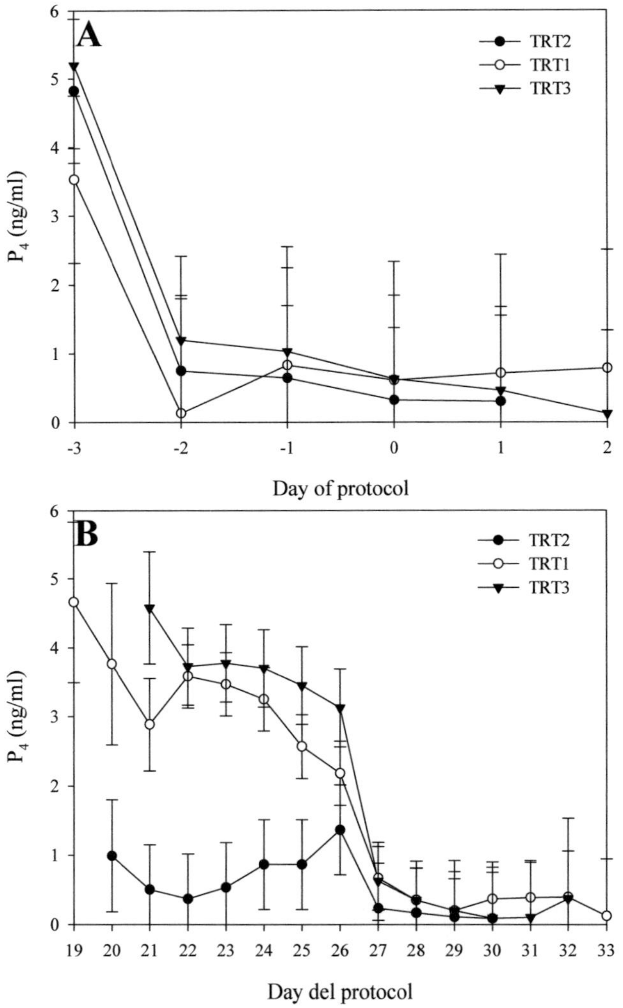

Fig. 4. Plasma P_4 concentrations by day of protocol during synchronization (A), and during resynchronization (B). Synchronization, TRT1: 8 ug GnRH (d-10), 150 ug PGF (d-3), heat detection every 12 h; TRT2: ½ Crestar ear implant (d-10 al -3), 8 ug GnRH (d-10), 150 ug PGF (d-3), 8 ug GnRH (d -1); and TRT3: 8 ug GnRH (d -10), 150 ug PGF (d -3), 8 ug GnRH (d -1). Resynchronization, TRT1: 8 ug GnRH (d 18), 150 ug PGF (d 25), heat detection every 12 h; TRT2: ½ Crestar ear implant (d 18 al 25), 8 ug GnRH (d 18), 150 ug PGF (d 25), 8 ug GnRH (d 27); and TRT3: 8 ug GnRH (d 18), 150 ug PGF (d 25), 8 ug GnRH (d 27).

3.2 Results and discussion

At synchronization, the percentage of cows AI was lower for the HDAI group compared to the TAI groups (80% vs. 100%, P<0.01; **Table 1**). On the contrary, the synchronization pregnancy rate (33%), the of cow AI (97%) and percentage of cows pregnant at resynchronization (31%), the cumulative pregnancy rate for both AI (56%), the pregnancy rate for natural service (50%) and final cumulative pregnancy rate (78%) were similar between treatment groups.

	TRT1[1]	TRT2[2]	TRT3[3]	Total
AI 1	80 (16/20)^{A}	100 (18/18)^{B}	100 (19/19)^{B}	93 (53/57)
PD 1	30 (6/20)	39 (7/18)	32 (6/19)	33 (19/57)
EL 1	3	0	0	3
AI 2	91 (10/11)	100 (11/11)	100 (13/13)	97 (34/35)
PD 2	18 (2/11)	36 (4/11)	38 (5/13)	31 (11/35)
PREG IA	47 (8/17)	61 (11/18)	58 (11/19)	56 (30/54)
NS	100 (9/9)	100 (7/7)	100 (8/8)	100 (24/24)
PD 3	44 (4/9)	29 (2/7)	75 (6/8)	50 (12/24)
PREG TOT	71 (12/17)	72 (13/18)	89 (17/19)	78 (42/54)

AI: artificial insemination, PG: pregnancy diagnosis, NS: natural service, EL: embryo losses;
A different from B, P<0.01;
[1]IACD. Synchronization: d0, 8 ug de buserelin (GnRH, Receptal®); d7, 150 mg cloprostenol (PGF, Preloban®, Intervet Argentina); d9, 8 ug GnRH; d10-12 heat detection + AI. Resynchronization: d18, 8 ug GnRH; d25, 150 ug PGF; d27 8 ug GnRH; d26-30 heat detection + AI;
[2]CRE. Synchronization: d0, 8 ug GnRH + ½ norgestomet ear implant during 7 days (CRE, Crestar®, Intervet, Argentina); d7, 150 mg PGF; d9, 8 ug GnRH; d10 TAI. Resynchronization: d18, 8 ug GnRH, ½ CRE implant during 7 days; d25, 150 ug PGF; d27 8 ug GnRH; d28 TAI;
[3]IATF. Synchronization: d0, 8 ug de GnRH; d7, 150 mg PGF; d9, 8 ug GnRH; d10 TAI. Resynchronization: d18, 8 ug GnRH; d25, 150 ug PGF; d27 8 ug GnRH; d28 TAI.

Table 1. Reproductive efficiency using three protocols for synchronization and resynchronization of estrus and ovulation in Mediterranean buffaloes.

4.1 Material and methods

Third and four trial

Lastly, in the third and forth field trials, we assessed the fertility obtained with a combination of GnRH, PGF and PIVD or EB, PGF and PIVD were used to synchronize and resynchronize ovulation in TAI programs in two commercial farms.

In the third field trial, 81 Mediterranean buffalo cows with a BCS of 3.79±0.27 (scale 1-5) from a farm in northeastern Corrientes Argentina (27° 20′ 33″ S and 58° 08′ 27″ W) were used in the study. Cows were randomly assigned to one of 2 TRT (**Figure 5**): 1) TRT1 (n=37; synchronization: d -10, 8 ug GnRH; d -3, 150 ug PGF; d -1 8 ug GnRH; d 0 TAI; resynchronization: d 18, 8 ug GnRH; d 25, ultrasound pregnancy diagnosis, open 150 ug

PGF; d 27, 8 ug GnRH; d 28 TAI), and 2) TRT2 (n=44; synchronization: d -9, 2 mg BE (BE®, Syntex, Argentina) and 1 g PIVD (Triu-B®, Biogenesis-Bagó, Argentina) for 7 days; d -2, 150 ug PGF; d -1 1 mg BE; d 0 TAI; resynchronization: d 19, 1 mg BE and 1 g PIVD for 7 days; d 26, ultrasound pregnancy diagnosis, open 150 ug PGF; d 27, 1 mg BE; d 28 TAI). Only 61 cows finished the experiment (**Table 2**). Synchronization pregnancy rate was higher in TRT2 group compared to TRT1 group (68% vs. 44%, P<0.03). However, resynchronization pregnancy rate (78%), percent of embryonic and fetal losses (12%), less and similar result, reports by Vale et al 1989, Campanile et al 2005, 2007. The final cumulative pregnancy rate without and with embryonic and fetal losses (93% and 85%) were similar between treatments.

In the forth field trial, 119 Mediterranean buffalo cows with a BCS of 3.17±0.11 (scale 1-5) from a farm in northeastern Corrientes Argentina (29° 42′ 20″ S and 59° 23′ 17″ W) were used in the study. Cows were randomly assigned to one of 4 TRT (**Figure 6**): 1) TRT1 (n=16); synchronization: d-10, 8 ug buserelina (GnRH, Receptal®, Intervet Argentina); d-3, 150 mg cloprostenol (PGF, Preloban®, Intervet Argentina); d-1, 8 ug GnRH; d 0 TAI; resynchronization: d18, 8 ug GnRH; d25, ultrasound pregnancy diagnosis (UPD), open cows 150 ug PGF; d27 8 ug GnRH; d 28 TAI; 2) TRT2 (n=39); synchronization: d-9, 2 mg estradiol benzoate (EB, BE®, Biogénesis, Argentina) and 1 g intravaginal P_4 releasing device for 7 d (PIVD, TRIU-B®, Biogénesis, Argentina); d-2, 150 mg PGF; d-1, 1 mg EB; d0 TAI; resynchronization: d19, 1 mg EB and 1 PIVD for 7 d; d26, UPD, open cows 150 ug PGF; d27 1 mg EB; d 29 TAI; 3) TRT3 (n=44); synchronization: d-10, 8 ug GnRH and 1 PDIV for 7 d; d-3, 150 mg PGF; d-1, 8 ug GnRH; d0 TAI; resynchronization: d18, 8 ug GnRH and 1 PIVD for 7 d; d25, UPD, open cows 150 ug PGF; d27 8 ug GnRH; d 28 TAI; and 4) TRT4 (n=20); synchronization: d-9, 2 mg de EB and 1 PIVD for 7 d; d-2, 150 mg PGF; d-1, 1 mg EB; d0 TAI; resynchronization: d19, 1 mg EB y 1 PIVD for 7 d; d26, UPD, open cows 150 ug PGF; d27 1 mg EB; d 28-32 AI detected heat.

4.2 Results and discussion

Only 104 cows finished the experiment (**Table 3**). Even though the synchronization pregnancy rate was similar between treatments (41%), more cows were resynchronized with the TAI protocols than with the HDAI protocol (100% vs. 67%, P<0.01). On the contrary, resynchronization pregnancy rate (57%), pregnancy rate to AI (76%), natural service pregnancy rate (30%), and final cumulative pregnancy rate (85%) were similar between treatments (P>0.13).

De Araujo Berber et al., (2002) and Ronci and De Rensis (2005) using a GnRH + PGF + GnRH + TAI protocol (Ovsynch) obtained higher pregnancy rates than those achieve by us in these field trials. The findings could be explained because they used weaned cows and most likely all were cycling. Conversely, Paul and Prakash (2005) and Warriach et al., (2008) reported lower pregnancy rates using an Ovsynch protocol. When De Rensis and Ronci, (2005) supplemented the Ovsynch protocol with P_4, pregnancy rates were similar to those obtained in our Ovsynch protocols that were supplemented with P_4. Presicce et al., (2005) using a protocol that combined a PIVD with EB and PMSG obtained higher pregnancy rates compared with an Ovsynch protocol alone, but this higher pregnancy rate is more likely due to the use of PMSG than EB.

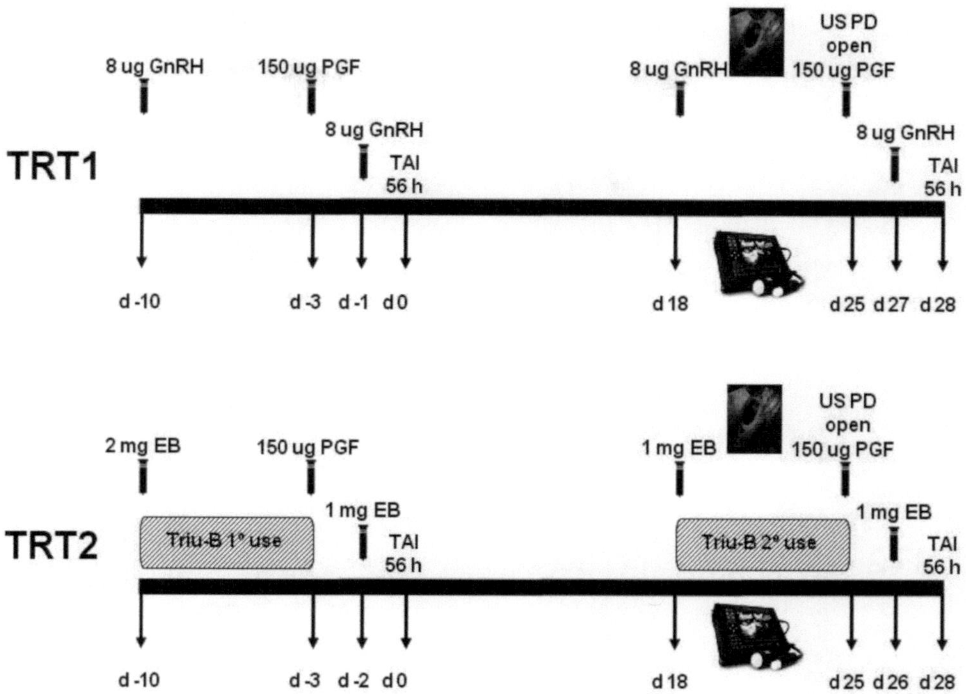

Fig. 5. Experimental design for studying fertility after synchronization and resynchronization of estrus and ovulation in buffaloes in field trial 3.

	TRT1[1]	TRT2[2]	Total
AI 1	37	44	81
NPD 1	3	3	6
PD 1	44% (15/34)[A]	68% (28/41)[B]	57% (43/75)
NAI 2	6	3	9
NPD 3	5		5
PD2	75% (6/8)	80% (8/10)	78% (14/18)
PREG AI	91% (21/23)	95% (36/38)	93% (57/61)
EL 50	13% (2/15)	11% (3/28)	12% (5/43)
PREG Final	83% (19/23)	87% (33/38)	85% (52/61)

PD: pregnancy diagnosis, EL: Embryo losses, NPD1: did not come to PD1, NAI2: did not come to AI2, NPD2: did not come to PD2;

A different form B, P<0.03;

[1]TRT1. Synchronization: d-10, 8 ug de buserelina (GnRH, Receptal®, Intervet Argentina); d-3, 150 mg cloprostenol (PGF, Preloban®, Intervet Argentina); d-1, 8 ug GnRH; d 0 TAI. Resynchronization: d18, 8 ug GnRH; d25, ultrasound pregnancy diagnosis, open cows 150 ug PGF; d27 8 ug GnRH; d 28 TAI.

[2]TRT2. Synchronization: d-9, 2 mg estradiol benzoate (EB, BE®, Biogénesis, Argentina) and 1 g P_4 intravaginal releasing device for 7 d (PIVD, TRIU-B®, Biogénesis, Argentina); d-2, 150 mg PGF; d-1, 1 mg EB; d0 TAI. Resynchronization: d19, 1 mg EB y 1 PIVD for 7 d; d26, ultrasound pregnancy diagnosis, open cows 150 ug PGF; d27 1 mg EB; d 28 TAI.

Table 2. Reproductive efficiency using two protocols for synchronization and resynchronization of estrus and ovulation in Mediterranean buffaloes.

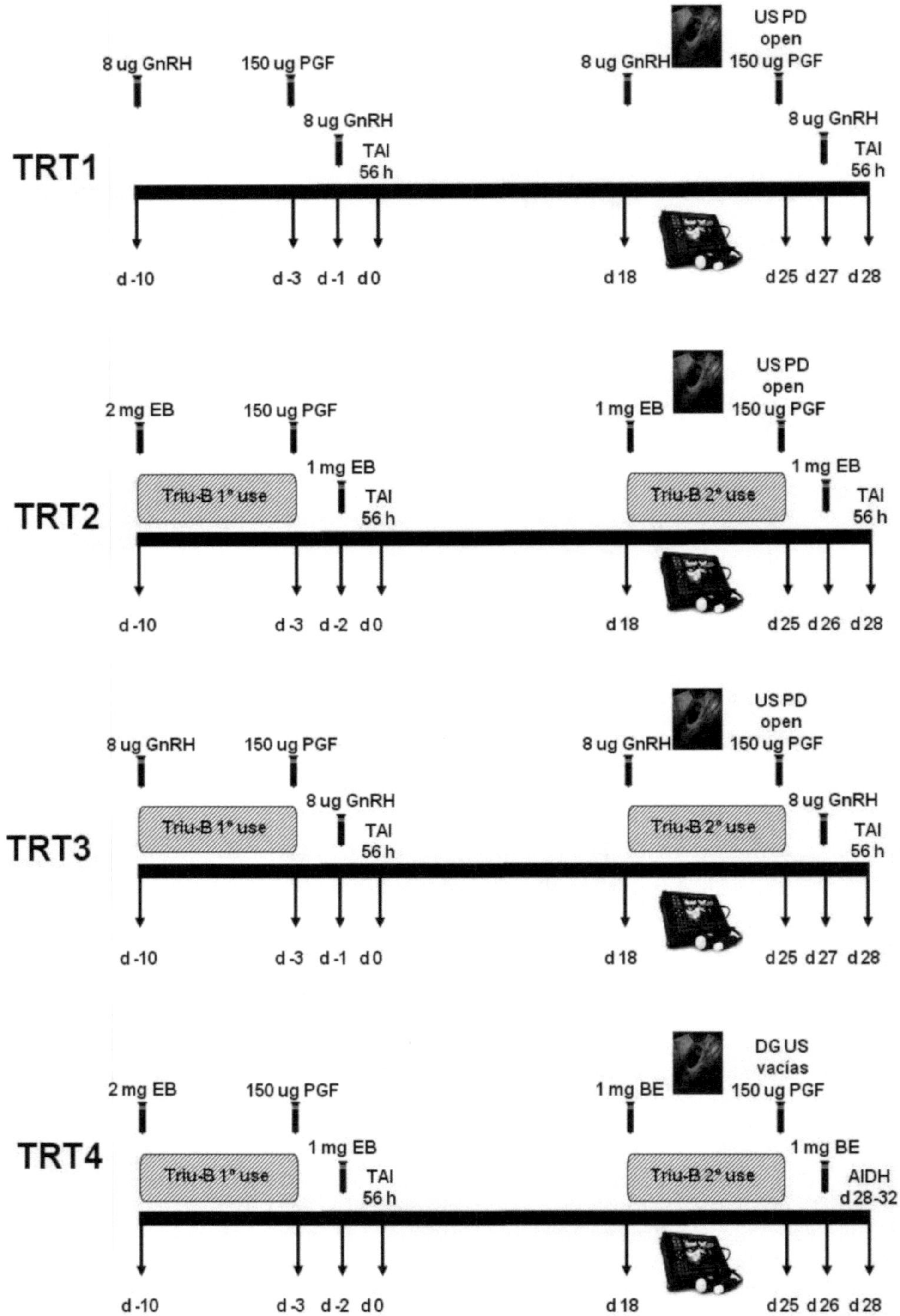

Fig. 6. Experimental design for studying fertility after synchronization and resynchronization of estrus and ovulation in buffaloes in field trial 4.

	TRT1	TRT2	TRT3	TRT4	Total
SYN	100 (16/16)	100 (39/39)	100 (44/44)	100 (20/20)	100 (119/119)
PD1	38 (6/16)	36 (14/39)	48 (21/44)	40 (8/20)	41 (49/119)
NAI2	2	5	3	0	10
RESYN	100 (8/8)[A]	100 (20/20)[A]	100 (20/20)[A]	67 (8/12)[B]	93 (56/60)
PD2	88 (7/8)	45 (9/20)	65 (13/20)	42 (5/12)	57 (34/60)
PREGAI	93 (13/14)	68 (23/34)	83 (34/41)	65 (13/20)	76 (85/109)
NS	100 (1/1)	100 (9/9)	100 (6/6)	100 (7/7)	100 (23/23)
PD3	0 (0/1)	22 (2/9)	33 (2/6)	43 (3/7)	30 (7/23)
NPD3	0	4	1	0	5
PREGT	93 (13/14)	77 (23/30)	90 (36/40)	80 (16/20)	85 (88/104)

SYN: synchronization, RESYN: resynchronization, PD: pregnancy diagnosis, NAI2: did not come to resynchronization, NPD3: did not come to PD3;
A different from B, P<0.0001;
[1]TRT1 Synchronization: d-10, 8 ug buserelina (GnRH, Receptal®, Intervet Argentina); d-3, 150 mg cloprostenol (PGF, Preloban®, Intervet Argentina); d-1, 8 ug GnRH; d 0 TAI. Resynchronization: d18, 8 ug GnRH; d25, ultrasound pregnancy diagnosis (UPD), open cows 150 ug PGF; d27 8 ug GnRH; d 28 TAI;
[2]TRT2 Synchronization: d-9, 2 mg estradiol benzoate (EB, BE®, Biogénesis, Argentina) and 1 g intravaginal P_4 releasing device for 7 d (PIVD, TRIU-B®, Biogénesis, Argentina); d-2, 150 mg PGF; d-1, 1 mg EB; d0 TAI. Resynchronization: d19, 1 mg EB and 1 PIVD for 7 d; d26, UPD, open cows 150 ug PGF; d27 1 mg EB; d 29 TAI;
[3]TRT3 Synchronization: d-10, 8 ug GnRH and 1 PDIV for 7 d; d-3, 150 mg PGF; d-1, 8 ug GnRH; d0 TAI. Resynchronization: d18, 8 ug GnRH and 1 PIVD for 7 d; d25, UPD, open cows 150 ug PGF; d27 8 ug GnRH; d 28 TAI;
[4]TRT4 Synchronization: d-9, 2 mg de EB and 1 PIVD for 7 d; d-2, 150 mg PGF; d-1, 1 mg EB; d0 TAI. Resynchronization: d19, 1 mg EB y 1 PIVD for 7 d; d26, UPD, open cows 150 ug PGF; d27 1 mg EB; d 28-32 AI detected heat.

Table 3. Reproductive efficiency using two protocols for synchronization and resynchronization of estrus and ovulation in Mediterranean buffaloes.

5. Conclusion

We can conclude from this series of field trials that the combination of GnRH, PGF and P_4 IVD or EB, PGF and P_4 IVD proved to be efficacious to synchronize and resynchronize ovulation in unweaned buffalo cows. Results from this work, show that a 75% pregnancy rate can be achieved during the first 28 days of the breeding season without heat detection and already taking into account early embryonic and fetal losses. Lastly, it is worth to point out that pregnancy rate achieved in all experiments with TAI protocols was numerically higher than that achieved with HDAI; hence these results indicate that TAI may be a very promising tool for genetic improvement in buffalo herds.

6. References

Awasthi Mk, Abhishek K, Kavani FS, Siddiquee, GM, Panchal MT, Shah RR. 2006. Is one-wave follicular growth during the estrus suckled a usual phenomenon in water buffaloes (bubalus bubalis)? Anim Reprod Sci. 92:241-253.

Awasthi Mk, Kavani FS, Siddiquee GM, Sarvaiya NP, Terashri HJ. 2007. Is slow follicular growth the cows of silent estrus in water buffaloes? Anim Reprod Sci. 99:258-268.

Barkawi AH, Hafez YM, Ibrahim SA, Ashour G, El Asheeri AK, Ghanem N. 2009. Characteristics of ovarian follicular dynamics throughout the estrous cycle of Egyptian buffaloes. Anim Reprod Sci. 110:326-334.

Campanile G, Neglia G, Gasparrini B, Galiero G, Prandi J, Di Palo R, D´occhio Mj, Zicarelli L. 2005. Embryonic mortality in buffaloes synchronized and mated by artificial insemination during the seasonal decline in reproductive function. Theriogenology. 63:2334-2340.

Campanile G, Di Palo R, Neglia G, Vecchio D, Gasparrini B, Prandi A, Galiero G, D´occhio, MJ. 2007. Corpus luteum function and embryonic mortality in buffaloes treated with a GnRH agonist, hCG and progesterone. Theriogenology. 67:1393-1398.

Chauhan FS, Sharma RD, Singh GB. 1983. Serum progesterone concentrations in normal cycling and sub oestrus buffaloes. Indian J Dairy Sci. 36:28-33.

De Araujo Berber RCA, Madureira EH, Baruselli PS. 2002. Comparison of two Ovsynch protocols (GnRH vs. LH) for fixed time insemination in buffalo (*Bubalus bubalis*). Theriogenology. 57:1421-1430.

De Rensis F, Ronci J. 2005. Conception rate after fixed time insemination following Ovsynch protocol with and without progesterone supplementation in cyclic and no-cyclic Mediterranean Italian buffaloes (*Bubalus bubalis*). Theriogenology. 63:1824-1831.

Kumar R, Jindal ED, Rattan PJS. 1991. Plasma hormonal profile during oestrus cycle of Murrah buffalo heifer. Indian J Anim Sci. 61:382-385.

Paul V, Prakash BS. 2005. Efficacy of the ovsynch protocols for synchronization of ovulation and fixed time artificial insemination in Murrah buffaloes (bubalus bubalis). Theriogenology. 64:1049-1060.

Presicce G, Parmegiani A, Senatore E, Estecco R, Barile VL, De Mauro G, De Santis G, Terzano G. 2003. Hormonal dymanics and follicular turnover in prepuberal Mediterranean buffaloes (bubalus bubalis). Theriogenology. 60:485-493.

Presicce G, Senatore E, Bella A, De Santis G, Barile VL, De Mauro G, Terzano G, Estecco R, Parmegiani, A. 2004. Ovarian follicular dynamics and hormonal profiles in heifers and mixed parity Mediterranean buffaloes (bubalus bubalis) following and estrus synchronization protocols. Theriogenology. 61:1343-1355.

Presicce GA, Senatore EM, De Santis G, Bella A. 2005. Follicle turnover and pregnancy rates following oestrus synchronization protocols in Mediterranean buffaloes (Bubalus bubalis). Reprod Dom Anim. 40:443-447.

Ronci G, De Rensis F. 2005. Comparison between Ovsynch protocols plus GnRH for fixed time artificial insemination in Buffalo cows. Proc 1° European Buffalo Congress, Salerno, Italia. p 248.

Vale WG, Ohashi, OM, Souza JS, Ribeiro HFL, Silva AOA, Nanba SY. 1989. Morte embrionária e fetal em búfalos (bubalus bubalis). Rev Bras Reprod Anim. 13:157-165.

Warriach HM, Channa AA, Ahmad N. 2008. Effect of oestrus synchronization methods on oestrus behaviour, timing of ovulation and pregnancy rate during the breeding and low breeding seasons in Nili-Ravi buffaloes. Anim Reprod Sci. 107:62-67.

3

Artificial Insemination of Sheep – Possibilities, Realities and Techniques at the Farm Level

Sándor Kukovics[1], Erzsébet Gyökér[2],
Tímea Németh[1] and Elemér Gergátz[2]
[1]*Research Institute for Animal Breeding and Nutrition*
[2]*Pharmagene-Farm Ltd, Biotechnical Research Station*
Hungary

1. Introduction

1.1 History of artificial insemination over the last 50 years

The state of artificial insemination in the sheep and goat industries has developed differently in Europe over the last couple of decades. The number of artificial inseminations in the sheep industry and the ratio of inseminated ewes increased sharply in East Europe, especially in the eastern part of Mid-Europe, during the 1950s and 1960s. The main reason for this increase could be due to the planned economy and certain central pressure from the state. The presence and the ratio of use of this method were much lower in other parts of Europe, and its development was rather slower.

Because of unfavourable economical circumstances, the profitability of the sheep industry fell in the eastern part of Europe and the number of sheep kept on big state and cooperative farms declined during the 1970s and the second half of the 1980s. With the changing economy in the early 1990s, the decline in sheep number continued. In Hungary, in particular, during the preparation period prior to accession to the EU, there was a sharp increase in sheep number, with the increasing trend lasting until the end of 2005. The trend has reversed since then, with a gradual and intensive reduction.

As the consequences of the use of artificial insemination (AI) with semen from imported breeding rams, wool production traits (fibre diameter, shearing, greasy wool weight and staple length among others) have steadily and gradually increased in Hungarian Merino flock. Artificial insemination centres were founded by the state between early 1950s and the end of the 1970s. Some regional sub-stations belonging to each county AI centres were supplying flocks from state and cooperative farms. Over this period, the state helped improve sheep breeding with the operation of AI centres. The number of inseminated ewes reached its peak in the mid 1960s, when 63% of ewes in the national flock were artificially inseminated with a relatively wide range, but from the end of this decade, the use of AI started to go back. In the Hajdu-Bihar County (east of the country) for instance, the number of inseminated ewes exceeded 85%, even in mid 1970s' (Kukovics, 1974; Jávor et al., 2006; Kukovics & Gergátz, 2009). From the mid 1970s, the state-owned artificial insemination centres started to close down, the number of rams kept for semen collection was reduced and the breeding animals were sold to various farms.

After this period privately-owned self-owned ram and artificial insemination units were established and took advantage of the sheep breeding state and cooperative farms.

Meanwhile, artificial insemination started to be more intensively used in Western Europe. The number of inseminated ewes and their ratio increased in breeding programmes where rapid genetic development was essential. One of these programmes was the French dairy Lacaune breeding system, where more than 82% of the nucleus part of the population (about 160 000 out of the 750 000 heads) were artificially inseminated by 1993 with semen mainly transported from several AI centres. During the previous thirty years, average milk production increased from 50 to 70 litres to 300 litres per ewe annually (Barillet et al., 1993). This trend did not change and the system expanded to other breeds in France, Spain and Italy (Jávor et al., 2006).

Since the beginning of the 1980s, the number of inseminated ewes has decreased noticeably in Hungary. As the whole economy of the country was reorganised and privatised from the early 1990s, the number of farms utilising AI as the breeding method has almost disappeared. Nowadays, less than 2 % of breeding ewes are inseminated artificially on about 15 to 20 farms out of the registered 6,900 sheep farms. Indeed, the relatively small size of flocks (about 150 heads of adult females) has an important role in the development of this situation. Almost twenty breeds are bred in the country, but AI is only used in limited numbers. The Merinos are the dominant breed in the country; however, very few farmers breeding Merino sheep use AI.

It was quite well known many years ago and even today that AI can not be carried out without special skills. Several hundred people were educated on artificial insemination (in the 1950s and 1960s up to the mid 1970s) in order to use this modern breeding method in the country.

The education of shepherds practically decreased in Hungary, and no one received even minimal skills in the AI of sheep and goats between 1986 and 1999. On behalf of the Hungarian Goat Breeders Association and the Hungarian Sheep Dairying Association, a series of indoor courses were organised for sheep and goat breeders in 1999 and 2000. The courses were carried out in the Biotechnical Research Station University of Western Hungary, in Mosonmagyaróvár. More than 60 people (shepherds and goat breeders) finished the three courses and took successful theoretical and practical examinations, receiving a certificate for their knowledge. Unfortunately, the organisation of further courses had to be stopped because of a shortage of funds needed to cover the costs of the courses. However, a couple of years later, special official courses were announced by the state in sheep and goat AI, but there was no interest until now.

At present, only a limited number of breeders are convinced about the importance and the value of AI. Most of the sheep and goat keepers have several numbers of breeding males for mating.

Until 2008, two officially certificated artificial insemination stations (Pharmagene-Farm Ltd, Mosonmagyaróvár, and Bakonszegi Awassi Corporation, Bakonszeg) were operating in the country; however, some research centres (universities and research institutes) had complete laboratories ready to offer services to various farms. In 2011, only one AI station remained active in Mosonmagyaróvár, and there was a new embryo transfer station officially certified in Budapest.

Unfortunately, not only is there a shortage of state-organised shepherds as well as a lack of educating inseminators (cattle and pig excluded), but there is also an absence of interest of the breeders association in forcing farmers to get knowledge and use artificial insemination.

The lack of interest, insufficient knowledge and education, absence of organisation, laziness, shortage of labour and low profitability can be found behind this symptom.
The director of Hőgyész State Farm, Béla Szüllő (Hungary), who supervised the breeding and production of more than 4,000 sheep stated in 1972, believed that the profitability of meat sheep farming could be achieved when 1.5 lambs could be utilised after one ewe annually (Kukovics, 1974). This level could be attained with the use of frequent lambing, utilisation of artificial insemination, and with the application of breeds with high prolificacy in crossbreeding programmes. That result was later confirmed by Kukovics & Jávor (2002) in their study.

1.2 The main factors affecting AI

There are several factors that could modify the effectiveness of artificial insemination and some of them are mentioned below.

1.2.1 The breed

In many publications, the ewe breed has been found to have a large effect on the pregnancy rate after artificial insemination. According to Hill et al. (1998), the wool type (strong wool - 67.6%; fine wool - 71.7%; fine medium and medium 73%) of Australian Merino affected the average pregnancy rate. In a Greek study (Karagiannidis et al., 2001), the conception rate rank of ewes was Chios, Vlachiki and (Vlachiki x Chios), with a significant difference between them. The pregnancy rate of Suffolk ewes was much lower (12%) than that of Finnish landrace (65%) in Irish studies (Donovan et al., 2001 and 2004), while the breed of the ram also had a significant effect on prolificacy after AI (Perkins et al., 1996; Donovan et al., 2001 and 2004; Anel et al., 2005).

1.2.2 Age of the ewe

The fertility rate in laparoscopic insemination gradually decreases from the age of 1.5 to 2.5 years (Anel et al., 2005), while it increases until 3.5 to 4.5 years of age in vaginal insemination.

1.2.3 The season of insemination

The season of insemination could have a strong effect on the results. According to Hill et al. (1998), the month of insemination exerted highly significant differences: it was 71.5% in March, April, or May and 67.6% in November, December, January or February. In the study of Anel et al. (2005), the season modified the conception rate after both laparoscopic and vaginal insemination (September-January 46.88 vs. 35.53%; February-June 43.96 vs. 29.79 %; July-August 38.95 vs. 22.72%), but the data of the first one were always higher.

1.2.4 The use of fresh, cooled, chilled, frozen semen

It is generally stated that the fertility of the semen decreases with cooling temperature. The use of freshly diluted semen could give the best result: 70 to 82 % (Donovan et al., 2001 and 2004) and 82.2% (Hill et al., 1998; Ehling et al., 2003). A similar level could be reached with cooled and stored semen /74-76% (Gergátz&Gyökér, 1997) and 56.7% (Fernandez-Abella et al., 2003) as well as with chilled and stored semen /between 37.5% (Fernandez-Abella et al., 2003) and 64.2-73.33% (Stefanov et al., 2006)/. The conception rate frozen-thawed semen was the lowest in all of the publications: 38 to 46% (Gergátz & Gyökér, 1997), 69.5 to 71.6%

(Hill et al., 1998), 29 to 52% (Donovan et al., 2001, 2004), and 42.86 to 53.33 % (Stefanov et al., 2006).

1.2.5 The labour
In the study of Anel et al. (2005), the results of laparoscopic (from 40.60 to 51.54%) and vaginal (from 23.85 to 43.16%) insemination highly depended on the technician who carried it out.

1.2.6 The year
Anel et al. (2005) reported that the level of pregnancy rate decreased for both techniques (from 62 to 44% for laparoscopic AI and from 38 to 31% for vaginal AI) between 1990 and 1997.

1.2.7 Time of insemination after oestrus synchronisation
The time of AI is especially important in the case of oestrus synchronisation. The best time of insemination could be 46 (Fernandez-Abella et al., 2003), 48 to 72 (Karagiannidis et al., 2001), and 58 to 63 (Donovan et al., 2001, 2004) hours after the pessary removal.

1.2.8 Dose of PMSG used
Hill et al. (1998) reported that the type and dosage of PMSG (Pregnant Mare Serum Globulin - 200 IU - 62.4%; 250 IU - 72.9%; 300 IU - 79.1%; 375 IU and above - 69.4%) had a significant effect on the conception rate in artificial insemination.

1.2.9 The extender used
The main aim of diluting is to enlarge the fertility and storing ability of ram semen (Mucsi, 1997; Sarlós, 1999; Gergátz, 2007) with additional energy. There are many kinds of extenders used for this reason (skimmed milk, Ivanov, Salamon, improved versions of them, etc. (Kukovics, 1974; Becze, 1982, Gergátz & Gyökér, 1997; Sarlós, 1999; Fernandez-Abella et al., 2003; Jávor et al., 2006), and most of the authors suggest materials. The semen used in any kind of artificial insemination is mainly diluted, and dilution is particularly important in the case of cooling, chilling and deep freezing of semen. The most common dilution rate is the 1:1 - 1:2 - 1:3 - 1:4, but in practice, a ratio higher than 1:8 is not really used (Fernandez-Abella et al., 2003; Gergátz, 2007).

1.2.10 Dose of inseminated semen
In general, the suggested dose of semen is 0.1 to 0.2 ml with about 50 to 100 million active spermatozoa. About 50 to 100 million spermatozoa is needed in one dose to vaginal insemination, but 25 to 50 million are suggested for cervical insemination and 15 to 20 million is enough for laparoscopic AI (Kukovics, 1974; Jávor et al., 2006; Gergátz, 2007). However, several scientists have used much higher numbers: 106 (Fernandez-Abella et al., 2003), 50 to 300 (Ehling et al., 2003) and 400 (King et al., 2004) million spermatozoa in one dose of semen.

1.2.11 The method (vaginal, cervical, cervico-uterinal or laparoscopic) used
The simplest method is vaginal insemination, which could result in the lowest conception rate. The use of cervical and trans-cervical methods could give much higher pregnancy

rates, but laparoscopic AI is the most effective one. However, it is also the most expensive and complicated method. Apart from the general trends, the publications show quite a wide range of rates: 31.25% (Anel et al., 2005) in vaginal, 18 (Yamaki et al., 2003); 42 (King et al., 2004); and 65-75% (Salamon & Maxwell, 1995; Donovan et al., 2001, 2004; Stefanov et al., 2006) in cervical; 69.6 to 76.4% (Szabados, 2006) in cevico-uterinal; and 44.89 (Anel et al., 2005), 64 (Yamaki et al., 2003), and 69 % (King et al., 2004) in laparoscopic insemination. It should be noted that these results are affected according to the semen used (fresh, cooled, chilled or frozen (Perkins et al., 1996; Moses et al., 1997).

1.3 Detection of ewes on heat and the number on inseminations

One of the key questions of artificial insemination is the detection of ewes on heat, the time of insemination following the selection, and the number of inseminations made. The main detection systems could be summarised as follows (Kukovics, 1974; Jávor et al., 2006):

I. Selection once a day (24 hours) in the morning (or in the afternoon)
(A) first insemination made immediately
(a) insemination every 24 hours
1. no further insemination
2. second insemination made without further selection
3. second insemination only in the case of when heat is detected
4. further insemination in the case that the ewe is still on heat
    4.1. no more than three inseminations
    4.2. further inseminations until the animal is on heat
(b) insemination every 8 to 12 hours
sub-points are the same as in point (a)
(B) the first insemination made 3 to 4 hours after selection or later
sub-points are the same as in point (A/a)
II. Selection every 8 to 12 hours
(A) insemination made right after detection
(a) no further insemination made
(b) further inseminations every 8 to 12 hours
sub-points are the same as in point I. (A/a)
(B) first insemination made 3 to 4 hours after detection or later
sub-points are the same as in point I. (A/a)

Since heat in ewes lasts 24 hours, in general, and is shorter in the case of yearlings, the first (I) method could have several limitations and so, the second (II) method is proposed and could be more effective.

Concerning the daily distribution of real heats, adjusted to the possibilities of practical life, the ewes on heat are detected between 6 and 7 hours in the morning as part of the so called "Mosonmagyaróvár insemination technique" (Gergátz, 2007). The first insemination is carried out between 10 and 11 am, and the second one between 3 and 4 pm. Because of the once daily detection, about 5% of the yearlings will be omitted from insemination at first, but 95% of them will be inseminated in the next heat.

Many opponents of artificial insemination declare that using this method, the level of pregnancy obtained naturally cannot be performed. The results of studies from the last decades have proved that the pregnancy rate of ewes selected and inseminated only once could reach 60 to 65%. The pregnancy rate of the ewes selected and inseminated twice during the same cycle could exceed 75% and reach 80 to 85%. With the use of three inseminations, 90 to 95% of pregnancy could be performed (Kukovics, 1974; Jávor et al., 2006; Gergátz, 2007).

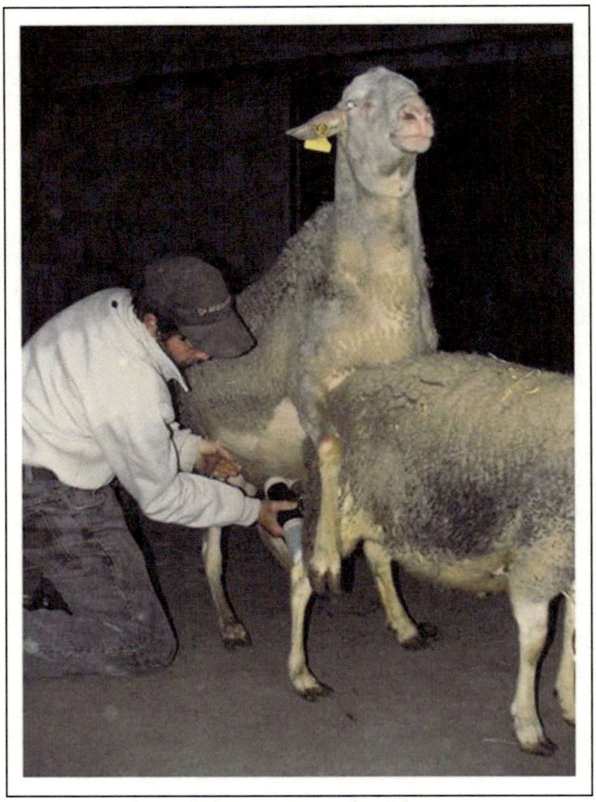

Fig. 1. Collection of semen at a farm (Photo: Németh, A.)

1.4 The costs of artificial insemination

It is rather difficult to estimate the costs of artificial insemination per average ewe on a farm. The following jobs and movements are involved: preparation of rams and ewes for AI, preparing equipments and tools for collecting semen and artificial insemination, collecting, qualifying, diluting and dosing semen, detecting and selecting ewes on heat, fixing animals to carry the AI, and finally performing the insemination, and cleaning the tools and equipments. These basically cover the expenditures of buying tools (and feeds) and the costs of labour. The use of oestrus synchronisation is an additional cost, even if it consists of several parts.

The cost of artificial insemination increased from 1.2 to 3.2 HUF/head to 2.5 to 4.5 HUF/head between 1966 and 1971 in the abovementioned Hajdú-Bihar County (Kukovics, 1974). This increase was the consequence of the intensive development of feed prices (especially the crops and concentrates). In order to evaluate current values (2010), these numbers should be multiplied by 100 to 500 (in 2011 1 Euro = 270 HUF approx.)

The estimated costs of artificial insemination change according to the method utilised, the places of semen collection, the labour/service company that is performing the job, the presence of oestrus synchronisation, and the handling of rams before the season, among others. Laparoscopic AI is the most expensive because it needs veterinary service and help. At the same time, vaginal, cervical or even trans-cervical insemination can be carried out by well-skilled shepherds, at a much lower level of costs, without significant losses in efficiency.

Due to reorganisation of the national economies of Mid-East European countries, state-owned AI centres have disappeared (Jávor et al, 2006) and most of the remaining sheep farms use rams for natural services. Shepherds educated on performing AI have either died or have left the sheep industry and the remaining ones do not want to work with it as it means extra work, attention and accuracy. AI is only used on very few farms nowadays and available data on expenditures of AI are rather limited or not published at all.

In Western Europe and the Western world, artificial insemination became a special service of companies, not really based on the skills of sheep owners and shepherds. At the same time, laparoscopic AI (LAI) has become the most popular, which can be carried out by veterinarians. Cervical and trans-cervical AI can also be provided by different veterinary and genetic companies.

Donovan et al. (2001) stated that cervical insemination was much cheaper than laparoscopic AI, but exact cost values were not given in the study. After out-of-season mating (May) of purebred and crossbred Lacaune ewes with oestrus synchronisation and induction, Gulyás et al. (2007) reported that the extra costs of using biotechnological methods were refunded with the good profits raised by selling lambs during Christmas time. According to an American presentation for sheep farmers, cervical and trans-cervical methods are easy to learn and use. Each sheep takes about two minutes to inseminate at a cost of $1.29, making it significantly faster and less expensive than laparoscopic surgical insemination (http://www.farmanddairy.com/news/ultrasound-and-artificial-insemination-techniques). The service charges of these companies are quite different, and most of them concerning only LAI do not cover all the costs. The service cost of LAI could be, for instance, GBP 10 to 15 per ewe (http://www.innovis.org) or GBP 10 to 25 per ewe plus indirect cost, which means the total costs could be around GBP 20 to 35 per ewe (http://www.trialanderroracres.com); or AU$ 15 to 30 per ewe (Genstock Animal Breeding Services, Australia - http://genstock.com.au) ; or NZ$ 15 to 30 (Genetic Gains Ltd and Premier Genetics Ltd, New-Zealand - http://genetic-gains.co.nz) , or the prepared semen could be ordered at the price of US$ 15 to 135 per straw (Super Sire Ltd - Pathway to Genetic Improvement - http://www.topRams.com). Apart from these, limited data are available about the real costs of AI. The service reports and offers discuss pregnancy rate levels and the charges.

2. Materials and methods

As mentioned above, less than 2% of the ewes kept in Hungary were artificially inseminated between 2000 and 2010; however, more than 63% of ewes were artificially inseminated in 1963. Examining the main characteristics of more than 6,900 sheep farms and about 500 goat farms, we observed that AI was utilised only on a limited number of sheep farms, and no goat farm practically used this breeding method.

2.1 The farms and the breeds kept

In order to study artificial insemination at the farm level, 11 sheep farms out of the less than 20 farms with available data were selected from 2003 to 2010. Twelve breeds and genotypes

of sheep were breed on the studied farms. The breeds kept on the various farms and the number of years when artificial insemination was utilised are summarised in Table 1.
On most farms, only one breed was kept, but three different breeds were bred on farm No. 2, 9 and 10, and two breeds on farm No. 11.
In the first farm, which was a corporation, a breeding project has been carried out since 1990 and purebred Awassi and crossbred Awassi (F_1, R_1, R_2, R_3, R_4) flocks have been reared. The majority of female sheep was artificially inseminated during 2003 to 2007, but because of low AI efficiency, natural insemination with breeding rams was used to get better pregnancy results. The farm was finally reorganised and sold in 2009, so the use of AI ended from 2008.
A breeding project was performed on the second farm, which was a state farm aiming to create a new synthetic breed and started operating from early 1970s. The Bábolna Tetra sheep breed was finally developed from the crossings of Hungarian Merino as well as 5 lines of Finnish Landrace and 3 lines of Romanov breeds, and it was officially accepted as a new breed in 1995. In addition to this, Ile the France and American Suffolk nucleus flocks were also developed on the farm, starting in 1988. The reorganisation and final selling of the farm and its sheep happened in 2009 and 2010, and it is currently a much smaller private farm.

Farm code	No. and name of breeds kept	No. of years
1	1: Awassi and Awassi crossbreds	5 (2003-2007)
2	3. Bábolna Tetra, Ile de France, Suffolk	8 (2003-2010)
3	1: Hungarian Merino	4 (2003-2006)
4	1: German Mutton Merino	6 (2003-2008)
5	1: Hungarian Merino	6 (2003-2008)
6	1: Lacaune	2 (2009-2010)
7	1: Lacaune	7 (2003-2010)
8	1: Lacaune	2 (2003-2004)
9	3: Hungarian Merino, German Mutton Merino, German Blackheaded Mutton Sheep	8 (2003-2010)
10	3: British Milksheep, Charollais, Hungarian Merino	5 (2005-2010)
11	2: British Milksheep, British Milksheep Crossbreds	8 (2003-2010)

Table 1. Number of breeds and the studied years on the farms

The other private farms were founded in the 1990s, when most of the cooperative and state farms were demolished, reorganised and the sheep were sold from them. The only exception was farm No. 7, which was a research station belonging to the University of West Hungary founded in 1982, and it is still a research station.
The use of AI stopped on farm No. 3 in 2007, and in 2009 in the case of farms No. 4 and 5 because of labour problems. On farm No. 8, the labour problem together with the low quality of AI made with transported semen led to the replacement of AI with the use of extra breeding rams.
On farm No. 10, only a small population of the sheep (purebred imported breeds) were artificially inseminated, and the AI started to be utilised in the nucleus part of the Merino flock only in 2007. On farm No. 12, the British Milksheep crossbred sheep (Hungarian

Merino x British Milksheep) were handled separately since 2007. On farm No.6, the use of AI was only started in 2009.

The results of AI were not possible to evaluate for year 2010 in the case of farms No. 6, 7, 10 and partly 11 because the lambing of artificially inseminated ewes started only in 2011 and was not finished before the time of data collection.

2.2 Data collection

Two surveys were carried out in late 2007 and at the beginning of 2011 in order to collect data of artificial insemination on the selected farms. Each farm was visited and the data was collected based on a questionnaire covering the following information:

- number of sheep kept,
- number of artificially inseminated ewes per breed and per year,
- number of progeny born and weaned after AI per breed and per year,
- method of selection and time searching ewes on heat,
- time and number of insemination,
- method of collecting and qualifying semen to use,
- level of dilution, kind of extender and the size of inseminating dose,
- method and use of oestrus synchronisation,
- method of insemination,
- fixing method of ewes during insemination,
- control of pregnancy and use of ram service after insemination,
- number of labour used over AI,
- cost of AI.

2.3 Processing of data

The methods of AI used on various farms were evaluated in details. The results of AI were studied on farm levels because of the farm difference in the number of breeds kept.

$$\text{Pregnancy rate (P\%)} = \frac{\text{lambed ewes}}{\text{inseminated ewes}}$$

$$\text{Lambing rate (L\%)} = \frac{\text{born lambs}}{\text{lambed ewes}}$$

$$\text{Weaning rate (W\%)} = \frac{\text{weaned lambs}}{\text{born lambs}}$$

The *pregnancy rate (P%)*, lambing rate (L%) and the *weaning rate (W%)* were calculated by farms and by breeds in every studied year. In the case of those farms where more than one breed was kept, the effects of breed and year were studied. In the case of farms where only one breed was kept, the effects of year were examined.

Chi-square test of SPSS 10.0 was applied to compare the breeds to each other and to compare the years by breed. Significant differences between breeds and years were determined at $P \leq 0.05$.

3. Results

The total number of sheep kept on various farms is summarised in Table 2. The size of flocks belonging to various breeds per farm changed over the studied period, the number of ewes mainly decreasing over the years. The numbers of artificially inseminated ewes per breed and per farm are presented in Table 3.

3.1 The tools of artificial insemination

The most important factors in artificial insemination are well-skilled labour (mainly shepherds or inseminators), well-prepared rams of good quality, ewes with good body condition, and the necessary equipments and tools.

Based on our study, at least one person per farm with proper skill in artificial insemination was working, and he was primarily the owner shepherd. There were technicians on farms No. 1 and 7. The animals were prepared (details presented later on) on each farm before the season.

The most important equipments and tools necessary for performing artificial insemination on farms are shown in Figure 2: artificial vagina, semen collecting glass with double wall (and warm water between the walls), warm water bath, thermometer, vaginal speculum (with different size for adult ewes and ewe hoggets), lamp for providing light into the vagina, pipettes, catheter, syringe and vaginal sponges or implants for oestrus synchronization. A microscope with relatively smaller capacity is also needed with a table and sheet object heater.

Farm code	2003	2004	2005	2006	2007	2008	2009	2010
1	1960	2120	2140	2200	2080	-	-	-
2	3138	2905	2753	2103	2251	2170	971	588
3	312	359	411	461	450	-	-	-
4	700	700	750	700	840	834	-	-
5	820	900	950	980	1050	960	-	-
6	-	-	-	-	-	-	1100	980
7	239	204	177	206	216	237	295	290
8	588	456	-	-	-	-	-	-
9	1160	1168	1183	1157	988	1060	968	940
10	-	-	430	450	470	460	460	450
11	420	390	350	380	380	350	345	340

Table 2. The total number of ewes kept on the studied farms between 2003 and 2010

Breed, farm code, year	Hungarian Merino				German Mutton Merino		German Blackheaded Mutton Sheep	British Milksheep		British Milksheep Crossbreds
	9	10	3	5	9	4	9	10	11	11
2003	446	-	274	160	438	640	174	-	420	-
2004	458	-	350	200	461	650	159	-	390	-
2005	477	-	385	220	476	690	171	33	350	-
2006	440	-	317	350	462	600	179	41	280	-
2007	522	118	-	165	319	650	147	31	280	70
2008	563	150	-	130	335	670	162	28	240	60
2009	498	150	-	-	288	-	182	41	235	60
2010	475	150*	-	-	310	-	155	70*	240*	65*

Breed, farm code, year	Charollais	Lacaune			Awassi	Bábolna Tetra	Ile de France	Suffolk
	10	7	8	6	1	2	2	2
2003	-	212	198	-	1960	1717	937	195
2004	-	196	127	-	2120	1379	996	245
2005	-	165	-	-	1760	1222	863	240
2006	-	151	-	-	370	1147	732	224
2007	11	167	-	-	50	1014	866	214
2008	8	127	-	-	-	1043	784	304
2009	16	245	-	297	-	311	310	242
2010	18*	255*	-	369*	-	286	186	107

* *lambing after AI made in 2010 started in 2011*

Table 3. Distribution of the number of inseminated ewes by breed and farms

Based on the results of our survey (visiting the eleven farms), all necessary tools and equipments were available. Moreover, officially-accepted artificial insemination stations were operating on farms No. 1 and 7, from where semen could be bought by other farms.

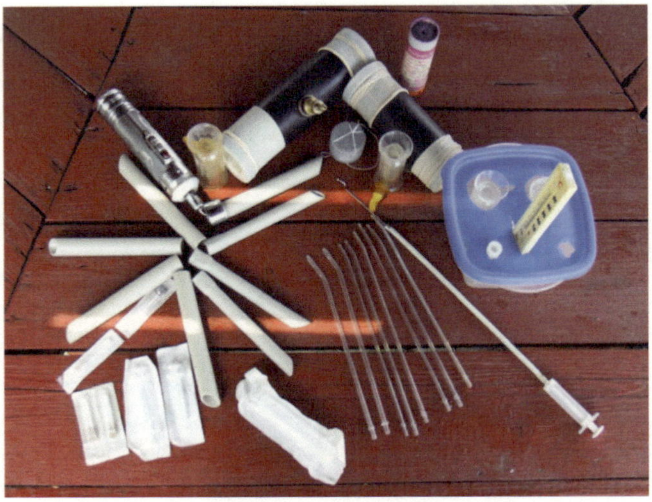

Fig. 2. The equipments and tools for artificial insemination (Photo: Kukovics, S.)

3.2 Preparing the animal for the mating (inseminating) period

The preparation of rams and ewes for the mating (inseminating) period was a common practice on all farms. In the case of rams, the level of nutrition started to improve at least four weeks before the planned season. Parallel to this, the training of the rams was also initiated and semen was collected at least two times a week. The quality of the semen was studied.

3.2.1 Preparing ewes and using oestrus synchronisation

Oestrus synchronisation and induction are highly recommended in the case of using artificial insemination. Yet these methods were not commonly utilised on the studied farms during the period under study. The nutritional method (flushing started four weeks before AI) was used on every farm in order to prepare the ewes for the mating period. The ram effect was not really used. However, on some farms, vasectomised rams were introduced to the flock of ewes, but it was not correctly planned. No other method (like reducing the length of light hours) was used on these farms.

Oestrus synchronisation and induction were used on only five farms (No. 1, 5, 6, 7 and 10). These methods were used during the main season and in spring time on farms No. 1 and 10 (only in the case of Merinos), only in spring on farms No. 5 and 7, and only in winter on farm No. 6.

During the first four years, the most popular product for oestrus synchronization was the "Eazy-bred" vaginal implant (produced in New Zealand), but since 2005 new purchases were not possible because of EU regulations. The vaginal sponge (Chrono-Gest) was used on the farms over the last 5 years of the studied period. There were significant differences among the farms in the size of PMSG dose. For example, on farm No. 1, 750 IU was administered in the first two years and 600 IU in the following years. 500 IU PMSG dose was used on farms No. 5, 6 and 7. On farm No. 10, 550 IU was utilised during the first three years, but because of too strong effects the dose was reduced to 425 IU over the last four years of the studied period.

3.3 Collecting and examining the semen

The semen was collected locally on most of the farms by the shepherd with appropriate skills, except for farm No. 8 where transported semen was used. Artificial insemination was carried out by the skilled shepherd, except for farm No. 1, where it was done by a veterinarian in the first two years and by a technician during the following years (Figure 1). Visual examination of the semen was performed before use on every farm, but three (No. 2, 6 and 11) out of the 11 farms used only this method. Following the visual study, microscopic and morphological examinations of the semen were also carried out on farms No. 1 and 7. Microscopic examination of semen together with the visual study was performed on the other six farms.

3.4 Diluting of semen

Several kinds of extenders are available for every day use, and in many studies, it has been demonstrated that the use of diluting liquids could help the survival of spermatozoa in the semen. Nevertheless, most shepherds thought that using un-diluted semen produced better results and was safer. Six (No. 2, 3, 4, 5, 9 and 11) out of the eleven farms did not use any kind of extender to dilute the semen before insemination. The 1:2 and 1:4 diluting ratios were used on the first farm and in the first three years on farm No. 10, where a 1:3-diluting ratio was used during the following three years. The 1:4 ratio was used on farm No. 5 (in 2003) and 1:8 on farms No. 6 and 7.

In the 1950s and 60s, one of the most popular extender was skimmed cow milk on farms. However, the Ivanov and the Salamon kinds as well as their improved versions were available after the late 60s and most of the shepherds carrying out the inseminations knew all of them and heard about several other ones. It was particularly interesting because more than half of the shepherds successfully participated in the AI courses mentioned above, and a few were even performing AI in cattle.

Three of the farms (6, 7 and 8) employed a special extender developed by the research station (farm No. 7). Semen diluted with this extender and cooled and kept at 2 to 4°C could be used successfully for 72 hours after collection. The improved Salamon kind of extender was used on farms No. 1 and 10.

3.5 Semen dose for insemination

In general, 0.2 ml was the most common dose of inseminating semen. It was used on seven (No. 1, 2, 3, 4, 5, 7 and 8) out of the 11 farms. Doses of 0.1 and 0.3 ml were used on farms No. 9 and 11, as well as No. 6 and 10, respectively.

3.6 Detecting ewes on heat for insemination

As the one of the most important factors of successful artificial insemination is selecting the ewes on heat, morning and afternoon selections were used on most farms (No. 1, 3, 4, 5 and 8). The selection was either only performed in the morning (No. 2, 7 and 9) or in the afternoon (No. 6 and 10) on the other farms. Midday was the selection time on farm No. 11 for the first 4 years, which was changed to the morning system during the following years.

The selection lasted half an hour to one hour during each part of the day. Vasectomised rams were used on farms No. 1 and 7 over the whole studied period. Entire rams with apron were used as teasing rams on five farms (No. 3, 4, 6, 9 and 10) and both kinds of rams were used on only one farm (No. 5). On farm No 2 and 8, vasectomised rams were used in the first four years, and entire rams with apron during the second four years, while on farm No. 11, the order was the reverse: the vasectomised rams were used in the second four years of the period.

3.7 The time and number of insemination

Two inseminations were used on most of the farms (No. 1, 2, 3, 4, 5, 6, 7 and 8) about 8 to 10 hours apart (morning-afternoon or afternoon-morning), but only one insemination was utilised on two farms (No. 9 in the morning and No. 11 in the afternoon). On farm No. 10, three inseminations (morning - afternoon - morning or afternoon - morning - afternoon) were carried out each year.

3.8 Performing insemination

For successful insemination, ewes have to be fixed and the rear part of their body should be lifted up. The rear legs of the ewes were lifted up and fixed by one labourer on the top of the barrier (Figure 3) in almost all of the studied farms. Farms No. 6 and 8 were the exceptions, where the labourer had to lift up the rear part of the ewes and hold them during the time of insemination.

This operation needs more than one labourer, therefore, one catcher and one inseminator should be used for this job as a minimum. On most of the farms, the inseminations were performed by the owner shepherd with one or two labourers to help him. On farms No. 1 and 7, technicians conducted the inseminations. There was only one catcher helping the inseminator on farms No. 5, 7, 9, 10 and 11. Two labourers caught and held the ewes on four farms (No. 3, 4, 6 and 8). On the first farm, 5 catchers helped the work of 2 inseminators during the first three years, and in the following two years only one inseminator with two labourers performed the job. On farm No. 2, the number of catchers decreased from two to one during the last three years and only one inseminator worked there.

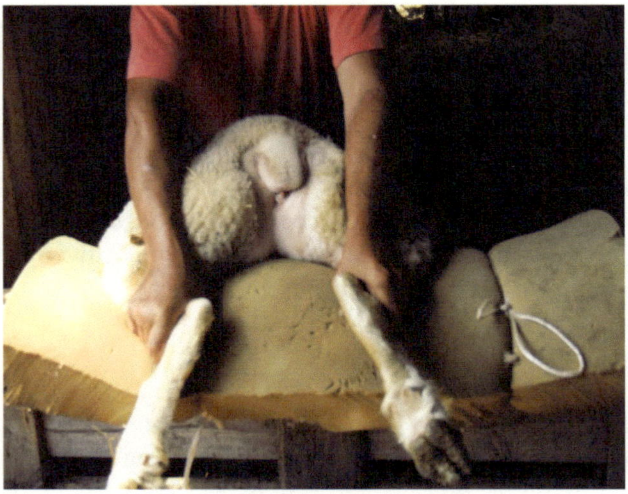

Fig. 3. The fixing of ewe for insemination (Photo: Kukovics, S.)

3.9 The place of semen deposition

The place of semen deposition is the other rather critical point of insemination. Traditional vaginal insemination was used on only one farm (No. 9) and only in the first three years of the studied period. They then changed to cervical deposition. Cervico-uterinal insemination was performed on farms No. 6, 7 and 10 (and sometimes on 11), while cervical insemination was used on other farms (Figure 4). Laparoscopic insemination was only used at the experimental level in the country. It was too expensive for farm practice.

Inseminating pipettes were available on all farms. The special catheter (Figure 1) for trans-cervical insemination developed by Tassy and Gergatz (Kukovics, 1974) were also used, which was utilised by most inseminators during the studied period. This catheter has a special bent tip that allows passage through the cervix and is made in different sizes for adult ewes and yearlings.

3.10 The pregnancy control

The results of lambing were too late to determine the effectiveness of artificial insemination. "State-of-the-art" pregnancy tests to determine the results of AI are important for profitable sheep farming. Yet, the level of pregnancy control in the case of inseminated ewes was rather low on the studied farms. The most up-to-date trans-rectal ultrasonography was used only on farm No. 1. Ultrasonography was performed within 60 days of AI in every studied year on farm No. 10, in the first 4 years on farm No. 7 and only in the first two years on farm No. 5.

The commonly used method to reach and keep pregnancy at the highest possible level was the post-mating with entire rams that started one cycle after the AI and lasted for two cycles. Farm No. 4 was an exception, where no post-mating was utilised. An interesting thing happened in the case of farm No. 7, where post-mating was not used during the second four years of the studied period.

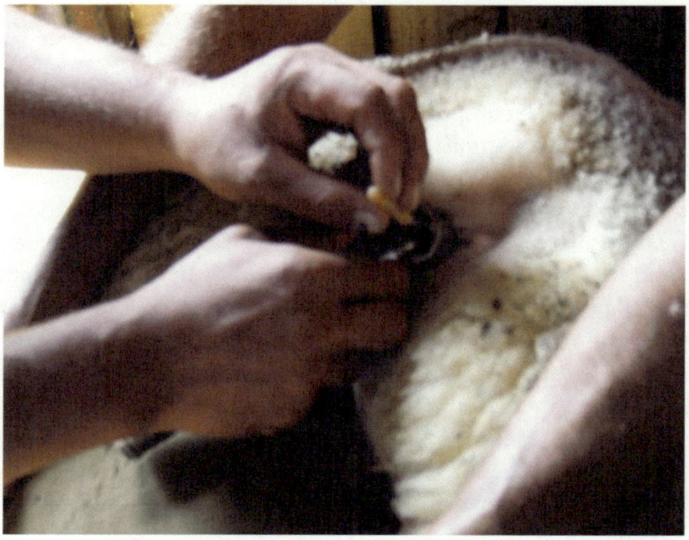

Fig. 4. The insemination (Photo: Kukovics, S.)

3.11 The results of artificial insemination

There were significant differences found among the studied farms and among the various breeds kept on various farms and also between the breeds within the farms. The pregnancy rate in general exceeded 80% and results over 90% were not exceptional at all. However, effects of farm, breed and year were observed on the results.

At least two or three breeds were kept on four farms (No. 2, 8, 10 and 11) and only one breed was bred on the other seven farms. Due to this, the results found in the case of four farms were evaluated separately, and the findings concerning the other seven farms were pooled together.

The pregnancy, lambing and weaning rate of the lambs were evaluated and the results are presented in the Tables from 4 to 10.

3.11.1 Farms breeding more than one breed

The pregnancy rate (P%) on farm No. 2 was different among breeds in 2004, where Suffolk ewes had a significantly lower value than the other two breeds (Table 4). In 2006, the pregnancy rate of Ile de France ewes was significantly higher than that of the other breeds. In 2005, 2008 and 2009, there were significant differences among all three breeds. In the Bábolna Tetra breed, the highest P% was measured in 2009, which was significantly higher than in the other years (except 2005 and 2010). The P% in 2008 was significantly lower than in the other years. In the Ile de France breed, the lowest P% in 2009 was different from the other values, like the values in 2007 and 2008. In the Suffolk breed, the P% of 2009 was significantly lower than in the other years (Table 4).

Significant effects of year were observed within the breeds in this trait, more than a 16%-range was found between the smallest and highest values in all three breeds; however, the biggest deviations were in the case of the Suffolk breed.

The lambing rate (L%) in the Bábolna Tetra breed varied between 1.6 and 2.0, while in Ile de France, the interval was narrower (between 1.2 and 1.4). In the case of the Suffolk breed, the L% changed every year (Table 4). It meant that the effect of the year was stronger in the Bábolna Tetra and Suffolk breeds than in the Ile the France. However, the differences reached the significant level ($P<5.0\%$) only between 2007 and 2009 and between 2004 and 2007 in the case of the first two years, respectively. Given that the lambing rate was a steady characteristic of the breeds, the comparison of these breeds was not justified (Table 4).

Breed and the year effect were equally found in the case of the weaning rate. Regarding the year effect, the smallest distance was observed in the case of Ile de France (less than 10%) and the biggest in Suffolk (more than 19%). The rate was 15.6% in the Bábolna Tetra breed.

The weaning % had an increasing trend from Bábolna Tetra to Suffolk via Ile de France in 2004, 2008, 2009, and the opposite trend was found in 2003. In the other years, the ranking of the breeds changed. The highest weaning % was measured in 2009 in the case of Bábolna Tetra (97.8%), while the most successful year was 2005 for the Ile de France and Suffolk breeds (91.1 and 93.2%, respectively). The weakest result in Bábolna Tetra was found in 2003 (82.2%), while this happened for Ile de France in 2010 (81.1%) and 2007 for the Suffolk (68.4%) breed. In most cases, there were significant differences among the data (Table 4).

Among the breeds kept on farm No. 9, the only differences were observed in 2004 and 2006, when the pregnancy rate of German Blackheaded Mutton was significantly lower than that of the other two breeds (Table 5).

In the Hungarian Merino breed, the P% of 2006 differed from those of the other years (except 2010), which differed from other previous years. In the German Mutton Merino breed, the data of 2006 differed from that of 2003, 2005 and 2007. In the German Blackheaded Mutton breed, there were no significant differences between 2003 and 2006 and from 2005 to 2010 (Table 5).

Breed, trait, year	Bábolna Tetra			Ile de France			Suffolk		
	P%	L%	W%	P%	L%	W%	P%	L%	W%
2003	82.2^{aA}	1.7	82.2^{aA}	81.4^{aA}	1.2	85.8^{bcA}	76.9^{aA}	1.4	86.4^{acA}
2004	86.1^{aB}	1.8	86.0^{aB}	83.3^{aA}	1.3	84.3^{acAC}	73.9^{bAB}	1.7	79.9^{bcA}
2005	87.3^{aBE}	1.7	94.2^{aC}	90.4^{bB}	1.3	91.1^{bcB}	66.3^{cB}	1.5	93.2^{acB}
2006	79.4^{aC}	1.7	83.7^{aA}	92.2^{bB}	1.2	88.7^{bcAB}	77.4^{aA}	1.4	85.4^{acA}
2007	79.7^{aAC}	1.6	88.5^{aD}	79.6^{aA}	1.3	87.1^{aA}	80.4^{aA}	1.2	68.4^{bC}
2008	73.1^{aD}	1.7	84.4^{aAB}	94.6^{bC}	1.3	83.3^{aAC}	79.6^{cA}	1.4	81.8^{aA}
2009	90.7^{aE}	2.0	97.8^{aDE}	84.7^{bD}	1.2	87.9^{aAD}	85.7^{C}	1.3	86.9^{aAD}
2010	86.7^{aABE}	1.9	82.3^{aA}	90.3^{aB}	1.4	81.8^{aA}	83.2^{aA}	1.5	82.1^{aA}

The different small letters in rows and the different upper case letters in columns mean significant differences (P≤0.05) per trait (pregnancy, weaning) among breeds and years.

Table 4. The result of AI on farm No. 2

The lambing rate (%) in Hungarian Merino varied between 1.5 and 1.7, while it was between 1.6 and 1.8 in German Mutton Merino. In German Blackheaded Mutton sheep, the lowest rate was 1.5 in 2009, while the highest 1.8 value was found four times (Table 5). The value of this trait exceeded the national average by 0.3 to 0.4 lambs in the case of Hungarian Merino. Additionally, German Mutton Merino and German Blackheaded Mutton sheep had a 0.2 to 0.3 advantage per lambing over the national average in the country.

Breed, trait, year	Hungarian Merino			German Mutton Merino			German Blackheaded Mutton Sheep		
	P%	L%	W%	P%	L%	W%	P%	L%	W%
2003	89.5^{aA}	1.6	96.4^{aA}	92.2^{aA}	1.7	95.9^{aA}	87.9^{aA}	1.8	96.7^{aA}
2004	92.4^{aAC}	1.6	97.4^{aA}	3.9^{aAB}	1.6	96.7^{aA}	85.5^{bA}	1.7	95.4^{aA}
2005	90.4^{aAC}	1.7	97.2^{aA}	93.1^{aA}	1.7	96.6^{aA}	91.8^{aAC}	1.8	95.3^{aA}
2006	97.5^{aB}	1.5	96.6^{aA}	96.3^{aB}	1.7	95.8^{aA}	89.9^{bAC}	1.8	94.9^{aA}
2007	91.4^{aAC}	1.7	4.9^{aAB}	92.8^{aA}	1.6	95.0^{aA}	95.2^{aBC}	1.8	93.0^{aA}
2008	93.1^{aC}	1.7	96.3^{aA}	93.7^{aA}	1.6	95.4^{aA}	94.4^{aBC}	1.7	94.3^{aA}
2009	94.6^{aACD}	1.7	96.6^{aA}	93.4^{aA}	1.8	95.3^{acA}	90.7^{aAC}	1.5	93.3^{bcA}
2010	96.4^{aB}	1.6	95.1^{aAB}	93.5^{aA}	1.7	95.3^{aA}	92.9^{aAC}	1.7	94.6^{aA}

The different small letters in rows and the different upper case letters in columns mean significant differences (P≤0.05) per trait (pregnancy, weaning) among breeds and years.

Table 5. The results of AI on farm No. 9

As this farm was one of the best, these data were very close to each other and their levels were close to the maximum of the genetic possibilities, yet the differences found among them originated from the breed characteristics. Of course, the year effects were also observed among these data, but the differences reached the significant level (P<5.0%) in only one case in German Blackheaded Mutton Sheep (2009 vs. 2003, 2005, 2006, 2007), in German Mutton Merino (2009 vs. 2004, 2007, 2008) and in Hungarian Merino (2006 vs. 2005, 2007, 2008, 2009).

In the weaning ratio of the period of 2003 to 2006, there were no significant differences in a breed between years and between breeds by year (Table 5).

In Hungarian Merino, only the ratio in 2004 differed from that of 2007 and 2010. In the other two breeds, there were no significant differences between years (Table 5).

The results from farm No. 10 keeping three different breeds are shown in Table 6.

The pregnancy rate of British Milksheep differed from Hungarian Merino in 2007 and from Charollais in 2009. In 2008, there were no significant differences. In British Milksheep, the pregnancy ratio of 2007 differed from that of 2009, but in the other two breeds, there were no statistical differences among the years (Table 6).

The lambing rate of British Milksheep was the highest among the breeds (between 1.9 and 2.6), while the lowest was in Charollais (between 1.4 and 1.8). In the Hungarian Merino, it varied between 1.5 and 1.7 (Table 6). Since the lambing rate was a steady characteristic of the breeds, the comparison of these breeds was not necessary. At the same time, the year effect was significantly lower in 2009 in British Milksheep compared to the other years and the difference also reached this level between 2007 and 2008. In the case of Charollais, the values of 2009 were significantly higher compared to those of the other two years.

The weaning ratio of British Milksheep differed from that of Hungarian Merino in 2007 and from Charollais in 2009. In 2008, there were no significant differences. In the weaning ratio of British Milksheep lambs, the year 2009 differed from the previous years, except 2008, while 2006 differed from all other years. In the other two breeds there were no statistical differences in weaning ratios among the years (Table 6).

Breed, trait, year	British Milksheep			Charollais			Hungarian Merino		
	P%	L%	W%	P%	L%	W%	P%	L%	W%
2005	97.0^{A}	2.5	73.4^{A}	-	-	-	-	-	-
2006	87.8^{A}	2.4	65.9^{AB}	-	-	-	-	-	-
2007	100.0^{aAB}	2.3	81.7^{aAC}	72.7^{acA}	1.5	100.0^{acA}	67.8^{bcA}	1.7	91.2^{bcA}
2008	89.3^{aA}	2.6	92.3^{aC}	100.0^{aA}	1.4	81.8^{aA}	76.0^{aA}	1.5	91.8^{aA}
2009	87.8^{aAC}	1.9	97.0^{aC}	93.8^{bcA}	1.8	85.2^{bcA}	70.7^{acA}	1.7	9.3^{acA}
2010	*	*	*	*	*	*	*	*	*

The different small letters in rows and the different upper case letters in columns mean significant differences (P≤0.05) per trait (pregnancy, weaning) among breeds and years.
**lambing started in 2011*

Table 6. The results of AI on farm No. 10

On farm No. 11, there were no significant differences in the years between the two breeds kept in P%. The pregnancy rate of British Milksheep in 2003 differed significantly from that of the other years. In the British Milksheep Crossbreds, there were no significant differences among the years (Table 7).

The lambing rate in purebred was higher than that in the crossbred population, varying between 2.0 and 2.4, while in crossbreds, it was between 1.9 and 2.4 (Table 7). In the case of crossbreds, the year 2009 was almost exceptional (P<5.0%; 2009 vs. 2007 and 2008), while in the case of purebred, the lambing rate of 2010 significantly differed from that of the years 2006 and 2007 (Table 7).

Breed, trait, year	British Milksheep			British Milksheep Crossbreds		
	P%	L%	W%	P%	L%	W%
2003	93.3^{A}	2.2	82.4^{A}	-	-	-
2004	88.5^{B}	2.1	87.8^{B}	-	-	-
2005	82.9^{CD}	2.1	92.1^{C}	-	-	-
2006	87.5^{BD}	2.0	94.9^{CD}	-	-	-
2007	78.6^{aCD}	2.0	88.9^{aBC}	78.6^{aA}	1.9	98.0^{bA}
2008	83.3^{aBD}	2.1	94.1^{aCD}	83.3^{aA}	2.0	93.9^{aA}
2009	83.0^{aBC}	2.3	96.7^{aD}	75.0^{aA}	2.4	98.2^{aA}
2010	85.7^{BC}	2.4	98.4^{D}	*	*	*

The different small letters in rows and the different upper case letters in columns mean significant differences (P≤0.05) per trait (pregnancy, weaning) among breeds and years.
**lambing started in 2011*

Table 7. The results of AI on farm No. 11

The weaning ratio of British Milksheep only differed from that of British Milksheep Crossbred in 2007. In British Milksheep, the ratio of weaned lambs in 2003 was significantly different from that of the other years, and 2010 from all other years. In British Milksheep Crossbred, there were no significant differences among the years (Table 7).

3.11.2 Farms with only one breed

Among the inseminating farms with one breed only, the Awassi farm's P% was significantly different among the years, except between 2003 and 2004. On farm No. 3, the lower pregnancy rate was found in 2005, which differed significantly from the other years, while only the values from 2003 and 2006 did not differ from each other.

On the P% on farm No. 5, the year 2005 was different from the other years. On farm No. 4, the values received from 2008 differed from those of 2005 and 2006. On farm No. 7, the rate in 2004 differed from that of 2003, 2006 and 2007, the value of 2005 was different from that of 2003, the rate of 2006 differed from 2007, and that of 2006 was different from those of 2004, 2005, 2008 and 2009. On farm No. 8, the P% was not significantly different from each other (Table 8).

The lambing rate of Awassi breed was steady at 1.3, the lowest among the breeds, and no year effects were observed. Small differences were found between the two Hungarian Merino populations, and the values of the "better one" sharply decreased over the last two years because of labour problem. German Mutton Merino had a constant lambing rate. In the Lacaune breed, the lambing rate varied between 1.4 and 1.6 on the three farms (Table 9), and minimal effects of year were observed in the case of farm No. 7.

Farm code	breed / year	2003	2004	2005	2006	2007	2008	2009
1	Awassi+Awassi crossbreds	37.3[a]	35.0[a]	45.0[b]	56.8[c]	80.0[d]	-	-
3	Hungarian Merino	83.2[a]	93.4[b]	67.0[c]	83.0[a]	-	-	-
5	Hungarian Merino	75.0[a]	67.5[ac]	78.6[ab]	62.9[bc]	66.7[a]	61.5[acd]	-
4	German Mutton Merino	84.4[a]	83.8[a]	87.0[ab]	86.7[a]	84.3[a]	81.0[ac]	-
6	Lacaune*	-	-	-	-	-	-	88.2
7	Lacaune*	95.3[a]	85.2[b]	81.8[b]	96.7[a]	97.6[a]	82.7[b]	79.6[b]
8	Lacaune	58.6[a]	66.1[a]	-	-	-	-	-

The different small letters in rows indicate significant differences (P≤0.05).
**The lambing after AI made in 2010 started in 2011*

Table 8. The pregnancy rate (%) on farms with one breed

Farm code	breed / year	2003	2004	2005	2006	2007	2008	2009
1	Awassi, Awassi crossbreds	1.3	1.3	1.3	1.3	1.3	-	-
3	Hungarian Merino	1.4	1.3	1.3	1.4	-	-	-
5	Hungarian Merino	1.5	1.5	1.5	1.4	1.2	1.2	-
4	German Mutton Merino	1.4	1.4	1.4	1.4	1.5	1.5	-
6	Lacaune*	-	-	-	-	-	-	1.5
7	Lacaune*	1.4	1.6	1.5	1.6	1.5	1.4	1.6
8	Lacaune	1.6	1.6	-	-	-	-	-

**The lambing after AI made in 2010 started in 2011*

Table 9. The lambing rate (%) on farms with one breed

Farm code	breed / year	2003	2004	2005	2006	2007	2008	2009
1	Awassi, Awassi crossbreds	94.5[a]	95.3[a]	94.8[a]	95.6[a]	96.2[a]	-	-
3	Hungarian Merino	96.6[a]	91.3[bd]	86.5[cd]	90.5[d]	-	-	-
5	Hungarian Merino	88.0[a]	89.8[a]	95.6[b]	97.4[b]	84.1[ac]	90.9[abc]	-
4	German Mutton Merino	89.3[a]	89.0[a]	89.3[ab]	90.9[a]	87.0[ac]	88.3[a]	-
6	Lacaune*	-	-	-	-	-	-	95.2
7	Lacaune*	53.0[a]	86.5[b]	84.8[b]	80.3[b]	85.5[b]	79.7[bc]	71.2[c]
8	Lacaune	89.8[a]	93.9[a]	-	-	-	-	-

The different small letters in rows indicate significant differences (P≤0.05).
**The lambing after AI made in 2010 started in 2011*

Table 10. The weaning rate (%) on farms with one breed

In the Awassi breed, there were no significant differences among years in the weaning rate. On farm No. 3, the W% was the highest in 2003, which was significantly different from the other studied years. However, the ratio in 2006 was close to the values found in 2004 and 2005. On farm No. 5, 2006 was the year most different from the others. On farm No. 4, the only difference observed was between 2006 and 2007, while on No. 7, the two terminal years (2003 and 2009) differed from the other years. On farm No. 8, there was no significant difference among years in the weaning rate (Table 10).

3.12 The cost of artificial insemination

Rather big differences were observed among the studied farms (Table 11). In most cases, these data were calculated by the owner of the farm and mainly covered the direct cost of semen collection and insemination, while other costs were not included. On some farms, the same level was calculated every year, while on others, the annual costs increased with the years. Apart from these, the use of oestrus synchronisation increased the costs by about 7 or above 8 euros per ewe.

In general, the average direct costs of artificial insemination per ewe could reach 0.4 to 0.5 euros, and in the case of oestrus synchronisation, the total costs could exceed 7 to 8 euros under present Hungarian circumstances.

Farm code	2003	2004	2005	2006	2007	2008	2009	2010
1	3.70*	3.70**	3.70**	3.70**	5.56**	-	-	-
2	0.74	0.74	0.74	0.74	0.74	0.74	0.74	0.74
3	1.48	1.67	1.85	1.85	-	-	-	-
4	0.37*	0.37*	0.37*	0.37*	0.37*	0.37*	-	-
5	0.74	0.74	0.93	1.11	1.11	1.31	-	-
6	-	-	-	-	-	-	0.37*	0.37*
7	3.70	3.70	3.70	3.70*	3.70*	3.70**	3.70**	3.70**
8	0.93	1.11	1.30	1.30	1.30	1.85	1.85	1.85
9	1.85	1.85	-	-	-	-	-	-
10	-	-	0.37*	0.37*	0.37*	0.37*	0.37*	0.37*
11		0.37	0.37	0.37	0.37	0.37	0.37	0.37

It was calculated on the changing rate of 1 euro = 270 HUF
In the case of oestrus synchronisation, the costs reached seven (*) or eight euros (**) per ewe.

Table 11. The estimated costs of artificial insemination (euro/ewe)

4. Conclusions

Apart from the fact that artificial insemination is used only on a limited number of Hungarian sheep farms, the effectiveness of this method was quite reasonable. Based on the results, the following conclusions can be drawn.

- Apart from the lack of officially-organised education of shepherds, there are some sheep owners and shepherds who can operate with the method of artificial insemination at a very good level (Kukovics & Gergazt, 2009).

- Artificial insemination of ewes can be performed with very high effectiveness on farms in every day practice mainly by shepherds. The reality is that AI does not need veterinary assistance, but maintaining the health of ewes needs veterinary control.
- The procedure of artificial insemination requires well-skilled shepherds with good practice and enough support.
- The breed of ewe has a significant effect on the pregnancy rate, which is consistent with the results of Hill et al. (1998), Perkins et al. (1996), Donovan et al. (2001 and 2004), Karagiannidis et al. (2001) and Anel et al. (2005). However, the results could be positively modified by the interest of the sheep owner.
- The dose of PMSG affected conception rate, similar to the findings of Hill et al. (1998). Thus, in some cases, the dose should be reduced in order to avoid too many lambs being born and higher lamb loss originating from the weakness of the lambs at birth.
- Most shepherds use fresh, locally collected, un-diluted semen with good results, and the importance of dilution is only realised by a small number of the shepherds.
- The year had a strong effect on the results of artificial insemination, in accordance with the results of Anel et al. (2005), but no trends could be discovered in the data. The environmental circumstances (available pasture and feed for instance) had stronger importance.
- The cost of artificial insemination depends on the farm, but in general, the direct cost was less than one euro per ewe. Of course, in the case of oestrus synchronisation and induction, these costs could reach 7 to 8 euros per ewe.
- The results of artificial insemination could easily be controlled by using ultrasonography (Egerszegi at al., 2008) at an early stage of pregnancy, but this method was only used on a small number of farms.

5. Acknowledgements

The authors would like to thank the owners and the representatives of the sheep farms for their excellent technical help in collecting the data and analysing the information needed for final evaluation. They are in alphabetic order: Attila Harcsa (Abbod Farm, Szendrő), Antal Kádas (Túrkeve), István Nagy and Imre Nagy (Ganna), László Nagy (Eger), Sándor Nagy (Bakonszeg Awassi Corporation, Bakonszeg), Zoltán Nagy (Harkakötöny), Mihály Sebők (Törtel), Ede Sipos (Móriczhida), Károly Szabó (Hajdúbagos) and Zoltán Szabó (Karcag).
The study was made by K-OVI-CAP BT within the framework of University of Debrecen Centre of Agriculture and Economic Sciences with the help of the Jedlik Ányos project supported by National Office of Research and Technology (NKTH)

6. References

Anel, L., M. Kaabi, B. Abroug, M. Alvarez, E. Anel, J.C. Boixo, L.F. de la Fuente, P. De Paz (2005). Factors influencing the success of vaginal and laparoscopic artificial insemination in Churra ewes: a field assay, Theriogenology, 63, 1235-1247.

Barillet, F., S., Sanna, D., Boichard, J.M., Astruc, A., Carta, S., Casu (1993). Genetic evaluation of the Lacaune, Manech and Sarda dairy sheep with Animal Model, Proceedings of 5th International Symposium on Machine Milking of Small Ruminants /Ed.: Kukovics, S./, Hungary, May 1993, 289-303.

Becze, J. (1982). Tanulmányok haszonállatok szaporításáról. (Studies on the reproduction of domestic animal breeds); Mezőgazdasági Kiadó, ISBN 963-231-114-0, Budapest

Donovan, A. , J.P. Hanrahan, T. Lally, M.P. Boland, G. P. Lonergan, D.J. O'Neil (2001). AI for sheep using frozen-thawed semen, ARMIS 4047 Project report, under the Research Stimulus Fund; OPARDF measure 5b, ISBN 1 84170 152 1

Donovan, A. , J.P. Hanrahan, E. Kummen, P. Duffy, M.P. Boland (2004). Fertility of the ewe following cervical insemination with fresh or frozen-thawed semen at natural or synchronised oestrus, Animal Reproduction Science, 84, 359-368.

Egerszegi, I., A., Molnár, P., Sarlós, F., Soós, J., Rátky (2008). Investigation of the follicular development and early Pregnancy in Hungarian Black Racka ewes by means ultrasonography - preliminary study (A tüszőnövekedés és korai vemhesség ultrahangos vizsgálata fekete racka juhokban - előkísérlet) AWETH 4. (2.) 311-318. 2008 I. Gödöllői Állattenyésztési Tudományos Napok, Gödöllő 12-13, (in Hungarian)

Ehling, C., P. Wirth, L. Schindler, K.-G. Hadeler, H.-H. Döpke, E. Lemme, D. Herrmann, H. Niemann (2003). Laparoscopical intrauterine insemination with different doses of fresh, conserved, and frozen-thawed semen for the production of ovine zygotes, Theriogenology, 60, 777-787.

Fernandez-Abella, D., M.O. Preve, N. Villegas (2003). Insemination time and diluting rate of cooled and chilled ram semen affects fertility, Theriogenology, 60, 21-26.

Gergátz, E. (2007). A juhok mesterséges termékenyítése; in: Házi emlősállatok mesterséges termékenyítése. (The artificial insemination in sheep; in Artificial insemination in domestic mammals); Szerk. (Edited) Tamás Pécsi; Pécsi Tamás, Mezőgazda Kiadó,Bp. ISBN 978-963-286-237-8

Gergátz, E., E., Gyökér (1997). Cervicouterinal Insemination method with cooled and deep frozen ram semen; 48. Annual Meeting of EAAP,Vienna, Book of Abstract, 319-325.

Gulyás, L., E., Gergátz, J., Végh, A., Németh (2007). A fogyasztási csúcsokhoz igazodó bárányelőállítás lehetőségei biotechnikai módszerek felhasználásával. (Possibilities of lamb meat production adjusted to consuming peaks using biotechnical methods). Acta Agronomica Óváriensis 49. 1.-29-42.

Hill, J. R., J. A., Thomson, N.R., Perkins (1998). Factors affecting pregnancy rates following laparoscopic insemination of 28,447 Merino ewes under commercial conditions: a survey, Theriogenology, 49, 697-709.

Jávor, A., S., Kukovics, Gy. Molnár (2006). Juhtenyésztés A-tól Z-ig (Sheep breeding to A to Z), Mezőgazda Kiadó, ISBN 963 286 275 9, Budapest.

Karagiannidis, A., S. Varsakeli, G. Karatzas, C. Brozos (2001). Effect of time of artificial insemination on fertility of progestegen and PMSG treated indigenous Greek ewes, during non-breeding season, Small Ruminant Research, 39, 67-71.

King, M.E., W.A.C. McKelvey, W.S. Dingwall, K.P. Matthews, F.E. Gebbie, M.J.A. Mylne, E. Stewart, J.J. Robinson (2004). Lambing rates and litter sizes following intrauterine or cervical insemination of frozen-thawed semen with or without oxytocin administration, Theriogenology, 62, 1236-1244.

Kukovics, S. (1974). A mesterséges termékenyítés eredményeinek értékelése, valamint a juh szaporaságának és gazdaságosságának néhány kérdése (The evalation of the results of artificial insemination and some questions prolificacy and profitability in sheep); Állattenyésztési Kutatóintézet (Research Institute for Animal Production) Herceghalom, research study report made for Ministry of Agriculture, p. 120.

Kukovics, S., E. Gergatz (2009). A juh mesterséges termékenyítése üzemekben (Artificial insemination of sheep on farm), In: Magyar Állatorvosok Lapja (Hungarian Veterinary Journal), 131, 21-26.

Kukovics, S., A., Jávor (2002). A világfajták szerepe a juh árutermelésben. (The role of world sheep breeds in commodity production), Magyar Juhászat + Kecsketenyésztés (Hungarian Sheep Farming + Goat Breeding), Vol. 11, No. 11, pp. 4-8.

Moses, D., A.G., Martinez, G., Iorio, A., Valcárcel, A., Ham, H., Pessi, R., Castanon, A., Maciá, M.A. de las Heras (1997). A large-scale program in laparoscopic intrauterine insemination with frozen-thawed semen in Australian Merino sheep in Argentine Patagonia, Theriogeneology, 48, 651-657.

Mucsi, I. (1997). Juhtenyésztés és - tartás (Sheep breeding and keeping), Mezőgazda Kiadó, ISBN 963912124, Budapest.

Perkins, N.R., J.R. Hill, R.G. Pedrana (1996). Laparoscopic insemination of frozen-thawed semen into one or bothuterine horns without regard to ovulation site in synchronised Merino ewes, Theriogenology, 46, 541-545.

Salamon, S., W.M.C. Maxwell (1995). Frozen storage of ram semen. I. Processing, freezing, thawing and fertility after cervical insemination, Animal Reproduction Science, 37, 185-249.

Sarlós, P. (1999). Kosspermatermelés, kosspermaminőség (Production of ram semen, quality of ram semen), Állattenyésztési és Takarmányozási Kutatóintézet, Herceghalom, Retrieved from <http://www.atk.hu/Magyar/Ubbs/juhtart/index.html>

Stefanov, R., E., Krumova, M., Dolashka, W., Voelter, Z., Zachariev (2006). Artificial insemination of sheep and cow with semen treated by Cu/Zn-superoxide dismutase from fungal Humicola lutea 103, World Journal of Zoology, 1 (1), 36-39.

Szabados, T. (2006). A cervikouterinális inszeminálás eredményességének vizsgálata juhászatokban /Study of effectiveness in cervico-uterinal insemination of ewes/; PhD thesis, University of Western Hungary, Faculty of Agriculture and Food Sciences, Mosonmagyaróvár, Hungary.

Yamaki, K., M. Morisawa, A. Ribadulla, J. Kojima (2003). Sheep semen characteristics and artificial insemination by laparoscopy, Tohoku Journal of Agricultural Research, 54(1-2), 17-26.

http://www.farmanddairy.com/news/ultrasound-and-artificial-insemination-techniques

http://genetic-gains.co.nz

http://genstock.com.au

http://www.innovis.org

http://www.trialanderroracres.com

http://www.topRams.com

4

Artificial Insemination in Dogs

Rita Payan-Carreira[1], Sónia Miranda[2] and Wojciech Niżański[3]
[1]*CECAV – Univ. of Trás-os-Montes and Alto Douro,*
[2]*Escola Universitária Vasco da Gama,*
[3]*Univ. Environmental and Life Sciences, Wrocław,*
[1,2]*Portugal*
[3]*Poland*

1. Introduction

In Artificial Insemination (AI) the semen is collected manually from a stud male and thereafter deposited (inseminated) in the female so that fertilization can occur in the absence of natural mating. Artificial Insemination, one of the earliest techniques for assisted reproduction in animals and humans, took longer to be implemented in dogs due to species-specific particularities. In past decades, progresses in the knowledge of canine physiology and new advances in canine semen technology allowed these services to become available worldwide. Hence, subsequent to the increase in the artificial insemination demand among dog breeders and owners and the broaden of the AI to preserved semen as a management tool in canine breeding, as through international exchange of frozen semen, inbreeding within breeds can be reduced. Therefore, with spread of canine AI dog, breeders now may select stud dogs from all over the world to improve their kennel′ genetics, without transport-associated stress to the animals. Also, it is possible to save semen from valuable dogs into sperm bank to be used in next generations, after their death or the peak of reproductive age. In addition, breeders also are aware of the sanitary benefits associated with AI. Avoiding direct contact between the male and female, AI also prevents the spread of sexually transmitted diseases, as those originated by *Brucella canis* or *Herpes virus* (Farstad, 2010; Linde Forsberg, 2005a).

Although the first reports on AI in dogs subsequent to the Spallanzani experiments (in late XVIII century) appeared by the end of the fifties, reporting the use of fresh semen, or in the sixties, the use of frozen semen, only in the nineties this technique was introduced into dog breeding practice, particularly in USA and Nordic countries (Foote, 2002; England & Millar, 2008). The reproductive physiology of this species and unfavourable response of the dog sperm to freezing were the two major constraints to the initial efforts to improve the AI technique in dogs (Linde Forsberg, 2005a). A lot of research was performed in those areas, especially in the northern Europe, to overcome these issues, generating a large amount of information and allowing technical development, in particular in the canine semen technology. Nowadays, as a consequence of the demand for reproductive technologies, in particular the AI with fresh or refrigerate semen, this is a current service offered in the small animal veterinary practice.

According to Linde-Forsberg (2001, 2005a), from all the AI in dogs performed by veterinarians today in Europe, about 50-55% is done with fresh semen, collected at the clinic, 10% with chilled semen and around 35-40% with frozen semen. However, at least in Portugal, the use of imported chilled semen is far most frequent than the use of frozen semen when compared to other countries in Northern Europe.

Research on AI in the domestic dog, along with other reproductive technologies, proceed worldwide, particularly on sperm survival at freezing and the identification of deleterious components to spermatozoa or fertilization, providing important information for the preservation of wild *canidae* semen that are currently threatened or endangered.

2. Indications for artificial insemination

Several main indications exist to perform AI in the dog (Linde Forsberg, 2005a; England & Millar, 2008; Farstad, 2010). In parallel, some ethical conditions must be discussed when facing the different interests of specific groups, namely dogs, breeders, owners and veterinarians.

Main indications for AI in dogs include both medical and breeding-management reasons (Table 1). As major potential advantage, AI may allow to reduce physical distances, the use of genetically valuable stud dog semen all over the word, fighting the stress of transportation of animals and inbreeding (Johnston et al., 2001; Linde-Forsberg, 2005a). It is also an important technique whenever physical and behavioural abnormalities in the male or female preventing natural mating (Table 2).

3. The ethics and role of artificial insemination in canine breeding programs

Performing canine AI may raise some ethical concerns, mostly to central institutions like the National Kennel Clubs or Veterinarian Orders or equivalent, in particular on what concerns the use of frozen semen and the need for intra-uterine insemination, mainly those involving surgical procedures. In fact, several countries (such as Norway, Sweden and the United Kingdom) refer to welfare concerns and discourage or even forbid the use of surgical procedures to obtain intra-uterine insemination (England & Millar, 2008; Linde-Forsberg, 2005b).

Ethical issues are seldom associated with the non-surgical process of artificial insemination *per se*. Most procedures used for semen deposition are neither detrimental to the bitch, nor interfere with animal welfare, and even allow protection against certain diseases. However, some attention may be given to the inbreeding of animals that may compromise health of following generations (England & Millar, 2008).

Restrictions to the use of AI in animals that never matted despite all physiological conditions met together to guarantee a successful mate, may respond to the ethical issue that demands for ruling out clinical reasons for AI, as an underlying unaware problem (congenital or behavioural) may exists. This concern is in fact previewed in the Fédération Cynologique International (FCI) breeding rules (http://www.fci.be/circulaires/102-2010-annex-fr.pdf). According to those rules, AI should not be performed in animals not having at least one previous litter registered from natural service. Furthermore, AI to be a recognisable breeding technique must be performed by veterinarian or a specifically recognisable technician, which skills will avoid complications or adverse effects, as well as stress or risks of welfare infringements towards the animals, in particular the female.

Potential benefits	Potential weakness
- Decrease stress, infectious deseases transmission, travel expenses - Semen collection without interruption of the male activity (show or training) - Splitting of an ejaculate to bred more females - Reduction of the costs with maintenance of stud dogs in a colony - Worldwide availability of the semen of a given dog - Allow early castration of working dogs while maintaining availability of their genes - Evaluation of semen quality prior to AI - Early detection of male reproductive pathologies - Semen preservation, so genetic material may be available in the future - Overcome problems associated with the refusal to breed (psychological or physical reasons, precocious ejaculation), inexperienced males - May overcome quarantine restrictions	- Induction of physical or psychological trauma during the AI process - Risk of performing AI for inappropriate reasons - Failure in careful clinical examination of the breeding animals - Potential risk for maintaining some disorders in a particular genetic line (hip dysplasia or anatomical abnormality of the reproductive tract) - Potential risk for introduction of inherited diseases or abnormalities - Potential overuse of a given male within a programme or breed - May allow confusion of parentage

Table 1. Main advantages and inconveniences for canine AI.

Factor	Cause
Female-dependent	- Male rejection - Aggression - Congenital abnormalities (e.g. presence of a vaginal septum; genital tract strictures, small vulva and vagina)
Male-dependent	- Reduced libido (due to local or systemic diseases, age, deficient breeding management, drugs) - Pain - Physical deficiency (such as inability to mount or to obtain penile erection, lumbar muscle problems, congenital abnormalities)
Associated to both male and female	- Inexperience - Male to female disproportion - Social and behavioural problems (dominant female, inversion of the social hierarchy)

Table 2. Main causes for refusal of natural mating.

The competence of the operator to perform the procedures is essential to avoid all technique-related ethical constraints to the use of AI in dogs. Before offering canine AI services, practitioners ought to specialised themselves, acquiring profound knowledge of the reproductive physiology and pathology of the species and the skills to collect semen and to inseminate the female without risking animal health or welfare.

4. Semen collection and evaluation

4.1 Semen collection in the dog

Semen collection in the dog is a relatively easy procedure, although requiring some training for optimization of the technique. Semen collection and evaluation is necessary to obtain good results in canine AI. Although practitioners are often asked to collect semen and perform AI without detailed semen analysis, every sample of semen collected should be evaluated (at least progressive forward motility, total sperm count and morphology) before it is used for artificial insemination or cryopreservation. Semen evaluation prior to insemination warrants the male potential fertility and consequently may predict the fertility potential for the AI. In addition, when preparing semen preservation, fertility certificate may be needed. In such cases andrological evaluation of the stud dog (breeding soundness evaluation or BSE) has to be performed. Semen collection should be performed before the physical exam or any stressful procedures on the stud, or can be booked to another day (Freshman, 2002; Johnston et al, 2001).

Semen can be collected from most dogs in the absence of a teaser, in a quiet and isolated room, where interruptions should be prevented, although the presence of a bitch would allow better ejaculates. In reluctant males, stimulating estrus scent can be provided by the presence of a female in estrus or by using frozen-thawed swabs or gauze sponges taken from vaginal secretions of estrus bitches (Freshman, 2002; Kutzler, 2005; Olson & Husted, 1986). Although possible, not everyone achieves the use of a chemical pheromone (methyl p-hydroxybenzoate, Aldrich Chemical, Milwaukee, WI) swabbed on the perineal area and tail of an anestrus teaser (Johnston et al., 2001; Kutzler, 2005).

Collection of semen should be prepared in advance, and interval between collections or between the natural mating and collection, should be registered, if the male is regularly used. Ideal intervals between collections are 2 to 5 days, whilst intervals longer than 10 days may result in an increased number of morphological abnormalities and decreased motility (Freshman, 2002; Johnston et al., 2001). In longer periods, it is advisable to perform one previous collection, if semen is to be chilled or frozen for shipment. If semen preservation is planned, semen extender should be prepared before the arrival of the animal (Freshman, 2002).

The most common method for semen collection in the dog is by digital manipulation, in the presence of a female. However, bitch presence, although desirable as it facilitates procedures, is not essential to accomplish the collection (Farstad, 2010; Linde Forsberg, 2005a). It should be noticed that when the collection is achieved in the presence of the bitch ejaculates present higher concentration.

The use of manual massage is the most commonly used technique (Farstad, 2010; Johnston et al., 2001; Linde Forsberg, 2005a), although in the past semen was collected from dogs using an artificial vagina. Nowadays, semen collection into a tube is commonly accomplished by penile massage and the use of a cone or plastic sleeve, a funnel or a special collecting vial (Linde Forsberg, 2005a). Briefly, the process is started with a massage of the dog prepuce at the level of the *bulbus glandis* until developing partial erection, followed by the quick retraction of the prepuce and penile expose. If the collector is right-handed, semen must be collected from the dog's left side, with the operator holding the dog's penis with the right hand and the collection container in the left hand. During pelvic thrusting, rigid vials should be kept at a distance from the penis, to avoid trauma. When pelvic movements are finished and the dog lifts its rear leg, a 180° backward rotation of the penis should be obtained and the erectile penis should then be directed into the collection cone or the funnel.

Some pressure may be applied with the thumb on the apex of the *glans penis*, at the level of the urethral process, to stimulate ejaculation. When a crystal clear fluid (prostatic fluid) begins to flow into the collection tube, you can gently slide the collection cone off the penis. Watch for semen to flow in the collection tube (Farstad, 2010; Linde Forsberg, 2005a).

Canine ejaculate consists of 3 fractions, with the first and third fraction consisting of prostatic fluid and the second being rich in spermatozoa (England et al., 1990) (Table 3). The first fraction, the presperm portion, is emitted in 0.5 to 1 minute and is colourless, with a volume range of 1-5 ml. It is expelled during first stage of erection, at the moment of the presence of evident copulatory movement of male. The second fraction, the sperm-rich portion, is also rapidly completed (1-2 minutes), and is grayish-white in colour, with a volume of 1-3 ml. It is expelled when thrusting movement of the male ceases and full erection is observed. The third fraction comes from the prostate and may be up to 30-40 ml; it may take up from 5 to 30 minutes to be completed (Günzel-Apel, 1994; Johnston et al., 2001).

Characteristics	1st fraction	2nd Fraction	3rd Fraction
Volume	0.1-2 mL (average 0.33 mL)	0.1-3 mL (average 1.17 mL) Sometimes larger volume	1-2 to >20 mL Quite variable depending on the animal.
Colour	clear or opaque	greyish-white, white, milky-white	clear, transparent
Consistency	watery	watery-milky, milky	watery
Character	prostate secretion with admixture of epithelial cells, urine, bacteria and sperm cells	sperm cells suspended in seminal plasma	prostate gland secretion
pH (average)	6.37	6.10	7.20
Duration	5-90 sec. (average 13.5 sec)	5-300 sec. (average 52.4 sec.)	60 sec-20 min. (average 6 min. 55 sec.)

Table 3. Main characteristics of the different fractions of the dog ejaculate.

Size of the dog	Volume of the ejaculate
< 20 kg	1-22.5 mL (average 5.38 mL)
> 20 kg	2-45 mL (average 12.75 mL)

Table 4. Variation on the volume of the ejaculate with the size of the dog (Dubiel, 2004)

In the dog, the volume of whole ejaculate varies between breeds (Table 4) mainly with animal size and is partially dependent on the volume of the third fraction collected, which constitute about 95% of the volume of the ejaculate in dogs (Farstad, 2010).

In most dogs, semen can be collected twice at 30 minutes interval (Farstad, 2010), although the second sample is usually slightly diluted.

Most often, artificial insemination with freshly collected semen is performed without fractioning the ejaculate, although for artificial insemination, only the second fraction is of interest (Thomassen & Farstadt 2009; Root Kustritz, 2003). Furthermore, it has been demonstrated the existence of detrimental effects on fertility when this fraction is not separated from the second one, particularly if semen will be processed as chilled or frozen. Consequently, ejaculate fractioning should always be accomplished, particularly separation of the third fraction. If the ejaculate has a very small volume, it may be diluted with semen extender, to facilitate its handling during insemination procedures.

4.2 Semen assessment

Semen assessment is an important part of the evaluation of fertility in males and it should be performed as routine element of prebreeding examination. Furthermore, semen evaluation ought to be completed before artificial insemination or sperm preservation. Semen should be assessed immediately after collection and it has to be handled carefully during all the procedures. Rapid changes of environmental temperature may be deleterious for spermatozoal motility and structure, and may also artifactually influence the results of examination. Any delay in semen assessment may decrease the percentage of motile sperm and simultaneously increase the percentage of dead sperm. It is advisable to keep all equipment necessary for semen collection and evaluation at the temperature near 37°C (Christiansen, 1984; Feldman & Nelson, 1996; Linde-Forsberg, 1991).

On table 5, the most frequent indications for routine semen evaluation are presented. Semen evaluation is also frequently performed in the absence of known reproductive pathology, upon request of the owner. In addition, it can be performed at a predetermined moment after the diagnosis of a clinical disease that may have negative reflects on the potential fertility of a male dog.

It should be notice that reliable *in vitro* estimation of the real fertilizing ability of sperm cells is not always possible. Usually, in males with aspermic (no ejaculate), azoospermic (no spermatozoa), or necrospermic (no motile spermatozoa) semen, the fertilizing potential may be excluded. When the quality of semen in a dog with history of unsuccessful matings is low, premises exist to exclude such male from the breeding programme. However, it should always be remembered that the semen characteristics should be recheck 2-3 times at 1-2 weeks intervals, to confirm the male infertility. On the other hand, good *in vitro* semen quality does not always prove the fertilizing potential of a particular dog.

Most frequent indications	Other situations, on request
- Semen evaluation before artificial insemination - Semen evaluation before/after chilling or cryopreservation - Clinical signs of a disorder of male genital organs - Whenever infertility or subfertility of a male is suspected	- New stud dog introduced to the breeding colony - Evaluation of young stud dog before first mating - In cases of serial unsuccessful matings of particular dog - Pathological lesions of male genital tract observed by the owner - Re-evaluation after the treatment of diseases of male genital tract

Table 5. Common reasons for canine semen assessment

The semen assessment performed once is not always reliable, because:

- Frequent matings or semen collections may temporary result in a decreased semen quality;
- After a prolonged sexual rest dogs may ejaculate many dead, immotile spermatozoa of abnormal morphology;
- In young inexperienced males and dogs which mated earlier only naturally, without experience on semen collection, the obtained semen sample may contain only the part of sperm-rich fraction.

4.2.1 Conventional assessment of semen

Different approaches are available to assess the quality of the dog semen that can be grouped in conventional and advanced techniques. The later, usually requires more sophisticated means for the semen assessment and the support of a technical equipment, while the former may be performed in an inhouse lab.

The conventional approaches to semen evaluation include macroscopical evaluation of the semen (volume and colour), but also the microscopical assessment, which will give the concentration and the number of viable cells in the ejaculate.

4.2.1.1 Macroscopic evaluation

Volume. The volume of the ejaculate may be assessed in the calibrated tubes used for semen collection. It mainly dependends on the size of the dog, the size of the prostate gland, the animal age, the frequency of semen collection, the level of erotisation, and the volume of 3rd fraction collected. A decrease of semen volume is observed in cases of benign prostatic hyperplasia, prostatic cysts, inflammatory lesions of prostate and testicles, inflammation of epididymis, vas deferens or urethra and at weak libido.

Colour. The colour of whole ejaculate depends on the volume of third fraction of ejaculate collected, on the concentration of spermatozoa per mL and the potential presence of non-germ cells in the ejaculate. When analysing the colour, one should be aware of the method of collection, as colour varies with the fraction to be analysed and the fact that analysis may been performed on the whole semen or on fractioned semen. The normal colour of whole ejaculate is greyish-white. Pathological colours include: green-greyish typical for the presence of the pus in semen; red or pink-specific for erythrocytes contamination (haemorrhages from urethra or corpora cavernosa, prostatitis); yellow specific for urine contamination; and brown, if in the presence of blood.

Any kind of semen contamination, such as hair or mud, exclude the specimen from further procedures including artificial insemination or semen preservation. It is therefore important to check the region of praeputial opening before semen collection and to clean it.

The presence of sediment consisting of sperm cells at the bottom of the tube is a normal feature if the semen is left for several minutes.

4.2.1.2 Microscopic evaluation

Motility. One of the most important step of conventional semen assessment is the subjective evaluation of progressively motile spermatozoa (Spz) under contrast-phase microscope. The optimal temperature for assessment of dog sperm cell motility is 39°C. A small drop of about 20 μL of semen is placed on in a pre-warmed slide and cover by the coverslip. The evaluation is performed under the objective of x20 to x40. If the highly concentrated sperm-rich fraction is collected separately, the semen should be extended with saline or Tris-buffer to a concentration allowing the observation of particular, single sperm cells. The assessment is based on the evaluation of the average percentage of progressively motile spermatozoa in a few different fields of the specimen. The normal dog semen contains at least 70% of progressively motile spermatozoa (Feldman & Nelson, 1996; Günzel-Apel, 1994).

A decrease in the percentage of motile spermatozoa may results from temperature shock, contamination with water, urine, blood or lubricants but also from long sexual abstinence and systemic or infectious diseases, such as brucellosis. Sperm agglutination is always pathological and is frequently found in cases of infectious diseases.

Concentration and total sperm count. The sperm concentration in whole canine normal ejaculate usually exceeds 80 x10^6 Spz/mL. If the second fraction of ejaculate is collected separately, the sperm cells concentration in sperm-rich fraction varies usually between 200-600 x 10^6 Spz/mL. It is generally assumed that the number of motile spermatozoa necessary for successful AI should be >150 x10^6 (Linde-Forsberg, 1991). Therefore, under normal conditions, the dog´s ejaculate contains far more sperm cells than those needed for a seminal dose, although sometimes, especially in miniature or toy breeds, ejaculate volume and the total number of sperm cells are relatively low (<100 x10^6 Spz/mL). The concentration of spermatozoa in semen volume is usually assessed by cytometric method on the haemocytometer, such as the Thoma, Thoma-Neu, Bürker or Neubauer chambers, with semen pre-diluted at 1:200. In order to find the sperm count *per* mL, the number of spermatozoa in the one or four large squares (depending of the chamber) is multiplied by 500 000. For the assessment of sperm concentration more sophisticated equipment could also be used, such as the spectrophotometer, flow cytometer or computer assisted semen analyser (Rijsselaere et al., 2005).

A large variety in the total number of spermatozoa *per* ejaculate is observed in different breeds. It varies between 50 x10^6 up to 1575 x 10^6 Spz (Linde-Forsberg, 1991; Oettle 1993). Small breeds do not produce as many spermatozoa as large breeds, as sperm cell production is related to the weight of the testicular tissue. The number of spermatozoa *per* ejaculate also varies according to age, testicular weight, sexual activity and the size of the dog (Amann, 1986). The total number of spermatozoa in the ejaculate may be decreased in young and older dogs and in inbred males. Apprehension, absence of the teaser bitch, painful prostate, spine rear limbs may also negatively influence the number of spermatozoa ejaculated.

Sperm morphology. The percentage of morphologically normal spermatozoa in canine semen should be greater than 70% (Günzel-Apel, 1994). The morphology may be assessed under contrast-phase microscope, but usually the evaluation is performed under light microscope on stained slides. Smears of undiluted or diluted ejaculate are examined microscopically for the presence of structural abnormalities of spermatozoa. The stains used include modified Giemsa stain (DiffQuik) and Spermac® stain. The semen is smeared on a glass slide in a similar manner to that of blood, air dried and stained. The semen may be also stained with a nigrosin-eosin stain. A drop of this stain is gently mixed with a drop of semen on a pre-warmed slide before being smeared, and allowed to air dry. Evaluation of sperm morphology should be completed microscopically using oil immersion, using an objective of x100 or x 125. A minimum number of 200 spermatozoa should be counted and evaluated for the presence of abnormalities. The percentage of cells with particular morphological defects and of normal cells are calculated. Traditionally sperm cells abnormalities are divided into primary defects - originating from abnormalities of spermatogenesis and secondary defects -

originating from abnormalities of semen maturation, transit through the ductal system and specimen preparation. According to another classification sperm abnormalities may be divided into major defects, negatively correlated with fertility, and minor defects, unassociated with fertility (Table 6) (Oettle, 1993).

	Primary spermatozoa defects	Secondary spermatozoa defects
Head	Macrocephalus, microcephalus, double, pointed, indented heads	Free, bent heads, swollen acrosomes, detaching acrosomes
Neck	Thickened, eccentric insertion	
Midpiece	Thickened, thinned, coiled, kinked, double midpiece	Bent midpiece, extraneous material surrounding midpiece, proximal, mid and distal cytoplasmatic droplets
Tail	Thin, double, triple tail.	Coiled, looped, kinked, folded, detached tail.

Table 6. Main defects of the dog spermatozoa

The acrosomal status, which is frequently assessed for the estimation of the quality of the frozen-thawed semen, may be evaluated with the use of eosin-nigrosin, Giemsa, Trypan blue, Bismarck brown, Rose Bengal or Spermac® stainings (Dahlbom et al. ,1997; Dott & Foster, 1972; Watson, 1975). When a spermatozoon presents more than one abnormality, it should be classified according to the most important abnormality or with the most prevalent one, if they have equal significance (Oettle, 1993).

'Live-dead' spermatozoa. The assessment of the percentage of live and dead spermatozoa is based on the assumption that dead spermatozoa possess disintegrated plasma membrane allowing eosin penetration. Thus the percentage of eosin positive cells stained with nigrosin-eosin stain is considered as percentage of dead cells. The normal dog semen consists of maximal percentage of 30% of dead sperm cells. The evaluation of the percentage of live and dead spermatozoa and the percentage of morphological defects may be performed on the same nigrosin-eosin stained slides.

4.2.2 Advanced semen assessment

In the past 2 to 3 decades, several strategies were developed to escape the subjectivity in the semen evaluation, related to the experience and skills of the observer, the method of specimen preparation, staining technique and number of cells evaluated, and wich is particularly important when the fertility potential of preserved sperm cells has to be ascertain. It is well documented that variations in results of the conventional evaluation of the same semen samples obtained by different observers and laboratories may reach 30-60% (Coetzee et al., 1999; Davis & Katz, 1992). Moreover, implementation of such methodologies, not routinely usable in the small to median veterinary clinics due to their costs, allows accurate comparisons between laboratories worlwide and minimizes occurence of large errors. Furthermore, advanced semen assessment is essential whenever the semen has to be preserved, in particular for freezing. Advanced semen assessment techniques are sumarized on table 7. In general, the results obtained with these methods are better correlated with the AI outcome than the results of traditional semen evaluation.

Tests	Aims	Procedure and Analysis	References
Hypo-osmotic swelling test.	Spz membrane integrity (indirect method)	Sperm incubation with hypo-osmotic solutions for 30 minutes at 37°C Spz with intact plasmalemma become swolled and show coiled tails	England & Plummer, 1993; Kumi-Diaka, 1993
Computer assisted sperm analysis [CASA]	Objective evaluation of sperm cell motility	Determination of motility parameters for individual spz Characterization of Spz movement according to the average velocity, the trajectory, the amplitude of movement and beat cross frequency. It allows identification of Spz subpopulations	Verstegen et al., 2001; Rijsselaere et al., 2003; Niżański et al., 2009
Zona pellucida binding assay	Assessment of sperm fertilizing potential	- ZP-binding assay (ZBA) using intact homologous oocytes - hemizona binding assay (HZA) using bisected hemizonae The number of spermatozoa bound to ZP is counted with contrast-phase microscopy. The number of bound Spz reflects its fertilizing potential	Hermansson et al., 2006; Kawakami et al., 1998; Rijsselaere et al., 2005; Ström-Holst et al., 2001
Fluorescent probes and flow cytometry	Membrane integrity and evaluation of live and dead cells	Combined use of several fluorescent dyes (i.e, propidium iodide PI and carboxyfluorescein diacetate, SYBR-14/PI) allow the identification of live cells Live cells activate fluorescence (deacylation) which is maintained intracellularly in intact membrane cells. Dead Spz are stained red due to the influx of PI through damaged plasma membrane.	Hewitt & England, 1998; Peña et al., 1998; Rijsselaere et al, 2005; P.F. Silva & Gadella, 2006
	Capacitation status	Fluorescent antibiotic chlorotetracycline (CTC), when bound to free calcium ions, is fluorescent. Combined with Hoechst 33258 allows also assessment of percentage of live cells and capacitation status Three classes of sperm cells may be assessed: uncapacitated and acrosome intact (F-pattern), capacitated and acrosome intact (B-pattern) and capacitated and acrosome reacted (AR-pattern)	Guérin et al., 1999; Hewitt & England, 1998; Petrunkina et al., 2004; Rota et al. 1999b

Tests	Aims	Procedure and Analysis	References
	Acrosomal status	Lectins conjugated with fluorescein isothiocyanate, such as Peanut Agglutinin (FITC-PNA) or Pisum Sativum Agglutinin (FITC-PSA). PNA labelling is specific for the outer acrosomal membrane whereas PSA is labelling acrosomal matrix. The absence of the fluorescence of the living sperm indicates an intact acrosome, whereas the presence of the fluorescence is indicative for acrosome disruption or acrosome reaction	Kawakami et al., 2002; Peña et al., 2001; Sirivaidyapong et al., 2000; P.F. Silva & Gadella, 2006
	Mitochondria	Rhodamine 123 (R123) is a potentiometric membrane dye used for the selective staining of functional mitochondria. It fluoresces only when the proton gradient over the inner mitochondrial membrane (IMM) is built up	Garner et al., 1997; Gravance et al., 2001
	Integrity of DNA structure	- Sperm chromatin structure assay (SCSA) with acridine orange (AO). - Terminal deoxynucleotidyl transferase-mediated nick end labeling (TUNEL) The SCSA is a flow cytometric method for identification of changes in the DNA status. AO shows green fluorescence when DNA is intact and red fluorescence when DNA is denaturated	Chohan et al., 2006; Bochenek et al., 2001; Garcia-Macis et al, 2006

Table 7. Concise description of the available advanced methods for sperm quality assessment.

5. Success rates for artificial insemination

The key-issues to obtain good results by using canine artificial insemination are:

- Proper timing of the insemination
- The use of adequate number of viable sperm cells *per* dose
- Good semen preparation and handling
- Adequate deposition of semen in the female reproductive tract

On next sections the major issues on timing the AI and available techniques of semen deposition on the bitch genital tract will be discussed.

5.1 Timing the moment for insemination

Obtaining successful pregnancies and adequate number of offspring per litter depends upon the correct timing for mating, as well as for insemination, particularly because bitches are mono-estrous, presenting usually one to two reproductive cycles per year. Although relationship among behavioral, hormonal and physiological events for the average bitch exists, considerable individual variation are also currently found on what concerns the duration of the estrogenic and early luteal stages (proestrus and estrus) and of the anestrus (Concannon et al., 1977; Concannon, 2004). The bitch usually presents a relatively long follicular phase and considerable variability exists in the onset of estrous behavior and acceptance of the male, making it difficult to determine occurrence of the LH surge and onset of ovulation in this species unless specific methods for timing the ovulation and estimating the fertile period are used (Linde-Forsberg, 1991). Furthermore, in this species, ovulation of immature oocytes (primary oocytes, before extrusion of the first polar body) determines the need for a maturation period in distal oviducts that may last for 96-108 hours (Concannon, 2004, 2010; Tsuitsui, 1989; Tsutsui et al., 2009); for most bitches, the secondary oocytes present a life span of 24-48h (Tsuitsui, 1989). Those particularities in the reproductive physiology may explain why the major cause for infertility in the bitch is the inappropriate breeding management (Goodman, 2001; Linde-Forsberg, 1991). Consequently, careful planning of mating time by timing ovulation is a key step in canine artificial insemination.

5.2 Vaginal cytology and progesterone blood levels

Determination of blood progesterone and the vaginal cell cornification on cytological specimens are the most widely used techniques (Linde Forsberg, 2003), to which recently has been added the vaginal endoscopy (that replaces the vaginoscopic exam) and the ultrasonographic follow-up of the follicular development and ovulation (England & Concannon, 2002; Hewitt & England, 2000; Fontbonne & Malandain, 2006; Levy & Fontbonne, 2007). These evaluations should be performed in sequence and with 2-3 days intervals for the majority of females (if the bitch has been reported to present short heat period, of about 6 to 9 days, is possible that daily evaluations may be needed).

On the vaginal cytology, epithelial cells of the vagina change their form in response to estrogen impregnation, and passes from small round cells with a clearly visible cytoplasm in non-estrogenic stages, to larger, cornified, angular shaped-cells with small pyknotic nucleus, almost to the point of disappearing, under the influence of estrogens (Figure 1). At beginning of estrus, vaginal cytology presents its maximum cornification index (>70%). By that time, serial blood sampling for progesterone determination should start to detect the initial progesterone rise (2-3 ng/mL) which correlates with LH surge, which in turn triggers ovulation within 2 days. On the day of ovulation (day "0" of the cycle) progesterone concentrations may vary between 4 and 10 ng/mL. The sudden increase in the number of round-shaped cells and of neutrophils reflects the onset of diestrus (Fontbonne & Malandain, 2006).

Progesterone semi-quantitative immunoenzymatic assays are available for clinical routines, but although rapids, these test lack accuracy. They give progesterone concentration according to a colorimetric scale for values corresponding to basal progesterone levels (0-1 ng/mL), intermediate levels corresponding to the LH surge (around 1-2.5ng/mL) and the ovulation periods (2.5 - 8ng/mL), and high progesterone levels (more than 8 or 10, depending on the kit). A recent study showed that, in dogs, semi-quantitative methods for progesterone determination are less accurate than the quantitative methods, in particular at intermediate plasma progesterone concentrations (Moxon et al., 2010). According to this study, the tested semi-quantitative assay estimated higher progesterone concentration than RIA (radioimmunoassay), which could suggest that the fertilization period had commenced earlier than it was actually the case. In addition to those assays, quantitative radio or chemiluminescent assays can also be used, even if not always available in the house lab, since cross-reactivity exist to the molecule between different species, for example with human progesterone.

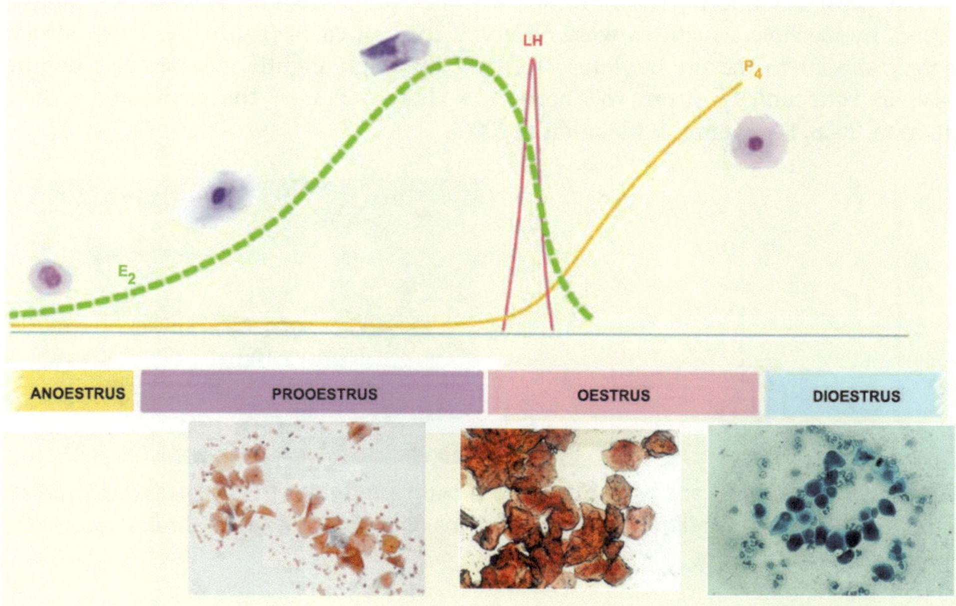

Fig. 1. Schematic representation of the major morphological changes of the predominant epithelial cell in the vaginal cytology during the dog estrous cycle. On the bottom, images of the vaginal péri-estrus cytological preparations stained with Harris-Shorr.

5.2.1 Ultrasound examination

Although ovarian ultrasound examination is a reliable and accurate method to determine ovulation in most domestic females, in the bitch fat accumulation in ovarian bursa that encloses the ovaries may difficult the value of the technique. In addition, several studies demonstrated that ultrasound images of the ovaries around ovulation are more difficult to analyze, due to the fact that ovarian follicles do not differ much in the immediate pre- and post-ovulatory period (England & Concannon, 2002), as not all dog follicles collapse at ovulation (Yeager & Concannon, 1996) and also because non-ovulated follicles frequently remain in the ovary (Wallace et al. 1992).

Consequently, follicular dynamics evaluation through ultrasonography (US) in dogs is still experimental and must follow a very precise protocol, which accuracy increase with the use of frequent examinations. In a recent study, Fontbonne (2008) reported that US was accurate enough to detect the occurrence of ovulation and obtain comparable numbers of ovarian structures between US examinations and macroscopic visual count on the surface of the ovaries after surgical removal, even if only one daily examination was performed. However, that author accepts that features of ovulation may be difficult to visualize in large breeds and in overweight animals. Pre-ovulatory follicles may present different aspects at US. Usually they appear as round to slightly triangular anechoic structures, sometimes slightly flattened, giving a honeycomb aspect to the ovary (Figure 2). At ovulation, different degrees of follicular collapse can be found in the US images, and usually a clear change of the ovarian echogenicity has been detected in a large number of bitches, giving the ovary a more homogeneous aspect (Fontbonne, 2008; Fontbonne & Malandain, 2006). Persistence of non-ovulatory follicular structures was perceived in US images after ovulation. Also, in the immediate post-ovulation period, until 24 hours after US changes of the ovaries at ovulation, hypoechoic structures were observed in most cases (Figure 2). These structures were very similar to the pre-ovulatory follicles, although slightly smaller, and tending to increase in echogenicity (from the border to the interior of the structure) with time (Fontbonne, 2008; Fontbonne & Malandain, 2006).

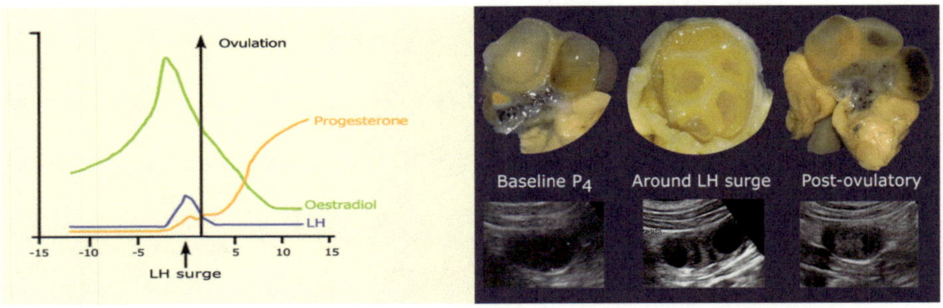

Fig. 2. Ultrasonographic scans of canine ovaries before and after LH surge and ovulation. US are compared with images of longitudinal sections of canine ovaries of similar stages of follicle developement.

5.2.2 Vaginal endoscopy

It is possible to use vaginal endoscopy to determine the fertile period although it does not allow accurate timing of ovulation. However, this method requires expensive equipment. Nevertheless, it may give a huge contribution to the vaginal evaluation and detection of anatomical abnormalities that may impair proper reproductive performance.

The fluctuation of estrogen and progesterone concentrations in the blood at consecutive stages of estrous cycle in the bitch results in specific morphologic changes of the vaginal mucosa. Analysis of these changes allows for exact assessment of the stage of the estrous cycle and for determination of the optimal insemination time (Goodman, 2001; Jeffcoate & Lindsay, 1989; Lindsay 1983). The observation of the cranial part of the vagina is performed for this purpose. The deep introduction of the tip of endoscope into the narrow part of the vagina close to the cervix (dorsal median postcervical fold) or paracervix, is of less diagnostic value (Pineda et al., 1973).

Vaginoscopic examination is performed using a rigid endoscope 3-4 mm in diameter, with diagnostic sheath and a length of 30-33 cm or longer. The examination should be done on the standing animal. Usually there is no need of administration of sedatives. The tip of the endosope is introduced at the beginning at angle of 45-60° cranially and dorsally. When the tip of the optics reaches the vagina it should be repositioned at horizontal axis.

During proestrus the increase of the estrogen concentration results in the oedema of the vaginal mucosa. Vaginoscopy reveals rounded folds in the vagina. The mucosa of the folds is turgid, pink in colour and with a smooth surface. Normally the bloody discharge is also visible in the vagina. Sometimes, periodic blood outflow from the cervix, through the paracervix may be observed. The lumen of the vagina is narrow, which can be appreciated when the endoscope is advanced cranially. At the last days of proestrus and at beginning of estrus, the decrease of estrogen concentration and increase of progesterone (P_4) level is noted. It results in the collapse of vaginal folds. Formerly turgid and smooth, the mucosa, becomes wrinkled and shrunked. Vaginal folds become smaller. Maximal intensity of shrinkage of vaginal mucosa is observed between 3 and 7-8 days of estrous cycle. This time the loss of fluid from the tissue of vaginal mucosa and submucosa is great and the shape of vaginal folds become angulated with sharp angles at the top of folds. As the result, the lumen of the vagina is wider in comparison to proestrus. During diestrus vaginal folds become flat and round. The mucosa is red and small petechia may be visible at places touched by the tip of the endoscope. This is due to the fact that epithelium of the vagina is thin and consists of only 2-3 cell layers in diestrus and anestrus. An opaque, thick mucus is sometimes visible on the surface of epithelium (Figure 3).

5.2.3 Proposed alternative methods

Other methods has been proposed to monitor the bitch oestrous cycle, such as serial reading of the electrical resistance of the vaginal mucus around the time of ovulation, using probes inserted into the vagina during the heat period (Fontbonne, 2008), or the crystallization patterns in anterior vaginal fluids (England & Allen, 1989) or in saliva (Pardo-Carmona et al., 2010), which have been found up not to present an acceptable reliabily in the identification of the canine ovulation.

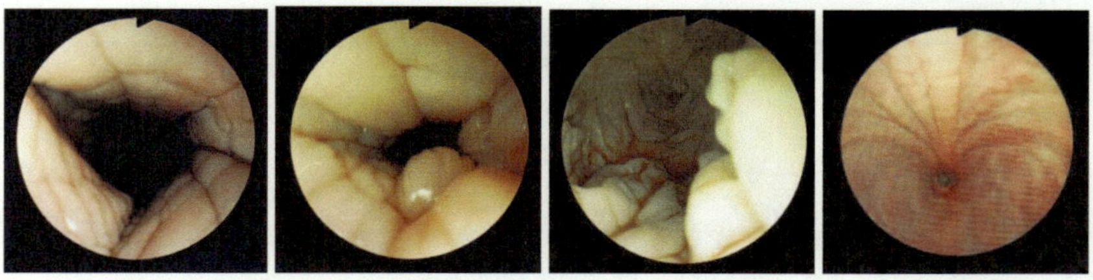

Fig. 3. Vaginal endoscopy of the bitch. [From left to right] Aspect of the vaginal folds at early proestrus, proestrus, estrus and diestrus.

5.3 The moment for insemination

In the bitch, when timing the day of ovulation as accurately as possible is essential to guarantee adequate fertility in natural mating systems, it becomes even more important to determine precisely when to inseminate bitches according to the sort of semen to be used (fresh, chilled or frozen semen), as usually semen longevity and sperm cells survival decreases with time. In addition, in frozen/thawed semen sperm cell capacitation is shorter due to secondary effects of the frozen procedure.

When fresh or chilled semen is used, insemination should be performed on the day of ovulation, and a second insemination must be schedule for 2 days later. On the contrary, when frozen/thawed semen is used, and considering the need of canine oocytes to mature in the oviducts, insemination should be performed 2 days after ovulation, and the second insemination 48h later (Figure 4). However, scheduling for the artificial inseminations may be slightly adjusted according to the experience of the operator, the place for semen deposition and the limitation on the number of inseminations. Consequently, regimes for canine AI may vary with authors (Root Kustritz, 2003). Table 8 condenses the available information on the AI schedules for fresh, chilled and frozen semen.

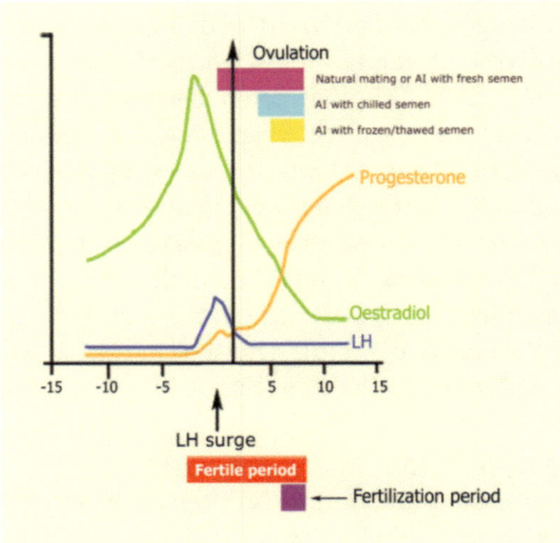

Fig. 4. Graphic representation of the fertile period and the ideal moment for canine AI according to the type of semen.

Semen	Dosis	Expected spz survival	Insemination schedule	Expected fertility
Fresh	150-200x10^6 spz/mL (extended)	4-6 days	- Every other day, when P_4 rise above 4ng/mL, up to 3 times. - Day 1 to 4 post-ovulation - P_4 levels between 8 and 15ng/mL	- 80-90% (either with transcervical or vaginal deposition)
Chilled	150 - 200x10^6 spz/mL (extended)	24-72hrs	- Breeding once or twice 2-4 days post ovulation (P_4 = 4 -10ng/mL). - Day 2 to 4 post-ovulation - P_4 levels between 8 and 15ng/mL	- 80-90% (either with transcervical or vaginal deposition)
Frozen	50 - 300x10^6 spz/mL (extended)	12-24hrs.	- Twice, at P_4 levels above 8ng/mL and estrus vaginal cytology - Day 5 to 7 post-ovulation - P_4 levels between 18 and 28 ng/mL	- 45% if vaginal deposition - 67 -84% if transcervical or intrauterine

Table 8. Artificial insemination schedules for dogs, according to the type of semen used.

If in the AI with fresh semen the success of the procedure is strongly related to the quality of semen used and the moment for AI (Table 9), when using chilled semen both the quality of semen and the site of semen deposition are important factors for success, whilst in the AI with frozen semen, the intra-uterine semen deposition is critical (Table 10).

	2AI, 48h apart				**Multiple AI**		**2AI, day 3 and 5 post LH surge**	
	Day 9-13 after bloody vaginal discharge		Eosinophilic index >80%		Eosinophilic index >80%		Progesterone measurements	
	n	%	n	%	n	%	n	%
Pregnancy rates	29	55.8[a]	33	66.0[ab]	37	78.7[b]	37	80.4[b]
Whelping rates	27	51.9[a]	31	62.0[a]	36	76.6[b]	36	78.3[b]
Length of pregnancy	63.7±1.4[a]		64.5±2.6[b]		64.4±2.4[b]		63.1±1.3[c]	
Number *per* group	52		50		47		46	

a,b,c – different superscript mean significant differences (P<0.05) between groups

Table 9. Success of canine AI with fresh semen according to the method used to timing AI (n=136) (Adapted from Nizański et al. 2005)

Semen	**Sperm deposition**	
	Intra-vaginal (n)	**Intra-uterine (n)**
Fresh	47.7 (1212)	62 (121)
Chilled	45.4 (348)	65.0 (40)
Frozen	36.7 (30)	55.5 (290)

Table 10. Comparison of whelping rates (%) in vaginal and intrauterine inseminations according to the type of dog semen (n=2041) (Adapted from Linde Forsberg, 2002a).

5.4 Insemination techniques

In dogs, during natural mating, occurs the projection of a considerable portion of the ejaculate into the uterus, through the cervical canal, during the coital tie (England et al., 2006; Thomassen & Farstad, 2009). When performing AI we should be aware that vaginal deposition *per se* will negatively influence sperm cell survival and their transport in the female genital tract, and therefore impairs ability to achieve normal whelping rates and/or litter sizes. However, deep vaginal insemination shows acceptable results when using fresh semen, and also to some extent for chilled semen. However, to obtain satisfactory success rates when using frozen/thawed semen, intra-uterine insemination is necessary.

As in other species, in dogs sperm cell number in the uterine lumen may be influenced by many factors, such as the moment of estrus, the type of breeding (natural mating or insemination) the method of insemination (intravaginal or intrauterine), the type of semen

(fresh, chilled or frozen) and sperm quality (total and progressive motility and sperm speed), besides some individual variations (Rijsselaere et al., 2004). However, despite the influence of the intrauterine *vs.* vaginal insemination on the success of the procedure, once intrauterine insemination is achieve, the exact place of semen deposition is not of the main importance for the sperm distribution within the uterus (England et al., 2006; Rijsselaere et al., 2004). Consequently, no potential differences or advantages exist between the vaginal endoscopic approach and laparoscopy when the intra-uterine insemination is intended, as no differences were found in the deposition of the semen in the uterine body or the cranial tip of the uterine horns (Fukushima et al., 2010). Nevertheless, abdominal laparoscopy or surgery is strongly discouraged on the basis of animal welfare issues, as non-healthy related invading procedure that should be avoided.
Based on the last two years inseminations performed at the clinic (with a global success rate of around 75%), using a comercial kit for progesterone determination, fresh semen and intra-vaginal deposition (2 AI, 48h apart), it was found that when inseminations were performed with progesterone levels above 8 ng/mL a higher success rate and a closer to predicted whelping dates were achieved (Table 11), comparing to inseminations at lower levels of progesterone (2.5-8 ng/mL). No diferences were found in the litter size between these groups, which were very similar in age and parity of the bitches.

Semen	Number of animals		Range of age (mean)	Progesterone at AI (ng/ml)	Days from last IA to whelping	Success rate (nº females whelped /inseminated)	Liter size (± SD)
Fresh	39	18	1-6 years (2.94 years)	2.5 to 8 ng/mL	63	66.6	6.33± 2.84
		12	1-6 years (3.23 years)	> 8 ng/mL	61	80.95	6.29 ± 2.26
Chilled	42		1-6 years (3.6 years)	>8 ng/mL	61	73.8	6.1 ±2.51

Table 11. Results for the AI procedures with fresh and chilled semen and 2 AI *per* animal, 48h apart.

Independently of the place for semen deposition, repeating the AI at 24-48 hrs intervals results in a significantly higher fertility: for fresh semen both the pregnancy rate and litter size present a significantly increase when multiple AI are performed (Linde-Forsberg & Forsberg, 1993), whilst for frozen semen the differences on the pregnancy rates are not significant, although litter size tended to increase with the number of inseminations (Linde-Forsberg, 2000, 2002a).

5.4.1 Deep vaginal insemination

Deep vaginal insemination is probably the widestly used method for insemination with fresh semen when the technique is performed by the breeder or in small budget clinics. For vaginal AI a simple plastic catheter of proper length may be used, to which a plastic disposable syringe containing the semen is attached. Or a commercial catheter in flexible latex tube presenting an inflatable balloon at the tip, like the Osiris gun, may be used; when inflated, this

kind of device has the advantage of increasing the probability for intrauterine transport of the semen and of preventing semen backflow (Farstadt, 2010; Linde Forsberg, 2005a).
Before AI procedures start, cleaning of the perineal area, in particular the peri-vulvar area, is needed. As transabdominal palpation is usually used to guide or ascertain the vaginal catheter position, the owner of the female should be instructed to bring the animal with an empty stomach, which facilitates the procedure (Linde Forsberg, 2005a).
The bitch is placed in a standing position on an examination table or on the floor (according to the size of the female). To avoid catheterization of the urethra (the urethral opening in the bitch is located at the pelvic brim), particular attention should be paid not to unintentionally introduce into the urinary bladder. The insemination catheter is carefully introduced in the vagina of the bitch, first steeply upwards until the pelvic brim has been passed, and then in a horizontal angle, when it is carefully pushed further ahead (Farstad, 2010). In alternative, the vulva may be elevated to just below the anus (as the bitch does when stimulated by the male dog) (Linde Forsberg, 2005a). At this point, the position of the AI catheter must be learn by palpation, and orientated. If the catheter is in the urinary bladder, the cranial part of the vagina and the cervix may be palpable above the catheter and also the tip of the catheter stands out more clearly, due to the thinner walls of the urinary bladder in comparison to those of the vagina (Linde Forsberg, 2005a). After certification that the catheter is correctly placed, it is moved onward through the cranial portion of the vagina delimited by the dorsal medial folds. In smaller or primiparous bitches this point can be difficult to overcome, and may not be possible to pass the catheter into the cervical fornix. Except for those females, the AI catheter should be further introduced until it reaches the paracervical area, which can be palpated as a 1- to 2-cm-long, firm structure that ends at the cervix (a firm, rounded to ovoid structure, freely movable). The semen is deposited once the catheter has been located in the paracervical area, close to the external *cervical os*.
During AI the bitch is held with the hindquarters up and head down, in an angle of 45-60°. This position facilitates transabdominal palpation of the cervix and ensures that the semen will not be expelled through backflow. According to earlier reports, the bitch should be maintained in the same position up to period of time varying from 5 to 20 min after AI. However, reducing the interval of elevated hindquarters to 1 min seems not affect fertility (Pinto et al., 1998). Also, feathering or stroking of the vulvar or perineal region is reported by several authors as form of stimulating the semen transport into the uterus, in an attempt to mimic the vaginal stimulation by the thrusting movements of the dog during natural mount. However, the contribution of such procedures to the exit of the technique has not been proven yet.

5.4.2 Intrauterine insemination

Intrauterine insemination may be performed by using non-surgical transcervical catheterisation (Linde-Forsberg, 1991; Linde-Forsberg and Forsberg, 1989, 1993; Linde-Forsberg et al., 1999) or by surgical semen deposition by laparotomy (Brittain et al., 1995; Günzel-Apel & Thiet, 1990) or laparoscopy (L.D.M Silva et al., 1995, 1996). The majority of European centers working on small animal reproduction prefer transcervical intrauterine insemination (TCI) due to reasons associated with animal welfare. However, catheterisation of uterine cervix in the bitch is a difficult procedure and demand skill and experience. The semen of lower quality, such as frozen-thawed or that collected from subfertile dogs have to be deposited intrauterine to assure satisfactory results of artificial insemination (Linde-

Forsberg et al., 1999; Thomassen et al., 2006). The conception rates after intravaginal insemination with frozen-thawed semen are significantly lower when compared with the results of intrauterine insemination.

5.4.2.1 The Norwegian or Scandinavian technique

The method of non-surgical transcervical intrauterine insemination was first time described in 1975 (Andersen, 1975). The technique has been adapted from the artificial insemination performed in foxes. Two catheters are used in this method - the outer plastic catheter and inner metal thin catheter. There are 3 sizes of the catheters, for small, medium and large breeds. The catheterisation should be made on standing animal. Sometimes there is no need for administration of sedatives, but usually a small dose of alpha-mimetic, such as medetomidine, is advisable for abdominal muscles relaxation. The outer plastic catheter should be introduced into the vagina. It should be advanced as far as is possible. In many bitches, especially those of larger breeds, the tip of the catheter passes into the cranial narrow part of vagina. However, in some smaller bitches the introduction of the outer catheter through the paracervix is difficult. It is necessary to palpate the end of the catheter and the cervix through the abdominal wall. The cervix is palpable at estrus as solid, ovoid structure. It is advisable to move the tip of the catheter ventrally towards the ventral region of abdominal wall. This procedure is helpful in palpation of the cervix. The inner metal catheter should be introduced through the plastic catheter. The cervix should be fixed between the thumb and other fingers and tilted to horizontal axis. The metal catheter is introduced into the cervical canal under the control of the position of the cervix by palpation through the abdominal wall (Andersen, 1975; Linde-Forsberg, 1991). This technique demands skill and experience. It is harder to perform uterine catheterisation in obese or nervous bitches and in giant breeds.

The scandinavian method of uterine catheterization is recommended for routine insemination of bitches (Ferguson et al., 1989; Günzel-Apel 1994; Linde-Forsberg, 1991, 1995). The use of this technique of insemination is especially advisable in cases when using of semen of lower quality due to male subfertility or sperm cryopreservation. Linde-Forsberg and Forsberg (1989) obtained 83.9% and 69.3% of pregnant bitches (data corrected for the stage of estrus) after insemination with fresh and frozen-thawed semen, respectively. The litter sizes were lower by 23.3%, when frozen-thawed semen was used in comparison to fresh semen. Rota et al. (1999a) reported 25% higher pregnancy rate after intrauterine semen deposition when using scandinavian technique than after vaginal semen deposition. On the basis of analysis of 327 inseminations Linde-Forsberg et al. (1999) concluded that success rate of scandinavian method and vaginal insemination with frozen-thawed semen was 84.4% and 58.9, respectively. Niżański (2006) proved that results of vaginal insemination with frozen-thawed semen are significantly lower in comparison with fresh semen, in spite of the use of modification of the technique of vaginal semen deposition, plasma addition and adjustment of the number of spermatozoa.

5.4.2.2 Endoscope-assisted vaginoscopic method (New Zealand method)

Intrauterine insemination of the bitch under the visual control of endoscopic equipment was first time described by Wilson (Wilson, 1993, 2001), using a rigid endoscope – cysto-uretroscope of the length 29 cm with diagnostic external sheath. The procedure is performed on the standing animal. Uterine catheterisation is made with the use of flexible catheter introduced into the working channel of the endoscope. The endoscope is introduced into the cranial narrow part of the vagina, while a flexible catheter is introduced cranio-dorsal into the external orifice of the cervical canal under the visual control performed through the endoscope. Usually it is not necessary to administer any sedatives.

The results for the intrauterine deposition of frozen-thawed semen when using this technique are quite satisfactory (Table 12). Wilson (1993), with the use of frozen semen, refers a pregnancy rate and litter size 83.3% and 7.5 puppies *per* litter, respectively. Niżański (2005) obtained whelping rates of 68.7% and 27.8%, when frozen-thawed semen was deposited by intrauterine vaginoscopic method and by vaginal insemination, respectively. Results obtained by Linde-Forsberg et al. (1999) were poorer in comparison with the Scandinavian method. However, vaginoscopic intrauterine insemination is currently considered as the practical, modern and useful tool in assisted reproductive techniques in dogs which may become in the future the routine method of insemination.

Insemination technique	**n**	**Whelping rate (n° females whelped/inseminated)**	**Litter size at birth (range)**	**Litter size at weaning (range)**	**Percentage of male pups/litter**
Intravaginal, using an infusion pipete	18	27.8^{a} (5/18)	3.0 ± 1.2^{a} (2-5)	2.6 ± 0.9^{a} (2-4)	51.5 ± 25.9^{a}
Intrauterine, using the endoscope	16	68.7^{b} (11/16)	4.9 ± 1.7^{b} (3-8)	4.6 ± 1.7^{b} (2-8)	54.7 ± 18.7^{a}

Different superscripts in the same column indicate significant difference ($p<0.05$)

Table 12. Whelping rate and mean litter size in bitches intravaginally or intrauterine vaginoscopically inseminated with frozen-thawed semen. AI were performed at 4th and 6th days of oestrous cycle.

Currently a large variety of rigid endoscopes of different brands is available. The most suitable are those of the length 30-35 cm with 30° or 0° view angle and the diameter of 3 mm or similar. Some companies market the equipment dedicated specifically for artificial insemination in bitches. The optics of endoscope should be used with outer sheath equipped with working channel allowing for introduction of flexible catheter of the diameter of 5-7 French gauge. The mechanism of Albaran is not useful in the endoscope for artificial insemination of bitches, as it is not practical and the diameter of the outer sheath becomes too large when it is attached.

The catheterization may be problematic in both toy and giant breeds. In the first case, the diameter of the equipment may be too large for introduction of the tip of optics near the uterine cervix, impairing visualization of external cervical orifice. In contrast, in giant breeds the length of the vagina may exclude the possibility to access the region of the cervix. One additional problem may be associated with the presence of the blood or mucus within the vagina. Sometimes the fluid present in the genital tract may cover the terminal lens of the endoscope making the observation impossible. Withdrawal the optics and cleaning of the lens is necessary in such cases. For better visualization of the vagina, especially within the cranial narrow part, insuflation with CO_2 made with insuflator or even with rubber bulb is advisable. Therefore the view of tissues is focused, sharper and clearer, which makes the procedure easier. The time necessary for catheterization is variable. It depends mainly on

the skill of the operator and on the anatomical features of the vagina, and varies usually between 0.5-3 minutes, but it may be longer. In nervous bitches the administration of small doses of sedatives, such medetomidine, is advisable, although in not too high doses, as the catheterisation should be done on standing bitch.
Currently the vaginoscopic method of intrauterine insemination appears to be advantageous and useful technique of semen deposition in the uterine lumen in bitches. The technique demands skill but it is practical and quick to perform for experienced operators. The visual control of introduction of the catheter into the uterus is the important advantage of the technique. The observation of the moments of semen deposition and control if there is no semen backflow is therefore possible. Moreover, it allows also uterine sampling when a female is suspected of infertility due to uterine disease (Thomassen & Farstad, 2009). For these reasons this method of intrauterine insemination is becoming more popular.

5.4.3 Surgical technique

Surgical insemination technique have been proposed once for frozen semen or when the bitch presents an anatomical obstruction that prevents the insertion of the catheter or endoscope. Both the laparoscopic approach and the laparotomy requires anaesthesia and good surgical skills. The semen is introduced into the uterus by puncture of uterine wall or incision with a scapel and passage of a tom cat catheter (Farstad, 2010; Thomassen & Farstad, 2009). However, in such methods, semen deposition is performed only once.
Some restrictions may exists to application of this method in different countries, that may compromise the registration of litters obtained without fulfilment of the legal requirements, such as previous evaluation of the situation or previous authorization of the local Kennel Club for the procedure. Furthermore, some ethical constraints have been raised regarding the use of surgical techniques for AI in dogs. Surgery is an invasive procedure, so it is unlikely to carry it out in the best interest of the animal, and the possibility of transmission of an undesirable trait in a particular animal genetic line should be kept in mind.

6. Rules and regulations concerning the import or export of sperm

Before implementing canine artificial insemination the owner and the clinician should be aware of the national or international regulations on semen import, if applicable, and of the local Kennel Club requirements respecting the use of canine AI and litter registration. In addition, procedures may differ between the use of national or imported semen. Consequently, attention should be paid well in advance to this matter.
In the absence of a specific national regulation, most Kennel Clubs follows FCI (*Fédération Cynologique Internacionale*) determinations for AI, transposed to the FCI International Regulation for Breeding (http://www.fci.be/circulaires/102-2010-annex-fr.pdf). To ensure that ethical issues are minimised, FCI recommends that AI should only be done in healthy dogs with proven fertility (article number 13). In addition, in the introductory section of this regulation, FCI specifically limit the use of dogs presenting diseases possible to be transmitted to following generations and those presenting major, eliminatory defects in regard to the breed standard. Furthermore, it presumes that the AI is performed by a Veterinarian, which should certify the quality of the dog semen (either for the fresh and the processed semen, the later being certified in a standard document to be released upon semen collection and preservation) and also to attest the Kennel club to the occurrence of an AI for a specific female. In both documents, correct identification of the animals (either the

male or female) is mandatory, and can be obtained through the use of a tattoo or a microchip. The time to submit the AI certificate may differ between national Kennel Clubs. In some countries the Club must be informed of the AI procedure within the first 2 weeks, whilst in others, only when the litter is to be registered.

Besides regulations on performing AI to a bitch, attention must be paid to issues concerning the semen collection and use. Besides the use of a recognisable male, with a certified pedigree, particular requirements may exist from national Kennel Clubs or the Official Agriculture entities, which may vary for chilled and frozen semen. In some situations the permit to import dog semen is required, which may or may not need to be accompanied by a DNA sample, and a health certificate that may include blood testing against the most important infectious or congenital canine diseases. Awareness of the latest official requirements is essential when considering semen international shipment. Additional information on the shipment regulations may be obtained throught the references Linde Forsberg, 2001, 2005b.

7. Conclusion

Demands for canine artificial insemination is growing worldwile together with an increase request for semen preservation in sperm banks. Furthermore, a tendency exists to increase the demands for the use of frozen/thawed semen over fresh semen AI, as part of breeding tools for genetic improvement. Nowadays is possible to achieve adequate whelping rates and litter sizes regardless of the type of semen used, as long as proper timing of AI and proper semen deposition are used. Client education and technical councelling must complete the AI services to be offered by specialized practicioners, in particular when breeding a problematic bitch.

8. Acknowledgments

The authors are greatly indebted to Dr Malgorzata Ochota for her valuable cooperation and thoughtful comments during language revision of this manuscript.

9. References

Amann R.P. (1986) Reproductive physiology and endocrinology of the dog, In *Current therapy in theriogenology.* 2nd edition, Morrow D.A. (ed), 523-538, W.B. Saunders Comp., ISBN 978-0721665801, Philadelphia.

Andersen K. (1975) Insemination with frozen dog semen based on a new insemination technique. *Zuchthygiene*, 10, 1-4.

Bochenek M., Smorąg Z., & Pilch J. (2001) Sperm chromatin structure assay of bulls qualified for artificial insemination. *Theriogenology*, 56, 557-567.

Brittain D., Concannon P.W., Flanders J.A., Flahive W.J., Lewis B.L., Meyers-Wallen V., & Moise N.S. (1995) Use of surgical intrauterine insemination to manage infertility in a colony of research German Shepherd dogs. *Lab. Anim. Sci.*, 45, 404-407.

Chohan K.R., Griffin J.T., Lafromboise M., De Jonge C.J. & Carrell D.T. (2006) Comparison of chromatin assays for DNA fragmentation evaluation in human sperm. *J. Androl.*, 27, 53-59.

Christiansen I.J. (1984) *Reproduction in the Dog & Cat.* Bailliere Tindall, ISBN 978-0702009181, London.

Coetzee K., Kruger T.F., Lombard C.J., Shaughnessy D., Oehninger S., Ozgür K., Pomeroy K.O., & Muller C.H. (1999) Assessment of interlaboratory and intralaboratory sperm morphology readings with the use of a Hamilton Thorne Research integrated visual optical system semen analyzer. *Fertil. Steril.* 71, 80-84.

Concannon P.W. (2004) Canine Breeding Management and Artificial Insemination: Techniques and Caveats, *Proceedings of the 29th World Congress of WSAVA*, Rhodes, Greece, 8-9 Oct. http://www.vin.com/proceedings/Proceedings.plx?CID=WSAVA2004&PID=8745&O=Generic

Concannon P.W. (2010) Reproductive cycles of the domestic bitch. *Anim Reprod Sci.*, Oct 8. [Epub ahead of print], doi:10.1016/j.anireprosci.2010.08.028.

Concannon P.W., Hansel W, & Mcentee K. (1977) Changes in LH, progesterone and sexual behavior associated with preovulatory luteinization in the bitch. *Biol Reprod.* 17, 604-13.

Dahlbom M., Andersson M., Vierula M., & Alanko M. (1997) Morphometry of normal and teratozoospermic canine sperm heads using an image analyser: work in progress. *Theriogenology* 48, 687-698.

Davis R.O. & Katz D.F. (1992) Standardization and comparability of CASA instruments. *J Androl.* 13, 81-86.

Dott H.M. & Foster G.C. (1972) A techniques for studying the morphology of mammalian spermatozoa which are eosinophilic in a differential 'live/dead' stain. *J. Reprod. Fert.* 29, 443-445.

Dubiel A. (2004) Plan badania psa reproduktora w kierunku płodności. (Andrological examination of the stud dog-in polish), In *Rozród psów,* ed. A. Dubiel, Wydawnictwo AR, ISBN 83-89189-49-6 Wrocław, 47-65.

England G.C. & Allen WE. (1989) Crystallization patterns in anterior vaginal fluid from bitches in oestrus. *J Reprod Fertil.* 86, 335-9.

England G. C. & Concannon P.W. (2002) Determination of the Optimal Breeding Time in the Bitch: Basic Considerations. In *Recent Advances in Small Animal Reproduction,* Concannon P.W., England G., Verstegen J. and Linde-Forsberg C. (Eds.), International Veterinary Information Service (www.ivis.org), Document No. A1231.0602.

England G.C. & Millar K.M. (2008) The ethics and role of AI with fresh and frozen semen in dogs. *Reprod Domest Anim.,* 43 (Suppl 2) 165-71.

England G.C. & Plummer J.M. (1993) Hypo-osmotic swelling of dog spermatozoa. *J. Reprod. Fert.* Suppl, 47, 261-270.

England G.C., Burgess C.M., Freeman S.L., Smith S.C., & Pacey A.A. (2006) Relationship between the fertile period and sperm transport in the bitch. *Theriogenology,* 66, 1410-8.

England G.C., Allen W.E. & Middleton D.J. (1990) An investigation into the origin of the first fraction of the canine ejaculate. *Res. Vet. Sci.* 49, 66-70.

Farstad W.K. (2010) Artificial insemination in dogs, In *BSAVA Manual of Canine and Feline Reproduction and Neonatology,* 2nd edition, England G. and von Heimendahl A. (Eds.). British Small Animal Veterinary Association ISBN 978-1905319190, Gloucester, UK.

Feldman E.C. & Nelson R.W. (1996) *Canine and Feline Endocrinology and Reproduction.* W.B. Saunders Comp., ISBN 978-0721636344, Philadelphia

Ferguson J.M., Renton J.P., Farstad W. & Douglas T.A. (1989) Insemination of beagle bitches with frozen semen. *J. Reprod. Fert.* Suppl. 39, 293-298.

Fontbonne A. (2008) *Ovulation, maturation ovocytaire et fecondation in vivo chez la chienne* (In vivo ovulation, oocyte maturation and fertilisation in the bitch). PhD Thesis, Institut des Sciences et Industries du Vivant et de l'Environnement (Agro Paris Tech).

Fontbonne A & Malandain E. (2006) Ovarian ultrasonography and follow-up of estrus in the bitch and queen. *WALTHAM Focus* 16 (2) 22-29.

Foote R.H. (2002) The history of artificial insemination: Selected notes and notables. *J. Anim. Sci.* 80(E. Suppl.) E22–E32

Freshman J.L. (2002) Semen Collection and Evaluation. *Clinical Techniques in Small Animal Practice* 17, 104-107.

Fukushima F.B., Malm C., Henry M., Gheller V.A., Serakides R., Neves M.M., Macedo S.P., Figueiredo M.S., Andrade M.E., Chaves M.S., Silva M.X., Rezende C.M. & Melo, E.G. (2010) Site of intrauterine artificial insemination in the bitch does not affect sperm distribution within the uterus. *Reprod Domest Anim.* 45, 1059-1064.

Garcia-Macias V., Martinez-Pastor F., Alvarez M., Garde J.J., Anel E., Anel L. & de Paz P. (2006) Assessment of chromatin status (SCSA®) in epididymal and ejaculated sperm in Iberian red deer, ram and domestic dog. *Theriogenology* 66, 1921-1930.

Garner D.L. & Johnson L.A. (1995) Viability assessment of mammalian sperm using SYBR-14 and Propidium Iodide. *Biol. Reprod.* 53, 276-284.

Garner D.L., Thomas C.A., Joerg H.W., DeJarnette J.M. & Marshall C.E. (1997) Fluorometric assessments of mitochondrial function and viability in cryopreserved bovine spermatozoa. *Biol. Reprod.* 57, 1401-1406.

Goodman M. (2001) Ovulation timing. Concepts and controversies. *Vet. Clin. North. Am. (Small Anim. Pract.)* 31, 219-235.

Gravance C.G., Garner D.L., Miller M.G. & Berger T.(2001) Fluorescent probes and flow cytometry to assess rat sperm integrity and mitochondrial function. *Reprod Toxicol.* 15, 5-10.

Guérin P., Ferrer M., Fontbonne A., Bénigni L., Jacquet M., & Ménézo Y. (1999) In vitro capacitation of dog spermatozoa as assessed by chlortetracycline staining. *Theriogenology* 52, 617-628.

Günzel-Apel A.R. (1994) *Fertilitätskontrolle und Samenübertragung beim Hund.* Enke/Gustav Fischer Verlag, ISBN 3-334-60512-4, Jena.

Günzel-Apel A.R. & Thiet W. (1990) Intrauterine deponierung von tiefgefriersperma nach laparotomie bei einer hundin. *Kleintierprax.* 35, 177-180.

Hermansson U., Ponglowhapan S., Linde-Forsberg C. & Ström-Holst B. (2006) A short sperm-oocyte incubation time ZBA in the dog. *Theriogenology* 66, 717-725.

Hewitt D.A. & England G.C. (1998) An investigation of capacitation and the acrosome reaction in dog spermatozoa using a dual fluorescent staining technique. *Anim. Reprod. Sci.* 51, 321-332.

Hewitt D. & England G. (2000) Assessment of optimal mating time in the bitch. *In Practice* 22, 24-33.

Jeffcoate I.A., Lindsay F.E.F. (1989) Ovulation detection and timing of insemination based on hormone concentrations, vaginal cytology and the endoscopic appearance of the vagina in domestic bitches. *J. Reprod. Fert.* Suppl. 39, 277-287.

Johnston S.D., Root Kustritz M.V., & Olson P.N.S. (2001) *Canine and Feline Theriogenology.* W.B. Saunders Comp., ISBN 978-0721656076, Philadelphia

Kawakami E., Hori T. &Tsutsui T. (1998) Changes in semen quality and in vitro sperm capacitation during various frequencies of semen collection in dogs with both asthenozoospermia and teratozoospermia. *J. Vet. Med. Sci.*, 60, 607-614.

Kawakami E., Morita Y., Hori T. & Tsutsui T. (2002) Lectin-binding characteristics and capacitation of canine epididymal spermatozoa. *J. Vet. Med. Sci.* 64, 543-549.

Kumi-Diaka J. (1993) Subjecting canine semen to the hypo-osmotic swelling test. *Theriogenology* 39, 1279-1289.

Kutzler M.A. (2005) Semen collection in the dog. *Theriogenology* 64, 747–754.

Lévy X. & Fontbonne A. (2007) Determining the optimal time of mating in bitches: particularities. *Rev Bras Reprod Anim*, 31, 128-134.

Linde-Forsberg C. (1991) Achieving canine pregnancy by using frozen or chilled extended semen. *Vet. Clin. North Am. (Small Anim Pract.)* 21, 467-485.

Linde-Forsberg C. & Forsberg M (1993) Results of 527 controlled artificial inseminations in dogs. *J Reprod Fert* Suppl 47:313-323)

Linde-Forsberg C. (2000) Fertility data from 2041 controlled artificial inseminations in dogs. *Advances in dog, Cat and Exotic Carnivore Reproduction* - Book of Abstracts. Oslo, Norway. Pg 120

Linde-Forsberg C. (2002a) What Can Be Learned From 2500 AIs in the Dog? *Proceedings of the 27th World Congress of WSAVA*, Granada, Spain, 3-6 Oct. http://www.vin.com/proceedings/Proceedings.plx?CID=WSAVA2002&PID=2685

Linde-Forsberg C. (2002b) Ethical aspects of artificial insemination (AI) in the dog. *Proc. 3rd EVSSAR Congress Liège*, pp 41-42.

Linde-Forsberg C. (2003) Artificial Insemination in the Dog: What Can Be Learnt From Results in the Field? *Proceedings of the 28th World Congress of WSAVA*, Bangkok, Thailand, 24-27 Oct. http://www.vin.com/proceedings/Proceedings.plx?CID=WSAVA2003&PID=6519&O=Generic

Linde-Forseberg C. & Forsberg M. (1989) Fertility in dogs in relation to semen quality and the time and site of insemination with fresh and frozen semen. *J. Reprod. Fert.* Suppl., 39, 299-310.

Linde-Forsberg C., Ström Holst B., Govette G. (1999) Comparison of fertility data from vaginal vs. intrauterine insemination of frozen-thawed dog semen: a retrospective study. *Theriogenology* 52, 11-23.

Linde Forsberg C. (2001) Regulations and Recommendations for International Shipment of Chilled and Frozen Canine Semen. In *Recent Advances in Small Animal Reproduction*, Concannon P.W., England G., Verstegen J. and Linde-Forsberg C. (Eds.). International Veterinary Information Service (www.ivis.org), Document No. A1209.0501.

Linde Forsberg C. (2005a) Artificial Insemination. In *ESAVS-EVSSAR Course Reproduction in companion, exotic and laboratory animal*, Nantes 12th-17th September 2005. Reference 5.1 (http://www.esavs.net/course_notes/reproduction1_05/artificial_insemination.pdf)

Linde Forsberg C. (2005b) Regulations and recommendations for international shipment of chilled and frozen canine semen. In *ESAVS-EVSSAR Course Reproduction in companion, exotic and laboratory animal*, Nantes 12th-17th September 2005. Reference 6.1 (http://www.esavs.net/course_notes/reproduction1_05/shipment_frozen_canine_seme.pdf)

Lindsay F.E.F. (1983) The normal endoscopic appearance of the caudal reproductive tract of the cyclic and non-cyclic bitch: post-uterine endoscopy. *J. Small Anim. Pract.* 24, 1-15.

Moxon R., Copley D. & England G.C. (2010) Technical and financial evaluation of assays for progesterone in canine practice in the UK. *Vet Rec.* 167, 528-31.

Niżański W. (2005) Comparisons of results of intravaginal and intrauterine insemination of bitches with frozen-thawed semen. *Electronic Journal of Polish Agricultural Universities* 8, 4, pp.6 (http://www.ejpau.media.pl/volume8/issue4/art-12.html)

Niżański W. (2006) Intravaginal insemination of bitches with fresh and frozen-thawed semen with addition of of prostatic fluid: use of an infusion pipette and the Osiris catheter, *Theriogenology* 66, 470-483.

Niżański W. & Klimowicz M. (2005) Skuteczność sztucznej inseminacji suk nasieniem świeżym przy zastosowaniu różnych metod wyznaczania terminu unasienniania (Success of artificial insemination with fresh semen with the use of different methods for determination of optimal insemination time in bitches). *Medycyna Wet.* 61, 75–81.

Niżański W., Klimowicz M., Partyka A., Savić M. & Dubiel A. (2009) Effects of the inclusion of Equex STM into Tris-based extender on the motility of dog spermatozoa incubated at 5 degrees C. *Reprod. Domest. Anim.* 44 (Suppl. 2) 363-365.

Oettl□ E.E. (1993) Sperm morphology and fertility in dog. *J. Reprod. Fert.*, Suppl. 47, 257-260.

Olsen P.N. & Husted P.W. (1986) Breeding management for optimal reproductive efficiency in the bitch and stud dog. In *Current therapy in theriogenology.* 2nd edition, Morrow D.A. (ed), W.B. Saunbders Comp., ISBN 978-0721665801, Philadelphia, 563-466.

Pardo-Carmona B., Moyano M.R., Fernández-Palacios R. & Pérez-Marín C.C. (2010) Saliva crystallisation as a means of determining optimal mating time in bitches. *J Small Anim Pract.* 51, 437-42.

Peña A.I., Johannisson A., & Linde-Forsberg C. (2001) Validation of flow cytometry for assessment of viability and acrosomal integrity of dog spermatozoa and for evaluation of different methods of cryopreservation. *J Reprod Fertil* Suppl. 57, 371-376.

Peña A.I., Quintela L.A., & Herradón P.G. (1998) Viability assessment of dog spermatozoa using flow cytometry. *Theriogenology* 50, 1211-1220.

Petrunkina A.M., Simon K., Günzel-Apel A.R. & Töpfer-Petersen E. (2004) Kinetics of protein tyrosine phosphorylation in sperm selected by binding to homologous and heterologous oviductal explants: how specific is the regulation by the oviduct? *Theriogenology* 61, 1617-1634.

Pineda M.H., Kainer R.A. & Faulkner L.C. (1973) Dorsal median postcervical fold in the canine vagina. *Am. J. Vet. Res.* 34, 1487-1491.

Pinto C.R., Eilts B.E. & Paccamonti D.L. (1998) The effect of reducing hindquarter elevation time after artificial insemination in bitches. *Theriogenology.* 50, 301-5.

Rijsselaere T., Van Soom A., Maes D. &de Kruif A. (2003) Effect of technical settings on canine semen motility parameters measured by the Hamilton-Thorne analyzer. *Theriogenology.* 60, 1553-1568.

Rijsselaere T., Van Soom A., Van Cruchten S., Coryn M., Görtz K., Maes D. & de Kruif A. (2004) Sperm distribution in the genital tract of the bitch following artificial insemination in relation to the time of ovulation. *Reproduction* 128, 801-11.

Rijsselaere T., Van Soom A., Tanghe S., Coryn M., Maes D. &de Kruif A. (2005) New techniques for the assessment of canine semen quality: A review. *Theriogenology* 64, 706-719.

Root Kustritz M.V. (2003) *Small animal theriogenology (The practical veterinarian).* Butterworth-Heinemann, ISBN 978-0750674089, Oxford, UK.

Rota A., Iguer-Ouada M., Verstegen J. & Linde-Forberg C. (1999a) Fertility after vaginal or uterine deposition of dog semen frozen in a TRIS extender with of without Equex STM Paste. *Theriogenology* 51, 1045-1058.

Rota A., Peña A.I., Linde-Forsberg C. & Rodriguez-Martinez H. (1999b) In vitro capacitation of fresh, chilled and frozen-thawed dog spermatozoa assessed by the chloretetracycline assay and changes in motility patterns. *Anim Reprod Sci.* 57, 199-215.

Silva L.D.M., Onclin K., Snaps F. & Verstegen J. (1995) Laparoscopic intrauterine insemination in the bitch. *Theriogenology* 43, 615-623.

Silva L.D.M., Onclin K., Lejeune B. & Verstegen J.P. (1996) Comparisons of intravaginal and intrauterine insemination of bitches with fresh or frozen semen. *Vet. Rec.* 17, 154-157.

Silva P.F. & Gadella B.M. (2006) Detection of damage in mammalian sperm cells. *Theriogenology* 65, 958-978.

Sirivaidyapong S., Cheng F.P., Marks A., Voorhout W.F., Bevers M.M. & Colenbrander B. (2000) Effect of sperm diluents on the acrosome reaction in canine sperm. *Theriogenology* 53, 789-802.

Ström-Holst B., Larsson B., Rodriguez-Martinez H., Lagerstedt A.-S. & Linde-Forsberg C. (2001). Zona pellucida binding assay- a method for evaluation of canine spermatozoa. *J. Reprod. Fertil.* Suppl 57: 137-140

Thomassen R. & Farstad W. (2009) Artificial insemination in canids: a useful tool in breeding and conservation. *Theriogenology*, 71, 190-199.

Thomassen R., Sanson G., Krogenæs A., Fougner J.A., Andersen Berg K. & Farstad W. (2006) Artificial insemination with frozen semen in dogs: A retrospective study of 10 years using a non-surgical approach. *Theriogenology* 66, 1645-1650.

Tsutsui T. (1989) Gamete physiology and timing of ovulation and fertilization in dogs. *J Reprod Fertil* Suppl. 39, 269-75.

Tsutsui T., Takahashi F., Hori T., Kawakami E. & Concannon P.W. (2009) Prolonged duration of fertility of dog ova. *Reprod Domest Anim.* 44 Suppl 2, 230-3.

Verstegen J., Iguer-Ouada M. & Onclin K. (2001) Computer assisted semen analyzers in andrology research and veterinary practice. *Theriogenology* 57, 149-179.

Wallace S.S., Mahaffey M.B., Miller D.M. Thompson F.N. & Chakraborty P.K. (1992) Ultrasonographic appearance of the ovaries of dogs during the follicular and luteal phases of the estrous cycle. *Am J Vet Res* 53(2): 209-215.

Watson P.F. (1975) Use of Giemsa stain to detect changes in acrosomes of frozen ram spermatozoa. *Vet. Rec.* 97, 12-15.

Wilson M.S. (1993) Non-surgical intrauterine artificial insemination in bitches using frozen semen. *J. Reprod. Fert.* Suppl. 47, 307-311.

Wilson M.S. (2001) Transcervical insemination techniques in the bitch. *Vet. Clin. North. Am. (Small Anim. Pract.)* 31, 291-304.

Yeager A.E. & Concannon P.W. (1996) Ovaries. In: *Small animal ultrasound*, Green RW (Ed.), Philadelphia: Lippincott Raven, 293-303.

5

Artificial Insemination in Pigs

Maes Dominiek, López Rodríguez Alfonso, Rijsselaere Tom, Vyt Philip and Van Soom Ann
Ghent University, Faculty of Veterinary Medicine, Salisburylaan 133, 9820 Merelbeke Belgium

1. Introduction

Artificial insemination (AI) of swine is widely practiced in countries with intensive pig production. In Western Europe, more than 90% of the sows have been bred by AI for more than two decades (Gerrits et al., 2005; Vyt, 2007). When compared with natural mating, AI is a very useful tool to introduce superior genes into sow herds, with a minimal risk of disease (Maes et al., 2008). The outcome of AI largely depends on the semen quality and the insemination procedure. In practice, fresh diluted semen for intracervical insemination is mostly used in pigs. Semen is obtained from boars on farms or from specialised AI-centres. The latter offer a diversity of breeds and genetic lines and distribute ready-to-use semen doses of constant quality to different sow herds.

Three important aspects should be considered. Firstly, only semen from healthy boars should be used, as diseased boars may ejaculate semen that is contaminated with pathogens. The semen from commercial AI-centres is shipped to a large number of sow farms. Contaminated semen could therefore lead to a rapid transmission of pathogens and to disease outbreaks in many different sow herds. Strict regulations and guidelines to prevent disease spreading are therefore implemented on porcine AI-centres. The second important aspect is the fertilizing capacity of the produced semen doses. The fertilizing potential of a semen dose is inherently linked to the quality of the spermatozoa itself (Tsakmakidis et al., 2010). Examination of the ejaculates is therefore necessary. A third important aspect of AI-centres is the semen processing procedure (Waberski et al., 2008). This is not only important to guarantee a low microbial presence but even more to obtain high quality sperm, namely viable spermatozoa in ready-to-use semen doses that can be used for several days. The dilution procedure and semen handling, the properties of the extender and the micro-environment for the sperm cells influence the survival and longevity of the spermatozoa.

The present chapter will review and critically discuss the different steps during the entire AI procedure in pigs, starting from the semen collection, dilution and processing, methods and technologies used to assess the semen quality, the storage conditions and the characteristics of the semen extenders that are required to maintain semen quality. A last part will focus on the different AI strategies.

2. Collection of semen, dilution and processing

Although automated semen collection systems have been developed (Barrabes Aneas et al., 2008), semen is mostly collected by the gloved hand technique from a boar trained to mount a dummy sow. Dummy sows should be solid in construction without sharp edges, and located in a quiet designated semen collection room with a non-slippery floor. A pre-warmed (38°C) collection container is used. The top of the container is covered with cheesecloth to filter out gel portion of the semen. The end of the penis is grabbed firmly with a gloved hand and the collection process is initiated with firm pressure to the spiral end of penis with the hand so that the penis cannot rotate. This process imitates the pressure applied by the corkscrew shape of the sow's vagina. Polyvinyl gloves can be used, not latex gloves as these are toxic for the semen (Ko et al., 1989). The first part of the ejaculate (pre-sperm) should be discarded. It is clear, watery fluid and does not contain sperm (~25 ml), but it may have a high bacterial count. The sperm-rich fraction should be collected (40-100 ml). It is very chalky in appearance and contains 80-90% of all sperm cells in the ejaculate. Once the sperm-rich fraction is complete, the remainder of the ejaculate is again more clear, watery fluid, and should not be collected (70-300 ml). After collection, the filter with gel should be discarded, and the collection container should be placed in warm water. The semen should be extended within 15 min. after collection. The ejaculation lasts up to 5 to 8 min, but may continue up to 15 min. About 100 to 300 ml of semen is collected. Semen collection from boars in AI-centres is performed approximately 2 times per week (Vyt et al., 2007).

The extension process should be done in a warm room with clean and sterile equipment. The extender is added to the semen, and cold shock should be avoided by diminishing the temperature gradually. A normal ejaculate usually contains enough sperm to inseminate 15 to 25 sows using conventional AI. Each dose should contain 2-3 billion spermatozoa in 80-100 ml.

3. Semen quality assessment

3.1 Assessment of the concentration of spermatozoa in the ejaculate

The number of spermatozoa in a semen dose is important for the fertilization process. On the other hand, AI-centres tend to dilute the ejaculates as much as possible to maximize semen dose production. Variation in the number of spermatozoa in an ejaculate has been described between different pig breeds *e.g.* Landrace, Duroc and Yorkshire (Kommisrud et al., 2002), which is a first factor influencing semen dose production. Not only differences in sperm number but also in sperm volume, ranging from 100 to 300 ml (Kondracki, 2003), influence sperm concentration. Individual variation within a breed is also very important (Johnson et al., 2000). Xu et al. (1998) demonstrated a difference in litter size of 0.09 to 1.88 piglets when inseminating sows either with $2*10^9$ or $3*10^9$ spermatozoa. Differences in litter size between both semen doses were largely dependent on individual variations between boars. Another study (Alm et al., 2006) using $2*10^9$ spermatozoa per dose mentioned not only a smaller litter size but also a lower farrowing rate at lower semen dose. In addition, several studies (Alm et al., 2006; Xu al., 1998) described lower fertility results when lower semen doses were used in boars with suboptimal semen quality. A general guideline for the number of good quality spermatozoa (Table 1) in a semen dose was set at $3*10^9$ spermatozoa per dose. According to the morphological or motility characteristics, the number of spermatozoa should be adapted (Martin-Rillo et al., 1996). By multiplying the total volume of the gel-free ejaculate (ml) times the sperm concentration per ml, the total sperm number is calculated. The volume is routinely measured by weighing the ejaculate considering 1 gram equal to 1 ml and the obtained total sperm numbers is a good indicator to evaluate spermatogenesis (Amann, 2009).The data above clearly indicate the importance of an accurate determination of the concentration of spermatozoa in the ejaculate.

3.1.1 Inspection of the raw ejaculate

Visual evaluation of the opacity of the ejaculate gives a rough idea on the sperm concentration. However, this method is crude and very subjective and therefore not suitable for AI-centres with large semen production.

3.1.2 Counting chambers

Different glass chambers are described to count cells in a known volume. Haemocytometers, such as the Neubauer, Thoma and Bürker chamber are reusable glass chambers with fixed volume used for counting immobilized spermatozoa in a grit. Other reusable glass chambers as the Mackler chamber are used for assessing concentration as well as motility (Tomlinson et al., 2001). Disposable chambers (Microcell^R, Leja^R) are commonly used in Computer Assisted Semen Analysis (CASA) since their small depth limits movement in the third dimension (Z-axis) when the sperm path is analysed (Verstegen et al., 2002). Haemocytometers are considered as the standard method for determining sperm concentration and have a lower coefficient of variation than disposable chambers (Christensen et al., 2005; Tomlinson et al., 2001). The concentration determined by the haemotocytometer however, was generally higher than the concentration determined using other chambers, especially with increasing concentration. Makler chambers were described as having higher standard deviations and more inconsistent results compared with the haemocytometer (Christensen et al., 2005; Tomlinson et al., 2001). Disposable chambers on the other hand, although they are also used for counting live cells, were reported to be more consistent and accurate (Mahmoud et al., 1997). The accuracy of different counting chambers is also dependent on the manner in which the chamber is filled. Thin, capillary-filled, disposable chambers are generally found to underestimate sperm concentration due to the Segre-Silberberg effect (Kuster, 2005). However, the variations between chambers when analysing sperm concentration seems to be technician and laboratory dependent (Christensen et al., 2005).

3.1.3 Photometry

Photometers (single wavelength) or spectrophotometers (multiple wavelengths) measure the optical density, *i.e.* the relative absorption and scattering of a light beam that is sent through a semen sample. The absorption and scattering is proportional to the sperm concentration. Next to the concentration of spermatozoa, the absorbance is also influenced by gel particles in the seminal plasma or the extender, by the quality of the sample cuvette, and the dilution of the sample (Knox, 2004). Photometry is commonly used in practice because it is fast and easy to perform (Woelders, 1991). Accurate dilution and a correct calibration curve are imperative to obtain proper results.

3.1.4 Flow cytometry

Several studies use fluorescent dyes that stain intact or damaged spermatozoa differently, and measure the distribution of dyes in the sperm cell population by a flow cytometer (Christensen et al., 2004; Ericsson et al., 1993). In that way, viability as determined by the percentage of intact cells as well as the concentration of spermatozoa in an ejaculate can be determined by using fluorescent microspheres. Since this technology can discriminate interference from gel particles, it has a low coefficient of variation (3.3%) (Christensen et al., 2004). However, the high costs and the dependence on qualified personnel make flow cytometry not the most suitable method for use in practice.

3.1.5 Other methods

Coulter counters, determining the number of particles within a known volume, can be used to assess spermatozoa concentration but discrimination of other particles with comparable size within the sample is difficult, resulting in a lower accuracy (Woelders, 1991). Other systems, *e.g.* computer assisted semen analysis (CASA) use image analysis to determine sperm concentration within counting chambers (Prathalingam et al., 2006; Verstegen et al., 2002). The accuracy of these systems depends not only on the optical properties and the software settings, but also on the kind of counting chamber that is used (Kuster, 2005). Nucleocounters are also used for determining sperm concentration, and they provide similar counts as those obtained with photometers (Camus et al., 2011; Hànsen and Hedeboe, 2003). In these devices, DNA is fluorescently labelled and counted by image analysis resulting in an accurate determination of sperm concentration.

The concern to obtain a correct estimate of sperm concentration led to a discussion on the accuracy of the different systems. Maes et al. (2010) did not find major differences between two types of colorimeters, the Bürker counting chamber, and the Hamilton Thorne Analyzer (Ceros 12.1) using two Leja chambers. Every system has its advantages and limitations. They concluded that in commercial porcine AI-centres, economic considerations such as purchase prices, labour, and high sample throughput are also important in the choice for one method or the other.

3.2 Morphology and viability assessment

The microscopic appearance of spermatozoa can give information on morphological abnormalities, cell membrane integrity and the acrosome. These are three important parameters that contribute to the fertilizing capacity of the sperm cells. Morphological abnormalities give an indication of aberrations in the spermatogenesis. Some malformations compromise the function of the cells and cannot be compensated for, therefore leading to culling of the boar. Abnormal shape of the head which carries the genetic material or abnormalities of the mitochondrial sheet which is important for the function of the flagella, are therefore called primary abnormalities. Remainders of cytoplasm, proximal or distal droplets, and small tail abnormalities are called secondary abnormalities and can be compensated for by the semen dose (Donadeu, 2004). Additionally, morphological anomalies (*e.g.* coiled tails) acquired by inappropriate handling of semen are called tertiary abnormalities.

Morphology can be assessed by staining techniques that do not require highly qualified personnel (Shipley, 1999). Normal morphology is correlated with fertility (Alm et al., 2006; Xu. et al., 1998), and should therefore be performed routinely in porcine AI-centres. Criteria for the maximum percentage of primary and secondary abnormalities in commercial porcine AI-centres were determined as 10% and 20%, respectively (Shipley, 1999). The percentage of spermatozoa with normal morphology should be at least 70% (Shipley, 1999). An overview of the criteria for use of porcine semen in artificial insemination is shown in Table 1.

Semen parameter	Requirement (%)			
	Kuster and Althouse, 1999	Martin-Rillo et al., 1996*	Shipley, 1999	Britt et al., 1999
Motility	> 70	60-100	> 70	>60
Abnormal morphology	< 20		< 20	
Normal acrosomes		<10		
Cytoplasmic droplets	< 15		< 15	
Proximal droplets		0-20		<20
Distal droplets		0-30		
Coiled tails		<5		
Primary abnormalities				<10
Secondary abnormalities				<20

* Recommendation for $2*10^9$ spermatozoa per dose

Table 1. Overview of the cut-off values for porcine semen quality in artificial insemination

Although several stains can be used, staining spermatozoa of farm animals for morphological examination is usually combined with membrane integrity assessment using a dye that is excluded by live cells, such as eosin (Figure 1). Therefore, besides being helpful for assessing sperm morphology, the eosin-nigrosin stain can be used to discriminate between live and damaged cells. This staining technique is widely used and is considered a simple and reliable technique that is easy to applyand its outcome correlates with fertility (Tsakmakidis et al., 2010).

Next to visual morphology assessment, automated CASA-systems were developed to obtain more objective information (Rijsselaere et al., 2005; Verstegen et al., 2002). Automated Sperm Morphology Analysis systems (ASMA) are able to locate the head of the spermatozoa and compare its morphology to internal standards. A disadvantage is the lengthy analysis which is required for each sample, and which is partly dependent on the contrast of the cells from the background necessary for the system to recognise the cell. The prolonged analysis time undoes the advantage of an objective measurement and renders the method not suitable for use in commercial AI-centres at the moment.

Several fluorescent dyes can also be used to assess cell membrane integrity and can be combined with flow cytometric analysis (Althouse and Hopkins, 1995; Woelders, 1991). The need for qualified personnel and a fluorescence microscope excludes the use of the latter stains from commercial AI-centres, although attempts have been made to incorporate this technology in the most recent generation of CASA-instruments. Next to staining methods, membrane integrity can also be evaluated by testing the osmotic resistance of the cells (Donadeu, 2004). The osmotic resistance of the porcine sperm cells was correlated with fertility results (Pérez-Llano et al., 2001). More advanced methods measure cell volume by detecting voltage changes when cells pass a capillary pore in a CASY 1 cell counter (Petrunkina al., 2004). Osmotic reactivity is a sensitive detection method of changes in plasma membrane, either in damaged cells or in capacitating cells.

Since the acrosome is important for the penetration of the oocyte, its integrity is considered vital for an optimal fertilising capacity. The acrosome integrity can be evaluated on the basis of its microscopic appearance, either by phase contrast evaluation of glutaraldehyde fixed spermatozoa or by various staining methods (de Andrade et al., 2007; Woelders, 1991).

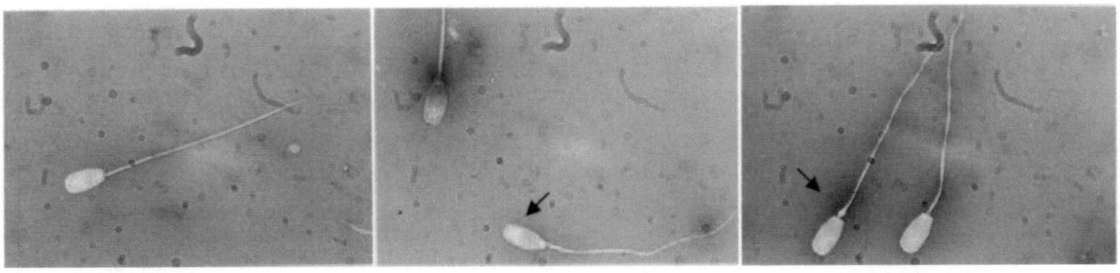

Fig. 1. Sperm morphology: spermatozoa with normal morphology, abnormal (narrow) head (primary defect) and proximal droplet (secondary defect) (arrows)

3.3 Motility assessment

Motility of spermatozoa has always been considered a primary requirement to fertilize eggs. Although the spermatozoa are brought to the fertilization site mainly by uterine contractions (Langendijk et al., 2002), sperm motility is required for penetration of the zona pellucida. Motility is known to be an important characteristic in predicting the fertilizing potential of an ejaculate (Gadea, 2005). Therefore, several methods have been used for motility assessment.

3.3.1 Visual motility estimation

The simplest way to evaluate sperm motility is by estimating the number of motile spermatozoa under a light microscope or using phase contrast microscopy. This method is subjective since it depends on the interpretation by an individual (Vyt et al., 2004b). It is however a cheap method and facilitates a high sample throughput which makes it popular in commercial AI-centres.

3.3.2 Computer assisted semen analysis (CASA)

Using digital image analysis, sperm cell tracks are analysed in different components (Rijsselaere et al., 2003; Verstegen al., 2002; Vyt et al., 2004b). CASA has major advantages: the method is objective, independent of the interpretation of the technician and gives detailed information on the sperm movement. This way, different motility patterns can be observed, *e.g.* progressive movement versus hyperactivity and even different subpopulations of spermatozoa within an ejaculate can be demonstrated (Peña et al., 2005; Rijsselaere et al., 2005; Verstegen et al., 2002). The detailed information given by the CASA-systems renders them also very susceptible to external influences on sperm movement, such as operator variability, semen handling and system settings are causes of inter-laboratory differences (Rijsselaere et al., 2003; Verstegen al., 2002). At the moment, CASA instruments have been validated for many animal species (Holt et al., 1994, 1996; Rijsselaere et al., 2003; Wilson-Leedy and Ingermann, 2007) which makes the method available for use in veterinary practice or commercial AI-centres. The high cost of the equipment compared to the alternative visual motility determination, is a restraint to the use of CASA in practice.

3.3.3 Sperm Quality analyzer (SQA)

The SQA systems convert variations in optical density into electrical signals to determine sperm concentration and motility. These electronic signals are analyzed by the SQA software algorithms and translated into sperm quality parameters. The effectiveness of different SQA systems for sperm analysis has been studied both in humans and animals, and different algorithms are needed for each species. A previous version of the SQA namely the SQA-IIC was consistent and suitable for the estimation of boar semen quality. There was a good correlation between the sperm motility index (SMI) obtained by SQA-IIC and several CASA parameters, especially with the percentage of motile sperm and with straight line velocity (VSL). However, the SQA-IIC is based on an old technology meant for human sperm analysis and the SMI values are based on overall information of the quality of the sperm, and do not discriminate between concentration, morphology and motility parameters. Recently, the SQA-Vp was introduced as an SQA device specifically designed for boars in which the sperm movement can be visualized on a screen and motility is given as percentage of motile sperm (López et al., 2011).

In pigs, a motility score of 60% motile cells, independent of the method of assessment, is required to be considered as a fertile ejaculate (Donadeu, 2004). Above 60% motile spermatozoa, no differences in farrowing rate and litter size were recorded (Donadeu, 2004). Apart from morphology, several attempts were made to correlate motility with fertility outcome. When using adequate numbers of spermatozoa per insemination dose ($3*10^9$), correlation with fertility outcome was hard to establish (Gadea al., 2004). At lower semen dose, motility was well-correlated with fertility parameters. In most studies involving pigs, the predictive effect of motility was evaluated using visual motility assessment. To increase the discriminating power of the motility estimation, objective motility assessment by CASA-measurements (Holt et al., 1997; Vyt et al., 2008) or motility of spermatozoa subjected to a percoll gradient (Popwell and Flowers, 2004) were used. These studies found motility to be positively correlated with fertility, especially with litter size.

3.3.4 Other sperm examination techniques

Sperm examination techniques requiring specialized knowledge and expensive equipment are not frequently used in commercial AI-centres. They are however used for research on porcine sperm. DNA fragmentation tests can be used to identify subfertile boars, but the study results are contradictory (Waberski et al., 2011; Boe Hansen et al., 2008). Some metabolic responses of sperm like resistance to oxidative stress (López et al., 2010) and *in vitro* fertilisation assays are also used for research purposes. The practical relevance of these techniques is limited due to the fact that most of the research on porcine semen is based on the semen from good performing boars (López et al., 2010). Subfertile or nonfertile boars are rapidly culled because of economic considerations, and therefore, there is a lack of information regarding sperm quality of infertile boars.

4. Storage of liquid semen

Frozen storage of boar semen still yields inferior fertility due to the loss of membrane integrity during freezing and thawing. Consequently, freshly diluted semen (liquid semen) is widely used for AI on the day of collection or in the following days. For storage of liquid boar semen, two factors are very important: the temperature of collection and storage, and the composition of the storage medium (Johnson et al., 2000).

4.1 Temperature of collection, transport and storage

A different composition of the phospholipids in the membrane of boar spermatozoa compared to bull spermatozoa, a low cholesterol/phospholipid ratio and an asymmetrical distribution of cholesterol within the membrane render boar spermatozoa very susceptible to cold temperatures resulting in increased permeability and loss of controlled membrane processes (De Leeuw et al., 1990). Hence, rapid cooling of ejaculates to 15°C or cooling below 15°C results in loss of viability or cold shock (Johnson et al., 2000). To avoid this cold shock, prediluted ejaculates are better left at temperatures above 15°C for several hours to induce cold resistance. In practice, semen is collected in isolated cans to avoid contact with colder surfaces and subsequent dilution is done in a manner in which temperature is diminished gradually. Two different protocols are normally used for this purpose: 1) One step dilution with either preheated diluter (~33°C) or diluter at room temperature or 2) a two steps dilution with first a 1:1 dilution with preheated diluter (~33°C), followed by a second dilution in either a preheated diluter or a diluter kept at room temperature (Waberski, 2009). After the final dilution, filling of commercial doses is done and the semen is allowed to cool down gradually to 17°C. When semen doses are to be transported, special precautions are taken to avoid temperature fluctuations (Green and Watson, 2002). Further storage of diluted semen is done at 17°C, at which temperature semen metabolism is reduced (Althouse et al., 1998), a condition necessary to extend storage time.

4.2 Storage medium

The storage media for liquid boar semen aim to prolong sperm survival, to provide energy to the cells, to buffer the pH of the suspension and to avoid the growth of bacteria (Vyt et al., 2004a). Therefore, porcine semen extenders contain ions to maintain the osmotic pressure of the medium, glucose as energy source, buffering systems to stabilize the pH of the extender and EDTA and antibiotics to prevent bacterial overgrowth (Johnson et al., 2000). The presence of glucose as the only energy source and the low oxygen content in the recipient in which diluted semen is stored stimulates the glycolytic metabolism. Consequently, the intracellular pH of spermatozoa is lowered which reduces their motility and enables them to survive several days at ambient temperature (Henning et al., 2009). Glucose also contributes largely to the osmotic equilibrium. The ions in the media for liquid boar semen are merely sodium bicarbonate and sodium citrate and are simultaneously used as buffer. In BTS extender, also KCl is added to prevent the potassium loss from inside the cells, and subsequent loss of motility due to Na-K pump inefficacy. Porcine spermatozoa are rather tolerant to minor changes in osmolality of the extender (Johnson et al., 2000). Iso-osmotic and slightly hyper-osmotic media are preferred for optimal preservation of fertilizing capacity (Weitze, 1990). Incubation in media below 250 mOsm and above 300 mOsm rendered irreversible damage to the membranes and subsequent loss of motility.

EDTA is added for its chelating properties. When Ca-ions are captured, the initiation of capacitation is inhibited (Watson, 1995). As a consequence, the fertilizing capacity of the spermatozoa is preserved. Depending on the composition of the extender, semen can be stored for 2 to 3 days in short-term extenders and up to five days or longer in long-term extenders (Johnson et al., 2000). Long-term extenders differ from short-term extenders mainly by the use of complex buffering systems (HEPES, Tris), mostly in addition to the bicarbonate buffering system, and by the presence of Bovine Serum Albumin (BSA). The latter has a positive influence on sperm survival due to the absorption of metabolic bacterial products from the extender. Cysteine is used as a membrane stabilizer (Johnson et al., 2000) inhibiting capacitation.

To prevent bacterial proliferation during storage, antibiotics are added to the extender. Bacteria originate mostly from the prepuce, thus depending on the semen collection technique, from semen manipulation or from the water used in the extender preparation (Althouse and Lu, 2005). Depending on the species, bacteria have deleterious effects on semen quality, namely depressed motility, cell death and agglutination (Althouse al., 2000), either by direct effect on the spermatozoa or by acidifying the environment. European legislation prescribes an antibiotic combination equivalent to 500 IU/ml penicillin, 500 IU/ml streptomycin, 150 mg/ml lincomycin and 300 mg/ml spectinomycin, for having a broad antibacterial spectrum and activity towards leptospira. In practice most commercial extenders use aminoglycosides, especially gentamycin (Althouse and Lu, 2005; Vyt et al., 2007). However, bacterial contamination should be first minimized by good hygiene and general sanitation by personnel (Althouse, 2008).

The extender-concentrates are diluted in distilled or de-ionized water. Next to the bacterial quality of the water, the electrolyte content, especially the absence of calcium ions, is an important characteristic for the water used to make the extender.

The comparison of different semen extenders has been subject of two kinds of studies: studies comparing different extenders *in vitro*, focusing on quality of semen after storage (De Ambrogi et al., 2006; Vyt et al., 2004a) and studies comparing fertility *in vivo* after insemination of semen stored for several days or stored in different extenders (Haugan al., 2007; Kuster and Althouse, 1999).

In vitro experiments showed no differences in cell viability between short-term and long-term extenders during 9-day storage (De Ambrogi et al., 2006). Motility remained unchanged within the first 72 hours, even in BTS-extenders, the most widely used short-term extender. Based on *in vivo* results, differences were noticed between different extenders but it was not always possible to relate these differences to the type of extender. Differences between long-term extenders were observed from day 4 of storage onwards (Kuster and Althouse, 1999). The limited number of extenders compared in each study makes it difficult to set up a ranking of the semen preserving quality of long-term semen extenders.

4.3 Storage of porcine semen in frozen state

As mentioned above, porcine spermatozoa are particularly sensible to low temperatures and to rapid cooling due to the specific composition of the cell membrane (De Leeuw al., 1990). Cold shock can be solved technically by inducing cold resistance, namely incubating sperm at ambient temperature for several hours (Watson, 1995), by contact with seminal plasma that has a protective effect on spermatozoa (Centurion et al., 2006), together with controlled freezing protocols. The variation in freezability of individual boar's semen is however more difficult to solve.

Semen extenders for frozen boar semen are completely different from extenders for liquid semen. The presence of egg-yolk, containing low density lipoproteins and cholesterol, has a protective effect on sperm membrane during cooling (Bathgate et al., 2006). Cryoprotectants, especially glycerol are added in low concentration to the medium in order to diminish membrane damage by freezing. Additionally, sugars and synthetic detergents are added, the latter having a modifying effect on the egg yolk inducing a better membrane stability of the cell membrane (Johnson et al., 2000). Thawing of the semen dose has been another point of concern. Thawing has to be fast in order to maintain sperm motility and acrosome integrity afterwards. Both processes *i.e.* freezing and thawing result in plasma membrane changes, explaining the variety of protocols available.

The fertility results with frozen semen have improved: cervical insemination results in a 75% farrowing rate and a litter size of 9.6 (Roca et al., 2003). Nevertheless, freezing and thawing are time consuming processes, restricting the use of frozen semen for specific indications, such as long transport times and conservation of valuable genetic material.

5. Insemination strategies

The management of AI is very important to determine the success of the procedure and the reproductive performance of the sows. Estrus control, timing and number of inseminations, the technique of AI, semen storage on farm and the use of new AI technologies, all require a specialized knowledge of pig reproductive physiology. The following measures could be taken to optimize the efficiency of AI on pig herds.

5.1 Boar stimuli

Correct timing of insemination requires careful detection of oestrus at regular intervals. Boar stimuli are important in promoting follicular development and expression of oestrus behaviour (Langendijk et al., 2006). Additionally, a high level of boar stimuli increases the frequency of uterine contractions, indicating a supportive role for passive sperm transport through the long uterine horns at the time of insemination. This effect can only be partially mimicked by a robot teaser boar which emits olfactory, acoustic and visual boar cues (Gerritsen al., 2005). Increase of oxytocin concentrations in peripheral blood plasma occurs in immediate response to boar presence and lasts for approximately 10 min (Langendijk et al., 2003). Therefore, exposure of sows to a boar during both back pressure testing and insemination is crucial.

5.2 Timing of insemination

Many studies have investigated time-relationships between oestrus, ovulation, insemination and fertilization using ultrasound testing. The key observation is that ovulation occurs at the beginning of the last third of oestrus regardless of the overall duration of oestrus. Precise prediction of the time of spontaneous ovulation in individual pigs has not yet been achieved. However, prediction of oestrus duration by observing the onset of oestrus after weaning has found broad acceptance in AI practice for calculation of the expected time of ovulation (Weitze et al., 1994). AI should be timed as close as possible to ovulation, preferably within 12 to 24 h before ovulation. The benefit of ultrasound testing of ovarian morphology for pig fertility management has been shown in practice (de Jong et al., 2009). Determination of the time of ovulation in relation to oestrus behaviour and AI management in representative numbers of sows on consecutive days has a great potential to provide short cuts in AI timing and to develop farm-specific strategies for improvement of AI management.

5.3 Use of new AI technologies

The development of techniques to inseminate with low numbers of spermatozoa in a small volume has increased insemination efficiency. This is particularly interesting when using spermatozoa of high value that are impaired, e.g. by freezing and thawing or sex-sorting. Post-cervical or intrauterine insemination with several devices has been developed to traverse the cervix and deposit sperm in the uterine body or posterior horn of multiparous sows. Compared to standard transcervical AI, post-cervical AI allows a threefold reduction in the numbers of spermatozoa to be inseminated, whereas deep intrauterine AI allows a 5 to 20 fold reduction (Vazquez et al., 2008). The use of post-cervical insemination varies among and within countries. Limits may arise from the use in sows only, skills needed for catheter handling, and the possibility of damaging cervical or uterine tissue. Semen encapsulation in a barium alginate membrane has been demonstrated to allow a single insemination (Vigo et al., 2009). Laparoscopy offers the possibility of inseminating a very low number of spermatozoa (i.e. 0.3×10^6) into the oviduct in anaesthetized pigs. However, the risk of polyspermic fertilization is substantial. Due to surgical intervention, its use is not appropriate in practice.

6. Conclusions

AI of swine is widely practiced and is a very useful tool to introduce superior genes into sow herds, with minimal risk for disease transmission. In practice, fresh diluted semen (3 billion spermatozoa in 80-100 ml) is mostly used for intracervical insemination .The success of AI is largely determined by the semen quality and the insemination procedure. Different parameters and techniques can be used to assess semen quality. Although more advanced technologies offer more accurate information, in commercial AI centres, semen quality is assessed based predominantly on concentration, morphology and motility using simple, cheap and practically easy-to-perform techniques. Critical issues for AI involve oestrus detection in the sow, timing of insemination and applying strict hygiene measures. Future developments will focus on new technologies to better assess semen quality in practice, to preserve semen for a longer time and to inseminate sows successfully using a lower number of spermatozoa using new AI techniques.

7. References

Alm, K.; Peltoniemi, O.; Koskinen, E. & Andersson, M. (2006). Porcine field fertility with two different insemination doses and the effect of sperm morphology. *Reproduction in Domestic Animals*, Vol.41, pp. 210-213, ISSN 0936-6768

Althouse, G. (2008). Sanitary procedures for the production of extended semen. *Reproduction in Domestic Animals*, Vol.43, pp. 374-378, ISSN 0936-6768

Althouse, G. & Hopkins, S. (1995). Assessment of boar sperm viability using a combination of two fluorophores. *Theriogenology*, Vol.43, pp. 595-603, ISSN 0093-691X

Althouse, G.; Kuster, C.; Clark, S. & Weisiger, R. (2000). Field investigations of bacterial contaminants and their effects on extended porcine semen. *Theriogenology*, Vol.53, pp. 1167-1176, ISSN 0093-691X

Althouse, G. & Lu, K. (2005). Bacteriospermia in extended porcine semen. *Theriogenology*, Vol.63, pp. 573-584, ISSN 0093-691X

Althouse, G.; Wilson, M.; Kuster, C. & Parsley, M. (1998). Characterisation of lower temperature storage limitations of fresh-extended porcine semen. *Theriogenology*, Vol.50, pp. 535-543, ISSN 0093-691X

Amann, R. (2009). Considerations in evaluating human spermatogenesis on the basis of total sperm per ejaculate. *Journal of Andrology*, Vol.30, pp. 626-641, ISSN 0196-3635

Barrabes Aneas, S.; Gary, B. & Bouvier, B. (2008). Collectis® automated boar collection technology. *Theriogenology*, Vol.70, pp. 1368-1373, ISSN 0093-691X

Bathgate, R.; Maxwell, W. & Evans, G. (2006). Studies on the effect of supplementing boar semen cryopreservation media with different avian egg yolk types on in vitro post-thaw sperm quality. *Reproduction in Domestic Animals*, Vol.41, pp. 68-73, ISSN 0936-6768

Boe-Hansen, G., Christensen, P., Vibjerg, D., Nielsen, M. & Hedeboe, A. (2008). Sperm chromatin structure integrity in liquid stored boar semen and its relationships with field fertility. *Theriogenology*, Vol.69, pp. 728-736, ISSN 0093-691X

Britt, J.H.; Almond, G.W. & Flowers, W.L. (1999). Diseases of the reproductive system. In: Straw B, D'Allaire S, Mengeling W, Taylor D (Editors), Diseases of Swine, 8th Edition, Blackwell Science Ltd, Oxford, pp. 903.

Camus, A.; Camugli, S.; Lévêque, C.; Schmitt, E. & Staub, C. (2011). Is photometry an accurate and reliable method to assess boar semen concentration?. *Theriogenology*, Vol.75, pp.577-583, ISSN 0093-691X

Centurion, F.; Echeverria, S.; Canul, N.; Ake, R.; Alfaro, M.; Santos, R. & Sarmiento, L. (2006). Influence of seminal plasma added to highly diluted semen on sperm motility of young boar feed with selenium and vitamin E. *Reproduction in Domestic Animals*, Vol.41, pp. 103, ISSN 0936-6768

Christensen, P.; Stryhn, H. & Hansen, C. (2005). Discrepancies in the determination of sperm concentration using Bürker-Türk, Thoma and Makler counting chambers. *Theriogenology*, Vol.63, pp. 992–1003, ISSN 0093-691X

Christensen, P.; Stenvang, J. & Godfrey, W. (2004). A flow cytometric method for rapid determination of sperm concentration and viability in mammalian and avian semen. *Journal of Andrology*, Vol.25, pp. 255-264, ISSN 0196-3635

De Ambrogi, M.; Ballester, J.; Saravia, F.; Caballero, I.; Johannisson, A.; Wallgren, M.; Andersson M. & Rodriguez-Martinez H. (2006). Effect of storage in short- and long-term commercial semen extenders on the motility, plasma membrane and chromatin integrity of boar spermatozoa. *International Journal ofAndrology*, Vol.29, pp. 43-552, ISSN 0196-3635

de Andrade, A.; de Arruda, R.; Celeghini, E.; Nascimento, J.; Martins, S.; Raphael, C. & Moretti, A. (2007). Fluorescent stain method for the simultaneous determination of mitochondrial potential and integrity of plasma and acrosomal membranes in boar sperm. *Reproduction in Domestic Animals*, Vol.42, pp. 190-194, ISSN 0936-6768

de Jong, E.; Vanderhaeghe, C.; Beek, J.; Van Soom, A.; de Kruif, A. & Maes, D. (2009). Ultrasonography of the ovaries in the sow: a helpful tool to determine the time of insemination. *Vlaams Diergeneeskundig Tijdschrift*, Vol.78, pp. 276-281, ISSN 0303-9021

De Leeuw, F.; Colenbrander, B. & Verkleij, A. (1990). The role membrane damage plays in cold shock and freezing injury. *Reproduction in Domestic Animals Supplement*, Vol.1, pp. 95-104, ISSN 0936-6768

Donadeu, M. (2004). Advances in male swine artificial insemination (AI) techniques. *The Pig Journal*, Vol.54, pp. 110-122, ISSN 1352-9749

Ericsson, S.; Garner, D.; Thomas, C.; Downing, T. & Marshall, C. (1993). Interrelationships among fluorometric analyses of spermatozoal function, classical semen quality parameters and the fertility of frozen-thawed bovine spermatozoa. *Theriogenology*, Vol.39, 1009-1024, ISSN 0093-691X

Gadea, J. (2005). Sperm factors related to *in vitro* and *in vivo* porcine fertility. *Theriogenology*, Vol.63, pp. 431-444, ISSN 0093-691X

Gadea, J.; Sellés, E. & Marco, M. (2004). The predictive value of porcine seminal parameters on fertility outcome under commercial conditions. *Reproduction in Domestic Animals*, Vol.39, 303-308, ISSN 0936-6768

Gerrits, R.; Lunney, J.; Johnson, A.; Pursel, V.; Kraeling, R.; Rohrer, G. & Dobrinsky, J. (2005). Perspectives for artificial insemination and genomics to improve global swine populations. *Theriogenology*, Vol.63, 283–299, ISSN 0093-691X

Gerritsen, R.; Langendijk, P.; Soede, N.M. & Kemp, B. (2005). Effects of (artificial) boar stimuli on uterine activity in estrous sows. *Theriogenology*, Vol.64, pp. 1518-1525., ISSN 0093-691X

Green, C. & Watson R. (2002). Adverse effect of winter overnight temperature on transported liquid boar semen. *The Veterinary Record*, Vol.151, pp. 302-303, ISSN 0042-4900

Hànsen, C. & Hedeboe, A. (2003). Determining concentration of raw semen: test of the nucleocounter SP-100, MiniTüb SDM5 and Coring 254. DanskeSlagterier, Landsudvalget for Svin, report 613

Haugan, T.; Gaustad, A.; Reksen, O.; Gröhn, Y. & Hofmo, P. (2007). Fertility results of artificial inseminations performed with liquid boar semen stored in X-Cell^{TM}vs BTS Extender. *Reproduction in Domestic Animals*, Vol.42, pp. 94-99, ISSN 0936-6768

Henning, H.; Petrunkina, A.M.; Harrison, R.A. & Waberski, D. (2009). Changes in responsiveness to bicarbonate under capacitating conditions in liquid preserved boar spermatozoa *in vitro*. *Society for Reproduction and Fertility Supplement*, Vol.66, pp. 79-80, ISSN 1470-1626

Holt, C.; Holt, W. & Moore, H. (1996). Choice of operating conditions to minimize sperm subpopulation sampling bias in the assessment of boar semen by computer-assisted semen analysis. *Journal of Andrology*, Vol.17, pp. 587-596, ISSN 0196-3635

Holt, C.; Holt, W.; Moore, H.; Reed, H. & Curnock, R. (1997). Objectively measured boar sperm motility parameters correlate with the outcomes of on-farm inseminations: results of two fertility trials. *Journal of Andrology*, Vol.18, pp. 312-323, ISSN 0196-3635

Holt, W.; Watson, P.; Curry, M. & Holt, C. (1994). Reproducibility of computer-aided semen analysis; comparison of five different systems used in a practical workshop. *Fertility and Sterility*, Vol.62, pp. 1277–1282, ISSN 1556-5653

Johnson, L.A.; Weitze, K.F.; Fiser, P. & Maxwell, W.M.C. (2000). Storage of boar semen. *Animal Reproduction Science*, Vol.62, pp. 143–172, ISSN 0378-4320

Knox, R. (2004). Practicalities and pitfalls of semen evaluation. *Advances in Pork production*, Vol.15, pp. 315-322, ISSN 1489-1395

Ko, J.; Evans, L. & Althouse, G. (1989). Toxicity effects of latex gloves on boar spermatozoa. *Theriogenology*, Vol.31, pp. 1159-1164, ISSN 0093-691X

Kommisrud, E.; Paulenz, H.; Sehested, E. & Grevle, I. (2002). Influence of boar and semen parameters on motility and acrosome integrity in liquid boar semen stored for five days. *Acta Veterinaria Scandinavica*, Vol.43, pp. 49–55, ISSN 0044-605X

Kondracki, S. (2003). Breed differences in semen characteristics of boars used in artificial insemination in Poland. *Pig News and Information*, Vol.24, pp. 119N-122N, ISSN 0143-9014

Kuster, C (2005). Sperm concentration determination between hemacytometric and CASA systems: Why they can be different? *Theriogenology*, Vol.64, pp. 614–617, ISSN 0093-691X

Kuster, C.E. & Althouse, G.C. (1999). The fecundity of porcine semen stored for 2 to 6 days in Androhep^{R} and X-cell^{TM} extenders. *Theriogenology*, Vol.52, pp. 365–376, ISSN 0093-691X

Langendijk, P.; Bouwman, E.; Kidson, A.; Kirkwood, R.; Soede, N. & Kemp, B. (2002). Role of myometrial activity in sperm transport through the genital tract and in fertilization in sows. *Reproduction*, Vol.123, pp. 683-690, ISSN 1470-1626

Langendijk, P.; Bouwman, E.G.; Schams, D.; Soede, N.M. & Kemp, B. (2003). Effects of different sexual stimuli on oxytocin release, uterine activity and receptive behavior in estrous sows. *Theriogenology*, Vol.59, pp. 849-61, ISSN 0093-691X

Langendijk, P.; Soede, N.M. & Kemp, B. (2006). Effects of boar stimuli on the follicular phase and on oestrus behaviour in sows. *Society for Reproduction and Fertility Supplement*, Vol.62, pp. 219-30, ISSN 1470-1626

López, A.; Rijsselaere, T.; Van Soom, A.; Leroy, J.L.; De Clercq, J.B.; Bols, P.E. & Maes, D. (2010). Effect of organic selenium in the diet on sperm quality of boars. *Reproduction in Domestic Animals*, Vol.45, pp. 297-305, ISSN 0936-6768

López, A.; Rijsselaere, T.; Bijttebier, J.; Vyt, Ph.; Van Soom, A. & Maes, D. (2011). Effectiveness of the sperm quality analyzer (SQA-Vp) for porcine semen analysis. *Theriogenology*, Vol.75, pp. 972-977, ISSN 0093-691X

Maes, D.; Nauwynck, H.; Rijsselaere, T.; Mateusen, B.; Vyt, Ph.; de Kruif, A. & Van Soom, A. (2008). AI transmitted diseases in swine: an overview. *Theriogenology*, Vol.70, pp. 1337-1345, ISSN 0093-691X

Maes, D.; Rijsselaere T.; Vyt, Ph.; Sokolowska, A.; Deley, W. & Van Soom, A. (2010). Comparison of five different methods to assess the concentration of boar semen. *Vlaams Diergeneeskundig Tijdschrift*, Vol.79, pp. 42-48, ISSN 0303-9021

Mahmoud, A.; Depoorter, B.; Piens, N. & Comhaire, F. (1997). The performance of 10 different methods for the estimation of sperm concentration. *Fertility and Sterility*, Vol.68, pp. 340–345, ISSN 1556-5653

Martin-Rillo, S.; Martinez, E.; Garcia C.;Artiga C. & De Alba, C. (1996). Boar semen evaluation in practise. *Reproduction in Domestic Animals*, Vol.31, pp. 519-526, ISSN 0936-6768

Peña, F.; Saravia, F.; Garcia-Herreros, M.; Nunes-Martinez, I.; Tapia, J.; Johannisson, A.; Wallgren, M. & Rodriquez-Martinzez, H. (2005). Identification of sperm morphometric subpopulations in two different portions of the boar ejaculate and its relation to post-thaw quality. *Journal of Andrology*, Vol.26, pp. 716-723, ISSN 0196-3635

Pérez-Llano, B.; Lorenzo, J.; Yenes, P.; Trejo, A. & Garcia-Casado, P. (2001). A short hypo-osmotic swelling test for the prediction of boar sperm fertility. *Theriogenology*, Vol.56, pp. 387-398, ISSN 0093-691X

Petrunkina, A.; Gröpper, B.; Günzel-Apel, A. & Töpfer-Petersen, E. (2004). Functional significance of the cell volume for detecting sperm membrane changes and predicting freezability in dog semen. *Reproduction*, Vol.128, pp. 829-842, ISSN 1470-1626

Popwell, J. & Flowers, W. (2004). Variability in relationships between semen quality and estimates of *in vivo* and *in vitro* fertility in boars. *Animal Reproduction Science*, Vol.81, pp. 97-113, ISSN 0378-4320

Rijsselaere, T.; Van Soom, A.; Maes, D. & de Kruif, A. (2002). Use of the Sperm Quality Analyzer (SQA II-C) for the assessment of dog sperm quality. *Reproduction in Domestic Animals*, Vol.37, pp. 158–163, ISSN 0936-6768

Rijsselaere, T.; Van Soom, A.; Maes, D. & de Kruif, A. (2003). Effect of technical settings on canine semen motility parameters measured by the Hamilton–Thorne analyzer. *Theriogenology*, Vol.60, pp. 1553–1568, ISSN 0093-691X

Rijsselaere, T.; Van Soom, A.; Tanghe, S.; Coryn, M.; Maes, D. & de Kruif, A. (2005). New techniques for the assessment of canine semen quality: A review. *Theriogenology*, Vol.64, pp. 706-719, ISSN 0093-691X

Roca, J.; Carvajal, G.; Lucas, X.; Vasquez, J. & Martinez, E. (2003). Fertility of weaned sows after deep intrauterine insemination with a reduced number of frozen-thawed spermatozoa. *Theriogenology*, Vol.60, pp. 77-87, ISSN 0093-691X

Shipley, C. (1999). Breeding soundness examination in the boar. *Swine Health and Production*, Vol.7, pp. 117–120, ISSN 1066-4963

Tomlinson, M.; Turner, J.; Powell, G. & Sakkas, D. (2001). One-step disposable chambers for sperm concentration and motility assessment: how do they compare with the World Health Organization's recommended methods? *Human Reproduction*, Vol.16, pp. 121-124, ISSN 0268-1161

Tsakmakidis, I.; Lymberopoulos, A. & Khalifa, T. (2010). Relationship between sperm quality traits and field-fertility of porcine semen. *Journal of Veterinary Science*, Vol.11, pp. 151-154, ISSN 1229-845X

Vazquez, J.M.; Roca, J.; Gil, M.A.; Cuello, C.; Parilla, I.; Vazquez, J.L. & Martínez, E.A. (2008). New developments in low-dose insemination technology. *Theriogenology*, Vol.70, pp. 1216-24, ISSN 0093-691X

Verstegen, J.; Iguer-ouada, M. & Onclin, K. (2002). Computer assisted semen analyzers in andrology research and veterinary practice. *Theriogenology*, Vol.57, pp. 149–179, ISSN 0093-691X

Vigo, D.; Faustini, M.; Villani, S.; Orsini, F.; Bucco, M.; Chlapanidas, T.; Conte, U.; Ellis, K. & Torre, M.L. (2009). Semen controlled-release capsules allow a single artificial insemination in sows. *Theriogenology*, Vol.72, pp. 439–444, ISSN 0093-691X

Vyt, Ph. (2007). Examination and storage of liquid porcine semen. PhD thesis, Ghent University, pp. 156, ISBN 978-90-586-4121-2

Vyt, Ph.; Maes, D.; Dejonckheere, E.; Castryck, F. & Van Soom, A. (2004a). Comparative study on five different commercial extenders for boar semen. *Reproduction in Domestic Animals*, Vol.39, pp. 1-5, ISSN 0936-6768

Vyt, Ph.; Maes, D.; Quinten, C.; Rijsselaere, T.; Deley, W.; Aarts, M.; de Kruif, A. & Van Soom, A. (2008). Detailed motility evaluation of boar semen and its predictive value for reproductive performance in sows. *Vlaams Diergeneeskundig Tijdschrift*, Vol.77, pp. 291-299, ISSN 0303-9021

Vyt, Ph.; Maes, D.; Rijsselaere, T.; Dejonckheere, E.; Castryck, F. & Van Soom, A. (2004b). Motility assessment of porcine spermatozoa: a comparison of methods. *Reproduction in Domestic Animals*, Vol.39, pp. 447-453, ISSN 0936-6768

Vyt, Ph.; Maes, D.; Rijsselaere, T.; Dewulf, J.; de Kruif, A. & Van Soom, A. (2007). Semen handling in porcine artificial insemination centres: the Belgian situation. *Vlaams Diergeneeskundig Tijdschrift*, Vol.76, pp. 195-200, ISSN 0303-9021

Waberski, D. (2009). Critical steps from semen collection to insemination. *Proceedings of the Annual Meeting of the EU-AI-Vets*, September 2009, Gent Belgium, pp. 66-69

Waberski, D.; Petrunkina A. & Töpfer-Petersen E. (2008). Can external quality control improve pig AI efficiency? *Theriogenology*, Vol.70, pp. 1346-1351, ISSN 0093-691X

Waberski, D., Schapmann, E., Henning, H., Riesenbeck, A. & Brandt, H. (2011). Sperm chromatin structural integrity in normospermic boars is not related to semen storage and fertility after routine AI. *Theriogenology*, Vol.75, pp. 337-345, ISSN 0093-691X

Watson, P. (1995). Cooling of spermatozoa and fertilizing capacity. *Reproduction in Domestic Animals*, Vol.31, pp. 135-140, ISSN 0936-6768

Weitze, K. (1990). The use of long-term extenders in pig AI - a view of the international situation. *Pig News and Information*, Vol.11, pp. 23-26, ISSN 0143-9014

Weitze, K.F.; Wagner-Rietschel, H.; Waberski, D.; Richter, L. & Krieter, J. (1994). The onset of oestrus after weaning, heat duration, and ovulation as major factors in AI timing in sows. *Reproduction in Domestic Animals*, Vol.29, pp. 433-443, ISSN 0936-6768

Wilson-Leedy, J. & Ingermann, R. (2007). Development of a novel CASA system based on open source software for characterization of zebrafish sperm motility parameters. *Theriogenology*, Vol.67, pp. 661-672, ISSN 0093-691X

Woelders, H. (1991). Overview of in vitro methods for evaluation of semen quality, *Proceedings of the second International Conference on Boar Semen Preservation*, KF Weitze and B Colenbrander (Editors), Paul Parey Scientific Publishers, Berlin and Hamberg, pp. 145-165

Xu, X.; Pommier, S.; Arbov, T.; Hutchings, B.; Sotto, W. & Foxcroft, G. (1998). In vitro maturation and fertilization techniques for assessment of semen quality and boar fertility. *Journal of Animal Science*, Vol.76, pp. 3079-3089, ISSN 0021-8812

6

Artificial Insemination in Swine

Eduardo Paulino da Costa[1], Aurea Helena Assis da Costa[2,3], Gustavo Guerino Macedo[3] and Emílio César Martins Pereira[3]
[1]*Federal University of Viçosa*
[2]*Germovet*
[3]*Post-graduation students from the first author*
Brazil

1. Introduction

The world population is 6.4 billion people approximately and is constantly growing. In this context, there is the expectation that it will reach 8.1 billion in 2030 and nine billion in 2050. In the next 25 years, this population growth will demand some 50% increase in food production. So, the world will be required some 53% increase in meat production, therefore elevating from 367 to 562 million tons. This will be necessary due the growth of the population and the increase of the per capita consumption, which is foreseen to reach 19.1Kg swine meat for inhabitant in 2030. So, the production of swine meat should present a growth around 20%, therefore reaching 155 million tons (Roppa, 2006). This growth is really happening, as considering that the world production of swine meat in 2010 reached 101 million tons, with projection of 133 million for 2019 (ABIPECS, 2011).

The increase of the productivity in the world swine confinement is happening along the last decades. According to data from ABIPECS (2011), China leads the world ranking by annually producing about 50 thousand tons of meat, as followed by the European Union, United States and Brazil (22,250, 10,052 and 3,170, respectively). This high production basically occurred by development and adoption of new technologies in practically all areas, such as genetics, nutrition, management, sanity and reproduction. Undoubtedly, in the reproduction area, the artificial insemination (AI) represents an enormous progress in production of swine. Since the beginning of the 70-ies, this technique provoked a great impact on increment of the swine production, especially in Europe and more recently in USA (Gerrits et al., 2005).

Initially, AI appeared in order to provide the genetic improvement of the animals and to solve sanitary problems. However, a significant improvement in both productive and economical aspects were later observed, as making possible an acceleration in diffusion of the desirable characteristics of the reproducers with high genetic value. This occurred due to AI great potential in making possible the use of biotechnologies such as those related to technology of the semen, preservation of embryos, and others.

The intracervical insemination (ICAI) is most used in the technified farms. Under the practical viewpoint, it is a simple and easily accomplished procedure. In this technique, the semen is deposited in cervix and the spermatozoids are transported until the ampulla of the uterine tube, the place where fecundation occurs (Rath, 2002).

More recently, new AI techniques in which the deposition of the semen is accomplished in uterus or in the uterine tube have been developed. So, there are intrauterine artificial insemination (IUAI), deep intrauterine artificial insemination (IUPAI) and the intratubal artificial insemination (IOAI) through laparoscopy. These new techniques are used in order to reduce the number of spermatozoids and the volume of the insemination dose. Many studies have been developed toward the improvement of those techniques, so that the spermatic concentration and the semen volume are maximally reduced, without negatively interfering in the reproductive efficiency. So, those techniques would make possible an increment in the genetic gain for reducing the cost of the dose and maximizing the use of the genetically superior males.

However, in spite of the relative simplicity of the AI in swine, there are several factors that direct or indirectly affect negatively the reproductive efficiency of inseminated sows. It is important to emphasize that many of those factors also interfere into reproductive efficiency of the sows submitted to natural mating.

In this chapter, the objective is to discuss the advantages, limitations and procedures of the AI. Besides, some important factors that direct or indirectly affect the reproductive efficiency of the swine herds.

2. The artificial insemination

According to the first reports, the use of AI in swine occurred in Russia and Japan (Ivanow, 1907; Nishikawa, 1964). Later, the AI diffusion was gradually happening in several countries. It is probable that the natural prolificacy of the swine species has delayed the development of the reproduction biotechnologies. However, the needs for genetic exchange and the sanitary pressures constituted a strong impulse for AI development.

In many countries, the AI growth is linked to expansion of the swine production at industrial scale. Considering the AI advantages, compared with the natural mating, the implantation of this one substantially facilitates the reproductive management of herds with high number of sows.

Most countries of the European Union adopt the AI at least in 60% of their females. In the last two decades, more than 90% swine females in the European west were artificially inseminated (Gerrits *et al.*, 2005). In Holland, for instance, more than 98% sows are artificially inseminated (Feitsma, 2009).

The AI use contributes for a larger sanitary control and hygienic cares in the matings. It also makes possible a better control of the semen quality due to rejection of inappropriate ejaculates. Besides those advantages, AI facilitates the management by the reduction of both time and work for mating. Another important aspect is the reproductive performance can be equal or superior to that obtained with the use of the natural mating.

This reproduction method presents great advantages compared to natural mating. In this context, the following advantages are distinguished: the genetic gains with the use of the genetically superior males, the reduction of the covering costs by female; and the decrease in the number of males in the farm. This last condition optimizes the use of the facilities.

Today, it is still possible to observe less technified farms that use the natural mating, which requires higher amount of males in a herd. This occurs because the male/female relationship for this condition to be a male for each 20 or 25 females, approximately. So, the producer will have higher expenses with facilities, feeding and medicines.

Despite all those advantages, however, the AI has some limitations in swine. In closed AI programs, in which the collection and processing of the semen are accomplished at the own farm, the investments in constructions and equipments are necessary for the installation of one semen production unit. In open programs, in which the doses are acquired from the centers external to farms, the main limitations are related to communication and to dose transports (Hansen, 2004).

Other limitations are also common in both programs, such as the need for maintaining the doses at temperature from 15ºC to 18ºC and the short storage period of the cooled doses (usually up to 72 hours). The reduced survival of the spermatozoids in the female genital organs is also a limiting factor. Besides those aspects, there are other factors such as the great variability in duration of the oestrum (from 12 to more than 96 hours) and at the moment of the ovulation among the swine females. However, the range of advantages obtained with AI undoubtedly overcomes the disadvantages of the same one.

2.1 Intracervical artificial insemination

The artificial intracervical insemination (ICAI) technique is the most used in technified farms. On the practical viewpoint, it is a simple and easily executed technology. The application of this technique optimizes the use of the males, which can supply up to 2,000 doses/year when under good management conditions (Bennemann et al., 2003).

In spite of this simplicity, a careful training of the employees and their understanding with reference to this technology are fundamentally important. Another relevant aspect is the way to implant the insemination technique in a farm. Since the year 1995, our work group already implanted ICAI in 69 farms at the states of Minas Gerais and Espírito Santo - Brazil. For this procedure, a transition period in the change of the natural mating to ICAI was defined. Our suggestion is the implantation to be partial, along approximately six months (transition phase). So, natural mating and inseminations occur weekly in the farm during this phase.

This condition makes possible to compare monthly the estrus replication between both methods. As soon the parturitions begin, the size of the litter will also be monitored. So, after approximately six months under evaluation, the decision for total implantation of the insemination is made. For this decision, the reproductive efficiency of the inseminated sows must be the same or superior to that of the sows submitted to natural mating.

The spermatic concentration required for ICAI are three billion spermatozoids. This concentration is important, as taking into account that in ICAI the semen is deposited in the cervix and its great part stays retained in the protuberances and cervical crypts. Then, these structures work as the first physical barriers to spermatic transport.

The swine specie is the only ones in which the volume of the insemination dose is as important as the spermatic concentration. In the other domestic species, the average or thin pallets (0,5 and 0,25mL, respectively) are generally used as containers for semen conditioning. In sow, the volume of the insemination dose used for ICAI is 80 to 100 mL. So, the semen recipients must have capacity to condition this volume. Very reduced volumes for ICAI can increase the rate of the estrus replication and/or to reduce the average number of pigs born by litter.

When the spermatozoids are deposited in the cervix, they are transported until the ampulla of the uterine tuba, where fecundation happens (Rath, 2002). For this condition, the spermatozoids find other physical barrier that is the uterutubal junction, which also works as spermatic reservoir (Langendijk et al., 2005).

Besides the barriers to be broken for the spermatozoid to reach the place of fecundation, other inconvenience of the insemination is the occurrence of seminal reflux. The inseminator' ability is fundamental to minimize the amount of reflux. However, only this ability has no effect, in case the inseminator is impatient. Besides, the time required for accomplishment of the insemination is an important factor. This makes sense, as considering that in the natural mating the penis introduced into female provokes the oxytocin liberation and, consequently, contributes to spermatic transport (Hafez, 2000). According to Langendijk et al. (2005), the IA pipette should remain in the animal'cervix during enough time for liberation of the oxytocin.

In this context, the recommendation by our work group is the insemination to be accomplished slowly, as maintaining the pipette fixed in cervix for approximately 10 minutes. Nowadays there are many available supports in the market, which are placed on the back of the sow for elevation and fixation of the pipette segment that is external to vagina, whereas the same one is fixed in the cervix. This way, the inseminator can inseminate other animals without the need for awaiting 10 minutes in each animal and later to begin IA in another animal.

In the ICAI technique, the semen is deposited in the first centimeters of the cervix. Due to anatomical characteristics of this structure, it acts as a natural barrier that hinders the arrival of the semen into uterus, therefore facilitating the occurrence of reflux through vagina.

The occurrence of reflux in the swine species is very common and it was observed in 100% animals inseminated by Steverink et al. (1998). According to those authors, the reflux presents differences in volume and in the spermatic concentration, according to each inseminated animal. However, some authors consider the reflux to be a physiologic event in the swine species. According to them, this reflux could only influence the fertility rate when the concentration of the insemination dose is equal or inferior to one billion spermatozoids, in 80 mL volume (Steverink et al. ,1998).

This spermatic concentration effect on fertility can be evidenced in the work by Watson & Behan (2002), When inseminating the females, those authors used three different spermatic concentrations (three, two and one billion spermatozoids) by ICAI and they concluded that the females inseminated with one billion spermatozoids presented low number of newborn piglets.

In a work carried out by our team, 120 females were inseminated by ICAI (Araújo et al., 2009), as being the semen reflux found in 100% females. The animals were observed up to 120 minutes after insemination. Some 100mL doses containing $3x10^9$ spermatozoids were used. The average volume of the reflux was 85.8mL, with a loss of 782.4 million spermatozoids by each IA. In this work, a relevant aspect is that insemination was carefully accomplished during a period of 10 minutes, by people highly expert in insemination. Surprisingly, animals with more than 105% reflux were observed, despite the cares previously mentioned, as indicating that secretions from the genital organs also constitute the volume reflowed. The reflux volume varied from 50 to 105%.

The ICAI allows for using the fresh, refrigerated or frozen semen. Concerning to fresh semen, it must be used immediately after its processing, without previous cooling. The cooling at temperature from 15° to 18°C is more used in both farm routines and insemination centers. It allows the maintenance of the spermatic viability for a period up to 72 hours.

Concerning to frozen semen, it was firstly used on the beginning of the 70-ies, as firstly with the insemination into uterine tuba and later with ICAI. There were progresses in using the frozen semen, due to researches accomplished with different cryoprotectors, conditioning packages, diluents, and freezing and defrosting curves. However, the use of the frozen semen in ICAI is still associated with the reduction from 10% to 20% in the parturition rate and from one to two piglets by litter, when compared to the use of refrigerated semen (Bernardi et al., 2005).

2.2 Intrauterine artificial insemination

In order to reduce the number of the spermatozoids/female/year, new techniques for artificial insemination were recently presented. Among them, the intrauterine artificial insemination (IUAI) through the use of the post-cervical probe is distinguished. This technique consists of deposition of the semen doses directly into body of the sow' uterus, from which the length is five to ten centimeters. The IUAI technique optimizes the semen production, as using low spermatic concentration by dose. This condition increases two to three times the number of doses by ejaculate.

The cost in maintenance of the semen donors includes the costs of the male acquisition cost, its depreciation, medicines, feeding and facilities. These expenses can represent 30 to 50% the total cost of the semen dose. In this sense, as higher is the number of the doses produced by each housed male, the higher will be the efficiency and lower the cost (Bennemann et al., 2003; Weber et al., 2003; Hansen, 2004). Whereas the traditional insemination requires one boar for each 100 to 150 female, one boar can attend up to 450 females in the intrauterine insemination, approximately.

Taking into account the better use of the ejaculate in IUAI, it is also distinguished the possibility to increase the selection intensity in the females production, by using the genetically superior males. Evidently, this condition would not be applied at commercial farms, from which the purpose is the production of animals for slaughter. In addition, this is a very useful technique for the researches with swine frozen semen, as taking into account that the IUAI, the spermatic volume and concentration are more reduced than in ICAI.

At first, IUAI is a higher perilous technique, as taking into account the impossibility to fix the cervix by hand, such as in cow or even retracting towards the outside of the vagina, as performed on goats and sheep. So, many technicians consider its implantation to be difficult in commercial farms. However, a work carried out by our group (Araújo et al., 2009) demonstrated the opposite. In this work, the ICAI techniques were compared to IUAI. ICAI was performed using a Melrose (Minitub®) pipette. IUAI was performed using an intrauterine catheter "Verona" (Minitub®). Despite the difficult passage of the pipette in 4.6% females submitted to IUAI, 100% of those females were inseminated (Table 1).

Description	Insemination technique	
	Intracervical	Intrauterine
Number of inseminations	120	480
Difficulty to introduce (n)	0^a	22^b

Table 1. Degree of dificulty to introduce the pipete in females for intracervical insemination (n=120) and intrauterine (n=480). A difference (P<0.05) was found between the insemination techniques by the chi-square test. Adapted from Araújo et al. (2009)

The difficult passage of the pipette in some animals is due to IUAI to be more invasive. In the present study, however, the catheter was introduced into uterus and the insemination happened successfully in all of the animals. However, Diehl et al. (2006) observed to be impossible the introduction of the catheter into uterus of 4.5% females. This difficulty probably occurred due to the short insemination time used by the authors (average: 2.3 minutes/insemination), especially in primiparous females, where there was higher number of animals in which there was difficulty in introduction of the catheter. In those cases, while the catheter is introduced, either inseminator's patience and the constant stimulation of the female by massage on lumbar area allow the success of the technique.

It is important to emphasize the possibility for occurrence of bleeding during the introduction of the insemination pipette, a condition verified by Watson & Behan (2002). This is due to factors such as the technical ability of the person responsible for insemination as well as the pipette type. Another interfering factor is the speed in introduction of the pipette, since as higher is the insemination speed as higher will be the bleeding possibility (Diehl et al., 2006). Besides those factors, the females with higher parturition number present larger development of the genital organs than the primiparas or nulliparas. Thus, it is easier the introduction of the catheter into cervix, therefore reducing the incidence of lesions.

However, the occurrence of bleeding during insemination does not affect the reproductive efficiency. This condition was verified by our work group, as the ICAI was compared with IUAI (Table 2). The presence of blood was observed in 1.6 and 7.7% of the animals inseminated via ICAI and IUAI, respectively. Nevertheless, this bleeding did not influence the estrum replication rate neither the total newborns by litter. Those results corroborate the by Watson and Behan (2002), who did not observe any deficit in the reproductive efficiency of the sows that presented bleeding after IUAI.

Insemination technique	Presence of blood	Number of Inseminations	Number of sows	Return to estrus rate[1]	Litter size per parity
Intracervical	Without	118	58	4.2	11.7 ± 3.2
	With[2]	02	02	0.0	9.5 ± 9.1
Intrauterine	Without	443	211	4.5	11.6 ± 3.1
	With	37	29	5.4	10.8 ± 4.3

Table 2. Return to estrus rate and litter size per parity with inseminations in the presence and absence of blood. Adapted from Araújo et al. (2009). No differences (P>0.05) found between the insemination techniques by the Chi-square test for return to estrus rate. No differences (P>0.05) between the insemination techniques (Duncan Test) for litter size mean per parity. [1]Return to estrus rate percentage of total number of inseminated sows for each insemination technique. [2]Not evaluated statistically due to the reduced number of occurrences.

The ICAI is known as technique presenting considerable vulvar reflux of the semen after AI. However, our work group (Araújo et al., 2009) verified that such a fact also happens with IUAI. In this experiment, we verified the semen reflux to occur in practically all animals, independent of the technique used (100 and 98% for ICAI and IUAI, respectively (Table 3). On the other hand, some works do not mention the presence of reflux in IUAI, perhaps because they only observed the first instants after AI (Benneman et al., 2004; Mezalira et al., 2005), differently of our work, in that the animals were observed until 120 minutes post IUAI, once the reflux does not occur right after insemination.

Insemination technique	Number of inseminations	Semen backflow rate (n)
Intracervical	120	100% (120)
Intrauterine	480	98% (471)

Table 3. Semen backflow in the inseminations according to the different insemination techniques. No differences (P>0.05) found between insemination techniques by the Chi-square test. Adapted from Araújo et al. (2009).

The occurrence of the semen reflux can have negative effects on the reproductive efficiency, such as the losses of spermatozoids. This condition is based on the fact that here is a minimum number of spermatozoids by dose, for the maximum reproductive efficiency. However, despite the high occurrence of semen reflux found by our work group, no negative effects occur in the return rate to estrum and in litter size (table 4).

Insemination technique	Backflow	Number of inseminations	Return to estrus rate	Litter size per parity
Intracervical	With	120	5.0%	11.56 ± 3.4
Intrauterine	With	471	4.0%	11.48 ± 3.3

Table 4. Return to estrus rate and litter size per parity in inseminations with backflow according to the different insemination techniques. No differences (P>0.05) found between the insemination techniques by the Chi-square test for the return to estrus rate. No differences (P>0.05) found between the insemination techniques by the F test for litter size per parity (Adapted from Araújo et al., 2009).

It is evident the spermatozoids number and the insemination dose volume are decisive factors for the volume reflux to interfere in the reproductive efficiency. In the experiment carried out by our group (Araújo et al.,2009), IUAI was compared with ICAI, as confronting two insemination volumes (100 vs. 50mL) and different concentrations of spermatozoids. Although the volume of the semen reflux has been similar among the treatments (P>0.05), the amount of spermatozoids of the reflux in females receiving IUAI was smaller (Table 5).

Insemination technique	Number of spermatozoids	Backflow volume in mL (%[1])	Total of backflow sptz in millions (%[1])	Number of backflows collected
Intracervical	$3x10^9$/100 mL	85.8 (85.8%)	782.4 (26.0%)[a]	23
Intrauterine	$1x10^9$/100 mL	83.2 (83.2%)	164.0 (16.4%)[b]	25
Intrauterine	$1x10^9$ /50 mL	41.5 (83.0%)	111.4 (11.1%)[b]	25
Intrauterine	$5x10^8$/100 mL	87.8 (87.8%)	80.5 (16.1%)[b]	28
Intrauterine	$5x10^8$/50 mL	45.3 (90.6%)	58.0 (11.6%)[b]	30

Table 5. Total number of spermatozoa during backflow in millions and number of backflows collected using the different insemination techniques. [1] Correspond to percentage in the reflux, as considering the volume or the total number of spermatozoids of the insemination dose. No differences (P>0.05) occurred between the insemination techniques by the Kruskal - Wallis test, concerning to the collected volume. There was difference (P<0.05) between the ICAI technique in relation to IUAI by the Kruskal - Wallis test, concerning to spermatic concentration. Adapted from Araújo et al. (2009).

This occurred because the semen is deposited at the third initial/medium of the uterus, as probably facilitating the fast progression of the spermatozoids toward the spermatic reservations, therefore allowing a high retention of cells in the genital organs (Dallanora et al., 2004).

Taking into account the advantages of IUAI, many researchers have been accomplished in the last years, in order to define the spermatic concentration and the ideal insemination volume for maximization of the results by using this technique. So, Dollanora et al. (2004) compared the use of ICAI (three billion spermatozoids at 90mL doses) with IUAI (1.5 billion spermatozoids at 60mL doses). Those authors obtained no differences between both treatments for the adjusted childbirth rate and total number piglets born.

When comparing ICAI (three billion spermatozoids in 100ML doses) with IUAI (1 billion spermatozoids in 50mL), Sumransap et al. (2007) verified there were no differences among the total number of spermatic cells in different segments of the genital organs from the most caudal area of the uterus until the ampulla of the uterine tuba. Thus, even with the reduced number of spermatozoids in the dose, IUAI provides the same number of spermatic cells in the spermatic reservoirs.

However, highly reduced concentrations of spermatozoids in the insemination dose (250 million) can reduce the size of the litter, by reducing the spermatic reserves (Mezalira et al., 2005).

The volume of the insemination dose is also a decisive factor in the reproductive efficiency of the herd. In this context, some works report that IUAI accomplished with highly reduced volume endangers the reproductive efficiency of the herd. This is evident in the work by Bennemann et al. (2005) who used IUAI with 500 million spermatozoids by dose, in volume of 20 mL (154 sows), as comparing with ICAI with three billion spermatozoids in 90 mL (144 sows). The farrowing rate did not differ between treatments. When using IUAI, however, a significant reduction occurred in the total number of born pigs.

The experience of our work group (Araújo et al., 2009) shows that the use of $5x10^8$ spermatozoids in 50mL can adequately substitute the traditional technique (ICAI) without endangering the reproductive efficiency of the inseminated animals (Table 6). It is probable that the use of the oxytocin in semen has contributed to those positive results. In works accomplished by our research group, the addition of 2.5 UI oxytocin at the insemination dose of 100 mL does not interfere in the physical parameters of the semen and morphological ones of the spermatozoids (Podda et al., 1999), as well as it does not endanger the replication rate of estrous. Additionally, the oxytocin in this preconized dose increases the size of the litter (Costa et al., 1999). With the physiologic role to promoting the contraction of the flat musculature of the uterus (Bevan, 1979), the oxytocin can facilitate the ascension of higher number of spermatozoids until the fecundation site, taking into account that only a small proportion of the spermatozoids deposited during natural mating or insemination reach the distal portion of the uterine tuba.

In spite of those positive results found in this experiment, in which the insemination was accomplished by the same employees who performed the insemination routine, we still did not implant the IUAI with $5x10^8$ spermatozoids/50mL in the routine of commercial farms. However, Since the year 2007, our work group implanted the IUAI with $1x10^9$ espermatozoids/100mL, by using two inseminations (at zero and 24 hours after the beginning of the estrus) in 100% primiparous and pluriparous females at four farms (total of 2.500 females). No nuliparous females exist in those farms. The primiparas are proceeding from other farm of the same company. It is important to emphasize that the inseminations are accomplished by employees of the farms. This condition reinforces our position that the IUAI technique can be accomplished at commercial farms by the own employees responsible for the gestation sector.

Insemination technique	Spermatozoid number	Farrowing rate ([1]n)	Estrus repetition rate	Number of newborns by farrowing
Intracervical	$3x10^9$/100 mL	90.0 (54)	10.0	11.5 ± 3,4
Intrauterine	$1x10^9$/100 mL	93.3 (56)	6.7	11.7 ± 3,4
Intrauterine	$1x10^9$ /50 mL	86.7 (52)	13.3	11.4 ± 3,2
Intrauterine	$5x10^8$ /100 mL	93.3 (56)	6.7	11.8 ± 3,0
Intrauterine	$5x10^8$ /50 mL	90.0 (54)	10.0	11.4 ± 3,6

Table 6. Farrowing, estrus repetition rates and total piglets born per farrowing in each insemination technique (60 females per treatment). [1]n: Number of animals which gave birth according to each insemination technique. No differences (P>0.05) occurred between the insemination techniques for farrowing and estrus repetition rates by the chi-square test. No differences occurred (P>0.05) between the insemination techniques for number of newborns by farrowing using Kruskal - Wallis test. Adapted from Araújo et al. (2009).

2.3 Deep intrauterine artificial and intratubal Inseminations

In the last years, many researches concerning to the deep intrauterine insemination (IUPAI) have been accomplished. In this technique, a low insemination volume (5mL) is used as well as reduced concentration of spermatozoids (200 million), without the need for surgical intervention (Vazquez et al., 2000). The objective of the researches accomplished until the moment is to turn this technique applicable (not endanger the reproductive efficiency of the herd, so that it can be commercially implanted at large scale. In addition, the use of reduced volume and low concentration of the sperm in IUPAI will favor the use of frozen semen and/or sexed.

The reduction of the semen volume used in IUPAI rather guarantees the optimization of the boar, as providing economical advantages to the farms. The possibility for using this technique is in line with the needs imposed by modern swine raise, which looks for reducing the insemination dose under use. This would provide a reduction in the male breeding stock and even in the frequency of using these ones.

It is considered that a great number of the spermatozoids are lost in ICAI process (Martínez et al. 2001). This occurs due to the semen reflux as well as to spermatozoid phagocytosis by the polymorphonuclear leucocytes. It is believed that approximately 1/3 of the spermatozoids by backflow in 2 hours after AI, due to those physiologic processes (Viring & Einarsson, 1981). After overcoming those obstacles, approximately 1×10^3 spermatozoids can be rescued at the caudal portion of the isthmus, a place where the spermatic cell stays until ovulation to occur (Mburu et al., 1996).

In this context, the IUPAI objective is the reduction of the spermatic flow inside the uterus, as reducing the seminal reflux and the phagocytosis rate on those cells (Vazquez et al., 2008). In addition, some physical barriers are transposed as the cervical folds and endometrial crypts. Thus, the insemination dose under use could be significantly reduced. So, Martínez et al. (2002) verified that IUPAI with 5×10^7 spermatozoids by dose (5mL) presents no differences in the gestation and parturition rates neither in the size of the litter, when compared with ICAI by using 3×10^9 spermatozoids (100mL). However, it is

important to emphasize that the control group (n=147) presented low rate for either parturition (83%) and for those born by litter (9.97), although those researchers used a high number of animals by treatment. Other aspect to be considered is that the estrum of the females submitted to IUPAI was induced, whereas the estrum of the control group was not.
The IUPAI technique consists of using a special pipette, which is fixed into cervix as in ICAI. Successively, a flexible catheter with 1.8m length is inserted through pipette along the cervical canal until reaching the final portion of the uterine horn. This technique provides the deposition of the semen in one of the uterine horns near the fertilization place.
The main IUPAI obstacle is the anatomical complexity of the sow´s genital organs. The cervical channel is characterized by presence of the cervical folds and uterine horns due to long length and naturally rolled. These characteristics delayed the development of a catheter for nonsurgical insertion in the uterine horns. So, Vazquez et al. (2005) report that, in 1999, they developed a nonsurgical catheterization technique for access to the uterus, by using a modified endoscope provided of flexible 1.35m optic fiber. Those researchers report the success in accomplishing this procedure.
Thus, the first accomplished IUPAI were based on the use of an endoscope at extremity of the insemination pipette, therefore allowing the visualization of either cervical channel and uterine horns. This technique associated with induction of the hormonal ovulation in sows has been making possible the deep deposition of the spermatozoid into uterus. It was demonstrated that the passage of the pipette associated with endoscope, along the cervical channel and uterine horn, is a simple process to be accomplished, as lasting 4.1 minutes on average (Martínez et al. 2001). Those authors show that the endoscopic IUPAI generates interesting results, such as parturition rates of 86.6%, 88.9% and 92.3%, by using 100, 20 or 5 x 10^7 spermatozoids in 5 mL of diluter, respectively. The average size of the litter was 9.41. Those data do not differ from ICAI (n=48) with 3 x 10^9 in 100mL. However, it is important to emphasize that the authors used a small number of animals (15, 18 and 13 females, respectively) for IUPAI. Besides, those animals were submitted to hormonal synchronization procedures, what could make unfeasible the use of this technique routinely in the commercial farms due to high cost.
The use of the endoscope represented a great progress in the procedure of the artificial insemination in swine. Due to deposition of the semen at proximities of the fecundation place, the IUPAI technique makes possible the use of the processed and weakened spermatozoids proceeding from cooling, freezing or sexing (Vazquez et al., 2005). However, the limitation of this technique is the cost of the equipment and its fragility. Thus, its use would not be applicable at field (Vazquez et al., 2005). From this verification, a number of researches were developed in order to eliminate the use of the endoscope in this procedure. This situation required the development of new IUPAI pipettes.
The proof of the IAIUP efficiency at field, without using the laparoscopy, was later confirmed by Martínez *et al.*, 2005b. This author demonstrated that the fertilization rate of the sows inseminated with 150 x 10^6 spermatozoids diluted into 5ml BTS did not differ from that when the animals were inseminated with 3 x 10^9 spermatozoids diluted into 100ml of the same diluent through IAIC. However, some 10.9 reduction in size of the litter were observed in the conventional IA for 9.8 piglets in IAIUP. Based on these results, the authors verified the IAIUP application in commercial farms to depend on the proof that this technique will not endanger the number of the piglets born by parturition.
With the progress of the researches, the number of spermatozoids used in IUPAI were twenty times reduced for refrigerated semen and up to six times for frozen semen, in

comparison with ICAI. In relation to volume, the decrease resulting from the use of IUPAI was 8 to 20 times lower compared to ICAI (Vazquez et al., 2008).

However, the recurring concern of the researchers refers to unilateral fertilization. Although small semen doses are only deposited in an uterine horn, the bilateral fertilization was proven in approximately 100% of the cases, according to either Martínez et al. (2002) who used the IUPAI with endoscopic catheter and Tummaruck et al. (2007) by using IUPAI with catheter without endoscope. Those authors did not find significant difference in the number of embryos found on each side. For this evaluation, they slaughtered the sows at approximately 60 hours after IUPAI. Then, they evaluated the washed of the uterine tuba and extremity of the horns.

However, a detailed study by Martínez et al. (2006) showed that, in sows ovulating spontaneously (without induced ovulation), the bilateral fertilization that is, in both uterine horns, is not 100% effective. For this confirmation, those authors used IUPAI with doses of 0.15×10^9 spermatozoids/ 20 mL. So, those researchers verified that 21% sows submitted to IUPAI presented unilateral fertilization. In addition, 15.8% sows presented partial bilateral fertilization. Those researchers also found differences regarding to the rate of normal embryos in the horn with less embryos, when comparing IUPAI with ICAI (2.95×10^9 spermatozoids/95mL). Corroborating with those authors, Buranaamnuay et al. (2011) demonstrated that, from a total of five inseminated animals, three presented unilateral fertilization. The animals were submitted to IUPAI procedure without laparoscopy, as using 1×10^9 defrosted spermatozoids.

Those contradictory discoveries suggest the mechanism in which the spermatozoid reaches the counterlateral horn still stays obscure and needs to be more studied, in spite of the evidences for trans-uterine and trans-peritoneal migration (Martínez et al. 2005a; Tummaruck et al. 2007).

The IUPAI will represent a great economical advantage to the farm, since it will reduce the costs with acquisition of males, ration, medicines, vaccines, management. Besides, it would guarantee a larger uniformization of both herd and litter. However, the high cost of the pipette for this procedure and the difficulties in execution of the technique still represent impediments for its implantation in commercial farms. To these factors are added the results still inferior in reproductive efficiency, when compared with ICAI and IUAI.

Thus, it is clear that IUPAI represents a technique with a promising future to be commercially used at the farms, since the costs are decreased and the reproductive efficiency is not endangered.

Another developed technique is the artificial intratubal insemination through laparoscopy (ITAI). This new technology attends the premise to use doses at much reduced spermatic concentrations and at small volumes. Above all in specific situations, when the use of frozen, sexed semen or the genetically modified semen is proposed, the low number of viable spermatozoids can be compensated by deposition of the close semen or the semen inside the uterine tuba, then obtaining satisfactory fertilization rates.

The ITAI allows the inseminator, with the aid of a laparoscope, to determine the time and the ideal place for deposition of the semen, as reducing the exhibition of the spermatic cells to adversities and positioning them close to the uterus-tubaric junction.

For execution of this technique (Vazquez et al., 2008), initially the animal is placed in Trendelemburg position (that is, dorsal decubitus with the head side lightly sloping) at 20° angle with the horizontal. Successively, an incision close to 1.5cm near the navel is accomplished. The borders of the incision are tractioned and a optiview trocar associated with a laparoscope is inserted into incision, as this being removed later. So, the access to the abdominal cavity is possible with laparoscope. The abdominal cavity is inflated with CO_2 and two lateral openings are accomplished in the hemi-abdomen for the access of the Forceps tweezers. Those tweezers aid in the manipulation and fixation of the uterine horns and uterine tubas for the introduction of the insemination needle. After accomplishing the procedure, the tweezers are removed and a small suture is necessary. The procedure takes approximately 15 minutes.

Laparoscopy is considered a less invasive technique than laparatomy for introduction of the semen into uterus or in the uterine tuba (Vazquez et al., 2008), since laparatomy can cause either higher stress to the animal and adherences at the postoperative period, therefore prejudicing the future inseminations (Fantinati et al., 2005).

The insemination by ITAI makes possible the use of doses as low as five million spermatozoids in 0.5mL (refrigerated semen) in each uterine horn, without affecting the efficiency of the fertilization and production of piglets, when associated with laparoscopy (Fantinati et al., 2005). According this author, however, this technique should be obligatorily accomplished in both horns, since the low concentration, the small volume and the deposition in a precise place impede the spermatozoid to migrate and reach the collateral horn.

Due to high number of spermatozoids introduced into uterine tuba (3-6 x 10^5) during ITAI, special attention should be taken with regard to polyspermy. The polyspermy is affected by the spermatozoid: oocytes proportion and by the insemination moment, as this one is related to modifications in the environment of the uterine tuba. In this context, Vazquez et al. (2008) verified the polyspermy incidence to be very low, when spermatic concentrations of $3x10^5$ and $5x10^5$ are used by dose or when the sows are inseminated before ovulation. Otherwise, when those animals are inseminated with 1 x 10^6 spermatozoids/dose or during the preovulatory period, the possibilities for polyspermy are increased. Thus, low spermatozoid concentrations ($3x10^5$) were shown to be effective when used before ovulation in ITAI, as opening possibility for use of the sexed and frozen semen.

When working with the dose of 5 x 10^6 spermatozoids/0.5mL in each horn in the laparoscopic IAITU and 3 x 10^9 in ICAI, Fantinati et al. (2005) obtained high fertilization rates of oocytes and developmental competence of the embryos, which were collected and cultivated *in vitro*. However, it is worth to emphasize that the females had the estrum induced with eCG and hCG.

Although this technique was commercially applied in sheep (Anel et al., 2006), in swine it is still limited to experimental assays. The highest difficulties for its commercial accomplishment are the need for personal training, structure and specialized equipments.

2.4 Some factors affecting the reproductive performance of inseminated females

Several aspects are able to interfere into results of the AI programs. However, it is important to emphasize that many of those factors also interfere in the reproductive efficiency of sows submitted to natural mating. The objective of this topic is to distinguish some important aspects in this context.

In the last 25 years, the AI in swine was expressively desenvolved, as contributing to genetic improvement of the herd and increase in production. During this period, a reduction in the number of spermatozoids by each dose, that passed from $6x10^9$ to up $5x10^4$. At the same time, the useful life of the semen increased considerably, as turning more flexible and practicable the process (Waberski et al., 2008).

The use of reduced spermatic concentrations in the insemination doses comes to encounter the premises of the swine confinement of the XXI century. To attend those requirements, however, it is necessary a high-qualified semen, therefore guaranteeing a high reproductive efficiency. In addition, to assure this condition, it is necessary an effective quality control and the monitorship of several factors that can interfere into results.

In this context, several factors are very important such as: the action of the pathogenic microorganisms, nutritional conditions, the age of the first mating, the lactation period, the seasonal influence and the management in detecting the estrus detection.

The reproductive efficiency of the artificially inseminated sows is extremely affected when a contaminated semen is used. The microbial contamination of the semen can result into reduced reproductive efficiency due to low seminal quality, precocious embryonic death, and endometritis (Guerín & Pozzi, 2005).

The forms of the semen contamination can be classified as being from animal origin or not. The contamination from animal origin is due to infection of the boar, proceeding from the testicles or other segments of the genital organs. In addition, a number of contaminations may occur by breathing secretions or feces, which happen during the collection process and semen processing. Otherwise, the contamination not arising from the boars can occur, in most cases inadvertently during manipulation of the semen by the person responsible for the collect. Another responsible factor would be the excessive and mistaken exposure of the material collected at the air, skin and breathing secretions. Besides those aspects, the semen can be also contaminated by the quality of the water used during the processing, the ventilation system, sinks and drains (Maes et al., 2008).

A second factor affecting the reproductive performance of the animals is feeding. The supply of a ration that is in perfect balance of nutrients is essential. For this reason, it is fundamental the producer to receive technical orientation of the professionals specialized in the animal nutrition area.

The age of the animal at the first natural mating is also an important factor that should be taken into account. Usually, the sows present the first estrus at the age of five or six months. However, it is not indicated those animals to be inseminated before the seventh or eighth month. On this occasion, they will be weighing approximately 130 to 140kg on average, as depending on the female' genetics, and they will be presenting the third estrus. This fact is based on verification by Martín Rillo et al. (2001) who confirmed that the length of the female' genital organs during the first natural mating is directly proportional to dimension of the animal. Additionally, those authors found correlation between the length of the vagina and the length of the uterus. They still verified a larger size of the litter in animals presenting more developed genital organs at the action of insemination.

Another factor affecting the reproductive efficiency of the inseminated female is the nursing period. In the past, it was consensus that a shorter nursing period would increase the number of piglet births by year and, consequently, larger number of parturition by year and consequently higher piglets/sow/year. However, this theory was mistaken, because based on survey of 79,729 parturitions, our work group observed that as longer is the length of the lactational period as larger is the size of the following litter (Table 8). Thus, lactational periods from 22 to 25 days result in approximately one more pig in the following litter, compared with periods from 8 to 13 days. This condition was verified either in primiparous and pluriparous sows (Costa et al., 2004).

Lactation length (days)	Primiparous		Pluriparous	
	N	LS	N	LS
8 to 13	1,074	10.34 ± 0.9[a]	3,513	10.70 ± 0.5[a]
14 and 15	2,911	10.41 ± 0.5[a]	13,951	11.16 ± 0.2[b]
16 and 17	2,249	10.46 ± 0.6[a]	16,095	11.15 ± 0.2[b]
18 to 21	2,987	10.68 ± 0.5[b]	24,069	11.34 ± 0.1[c]
22 to 25	1,186	11.43 ± 0.8[c]	8,692	11.87 ± 0.3[d]
Total	10,867	10.86 ± 0.3	68,862	11.44 ± 0.1

Table 8. Average of litter size (LS) of primiparous and pluriparous sows submitted to different lactation lengths and respective parity number (N). Averages with different letters in the same column differ ($P<0.05$) by the Duncan test (Costa et al., 2004).

According to Koketsu *et al.* (1997), the uterine retrogressive development is not essential for establishment of the next gestation. In sow, however, the complete recovery of the endometrium happens between the second and third postpartum week (Hafez, 2000). This explains (Table 8) the influence of the nursing period on size of the litter only from 18-21 days under nursing in primiparous sows.

In pluriparous sows, however, a nursing from 14 to 15 days shows a significant increase in size of the litter, as compared with the precocious weaning (8-13 days), whereas primiparous females did not present this condition. Those results show the *post-partum* recovery to be less efficient in primiparous gilts, probably due to higher weakening of those animals. According to Koketsu et al. (1997a,b) the adverse effects of a short nursing period on the subsequent reproductive efficiency is less intense in females that maintain high ration consumption during nursing.

So, the uterine involution could be the main factor responsible for the low embryonic survival and, consequently, the reduced size of the litter in females submitted to the precocious weaning (Allrich et al., 1979; Foxcroft and Aherne, 2000; Machado et al., 2000). Associated the those factors, the presence of lochia can hinder the embryonic implantation and provoke the death of the embryos (Grunert and Birgel, 1982).

Our work group also evaluated the influence of the nursing period on the weaning-insemination interval (Table 9). Those discoveries demonstrate that a nursing period of 22 days at least provides a shorter weaning-insemination, interval, then decreasing the unproductive days of the sow.

Lactation length (days)	Primiparous		Pluriparous	
	N	WCI	N	WCI
8 to 13	1,074	5.63 ± 0.5[a]	3,513	4.94 ± 0.8[a]
14 and 15	2,911	5.43 ± 0.3[b]	13,951	4.60 ± 0.1[b]
16 and 17	2,249	5.07 ± 0.3[c]	16,095	4.44 ± 0.1[c]
18 to 21	2,987	4.80 ± 0.3[d]	24,069	4.38 ± 0.1[d]
22 to 25	1,186	4.67 ± 0.5[e]	8,692	4.31 ± 0.1[e]
Total	10,867	5.11 ± 0.2	68,862	4.54 ± 0.8

Tabela 9. Weaning-conception interval (WCI, average ± standard deviation) in 79,729 parturitions in pluriparous and primiparous sows with lactation periods of different lengths. (Amaral Filha et al., 2004). Averages with different letters in the same column differ ($P<0.05$) by the Duncan test.

Another aspect that should be observed in artificial insemination programs is the thermal condition of the environment to which the animal is submitted. The high temperatures reduce the efficiency of the heat loss, as making the animal to enter a hyperthermal state. This condition leads to embryonic mortality at the initial gestation stage. A survey accomplished with 100,934 parturitions in a tropical climate area shows the size of the litter to be significantly smaller in the hottest months of the year (Table 10). In the same way, in temperate area (Mediterranean conditions), the efficiency of the IA (parturition rate and litter size) is lower in summer-autumn season. Additionally, the administration of exogenous hormones (eCG and hCG) in the attempt to improve the ovulation rate proved to have no effects during this period (Bolarín et al., 2009).

However, when the environmental temperature becomes a restrictive factor for the embryonic viability, there are some alternatives to minimize the thermal effect. The ventilation, the floor cooling and the use of nebulization could partially reduce the adverse effect of the temperature on sow. This practice is applicable, mainly in tropical countries where the hangars for animals are open and exposed to adverse effects of the climate. Adult animals can have their critical temperature increased, that is, their resistance to heat is increased up to 2°C when they are submitted to ventilation from fans within facilities (Nääs, 2000).

Another aspect to be considered in AI is the efficiency in detecting the estrus. For the obtainment of indexes compatible with the goals established by the reproductive program, it is necessary to observe the IA ideal moment, as considering both estrus and ovulation. This condition is important, since a long IA - ovulation interval reduces the gestation rate, the embryonic survival and the litter size (Spencer et al., 2010).

The insemination protocol (AI moment) is defined as a function of the estrus beginning. Thus, more important than to find a sow under estrus is to detect the beginning of the same one. However, even with a good management in detection of the estrus, many times the beginning of this one is not characterized, taking into account that it might have happened during night. This fact can be the responsible for the highest incidence of the estrus detected at the beginning of the morning and not during afternoon. In a study conducted by our work group (Pinheiro, 2000), we verified that 16.66% of the estrus were initially detected at 15:30 hours. However, at 7:30 and 23:30 the estrus were detected in 44.44 and 38.88% of the animals. Therefore, 83.24% initial detections of the estrus occur in the morning, taking into account there is no routine at the farms for night detection.

Considering the importance of the initial detection of the estrus, it is worth to emphasize that some animals do not accept promptly the natural mating even when they are in estrus. However, when insisting with detection incentive, the animal presents the immobility reflex. So, it is very important a careful detection, mainly in females that already present modifications such as the vulva edema.

When the gilts are housed in stalls, the introduction of the teaser is recommended in those stalls, on the beginning of the morning and on the end of the afternoon, in order to detect the females in estrus. Those females presenting immobility to natural mating, a behavior known as reflex of tolerance to male (RTM), are considered to be in estrus. However, special attention should be given when RTM does not occur in females that already present modifications such as the vulva edema. In this case, we recommend to take the female to stall of the teaser it can be carefully evaluated.

Though, the management of the estrus detection in primiparous and pluriparous females are differentiated. After weaning of the litter, the females are housed in collective stalls or individual cages. Usually, the beginning of the estrus happens from the third and fourth day after weaning. However, RTM should be made already at the following day after weaning, at the beginning of the morning and final of the afternoon. This procedure is important, taking into account that some sows can advance the beginning of the estrus, in other words, at the first or second day after weaning.

When the females are housed in cages, the teaser is conducted in the corridor of the hangar, so he has contact with the sow. At this moment, an employee stimulates the sow by pressuring the back or even mounting on the same one. From the third day from weaning, the females presenting no characteristic behavior of estrus should be individually taken to the stall of the teaser. For standardization either in gilts and primiparous and pluriparous, the zero hour of the estrus is the moment at which the female presents RTM for the first time.

Another procedure used in practice for detection of the estrus is the reflex of tolerance to the man (RTH). This reflex is the result of the man-animal interaction, without the presence of a male. However, the results are various and inconsistent. A study carried out by our work team (Pinheiro, 2000) showed that 23% sows in estrus do not present RTH. For this study, the estrus was confirmed by RTM, besides the occurrence of ovulation that was confirmed by ultrasonography. The detection of the estrus was accomplished at 8hrs intervals (7:30, 15:30 and 23:30). The RTH reflex was accomplished before RTM, as considering that many sows in estrus can present positive RTH after they were previously sensitized by the contact with male.

We also verified that 44% females, which were in estrus, presented very short RTH (less than 16 hours). Those considerations were corroborated by DIAS et al. (1999), who found a very varied RTH period. Those researchers observed that 11% animals presented no RTH and 26.5% presented it for a period lower than 16 hours. Also SOEDE (1996) found that 18% animals presented RTH for 16 hours or less and many animals presented a discontinuous or very short symptomatology. Thus, considering the mentioned aspects, RTH should not be considered as an efficient procedure in the estrus detection.

3. Conclusion

The artificial intrauterine insemination (IUAI) allows for better use of the ejaculates, compared with the intracervical artificial insemination ICAI). This condition is possible, as taking into account that a lower spermatic concentration can be used in the insemination dose. The IUAI technique can be used at commercial farms in substitution to ICAI without endangering the reproductive efficiency.

In spite of the progresses and refinement of the different artificial insemination techniques, the deep intrauterine insemination (IUPAI) is a promising procedure. In this context, the possibility for using the insemination doses with small volume and reduced spermatic concentration will optimize the use of the males, as providing economical advantages to the farms. In addition, the use of the reduced volume and low spermatic concentration in IUPAI will allow progresses in the use of frozen semen.

However, the high cost of the pipette for this procedure and the difficulties in execution of the technique still represent impediments for its implantation in commercial farms. The results still inferior in the reproductive efficiency, when compared with ICAI and IUPAI, are added to those factors. Thus, it is evident that IUPAI is a technique with promising future to be used commercially at the farms, since the costs are decreased and the reproductive efficiency is not endangered.

The appropriate procedure of the artificial insemination is not the only factor determining the obtainment of desirable results in the reproductive efficiency. Thus, special attention must be to factors that can, direct or indirectly, influence the results.

4. Acknowledgement

The authors thank the company GERMOVET - Biotechnology in Animal Reproduction, for the support.

5. References

ABIPECS 2011 http://www.abipecs.org.br/pt/estatisticas/mundial/producao-2.html

Allrich, R.D.; Tilton, J.E.; Johnson, J.N. & Slanger, W.D. (1979). Effect of lactation lenght and fasting on various reproductive phenomena of sows. *Journal of Animal Science*, Vol. 48, No. 2, pp. 359-362.

Amaral Filha, Wald'ma Sobrinho ; Costa, E. P. ; Costa, A.H.A. ; Carvalho, F.F.; Santos, A.K., Silva, A.F. . Impact of the length of lactation period on the weaning-conception interval in sows.. In: 15 International Congress on Animal Reproduction, 2004, Porto Seguro. Abstract of 15 International Congress on Animal Reproduction, 2004. p. 322.

Anel, L., Alvarez, M., Martinez-Pastor, F., Garcia-Macias, V., Anel, E. & de Paz, P. (2006). Improvement strategies in ovine artificial insemination. *Reproduction in Domestic Animals;* Vol. 41, No. 2, pp. 30–42.

Araújo, E.B.; Costa, E.P.; Costa, A.H.A.; Lopes, F.G.; Macedo, G.G. & Paula, T.A.R. (2009). Reproductive performance of sows submitted to intrauterine insemination. *Brazilian Journal of Animal Science,* Vol. 38, No. 8, pp.1460-1467, ISSN 1516-3598.

Bennemann, P. E.; Wentz, I. & Bortolozzo, F.P. (2003). Avaliação do Custo de Doses Inseminantes em Centrais de Inseminação Artificial de Suínos em Sistema Aberto. *Proceedings of XI Congresso Brasileiro de Veterinários Especialistas em Suínos (ABRAVES)*, Goiânia/GO, setembro, 2003.

Bennemann, P. E.; Milbradt, E.; Diehl, G. N.; Schimidt, A. C. T.; Bernardi, M. L.; Wentz, I.; Bortolozzo, F. P. (2004). Reproductive performance of sows submitted to intrauterine insemination at different pre-ovulation intervals. *Animal Reproduction.* v. 1, n. 1, p. 106 - 110.

Bennemann, P.E.; Koller, F.L.; Bernardi, M.L.; Wentz, I.; Bortolozzo, F.P. (2005). Efeito da inseminação artificial intra-uterina com 500 milhões de espermatozóides na taxa de prenhes e tamanho da leitegada em fêmeas suínas. *Proceedings of XII Congresso Brasileiro de Veterinários Especialistas em Suínos (ABRAVES)*, Fortaleza/CE, outubro, 2005.

Bernardi, M.L.; Bortolozzo, F.P.; Wentz, I. (2005). Emprego de sêmen congelado na inseminação artificial de suínos. In: *Inseminação Artificial na Suinocultura Tecnificada* Bortolozzo, F.P.; Wentz, I. pp. 159 - 179. Editora Pallotti, Porto Alegre/RS.

Bevan, J.A. (1979). Introdução aos princípios de ação das drogas, In: *Fundamentos da Farmacologia,* Editora Harper e Row do Brasil, pp. 24-29, São Paulo, 1979.

Bolarín, A.; Hernández, M.; Vazquez, J.M.; Rodriguez-Martinez, H.; Martinez, E.A.; Roca, J. (2009). Use of frozen-thawed semen aggravates the Summer-autumn infertility os artificially inseminated weaned sows in the Mediterranean region. *Journal of Animal Science,* Vol. 87, (August 2009), pp. 3967-3975, doi 10.2527/jas.2009-1941.

Buranaamnuay, K.; Panyaboriban, Y.; Tummaruk, P.; Techakumphu, M. (2011). Fertilization rate and number of embryos on day 2 after intrauterine and deep intrauterine insemination using frozen-tawed boar semen in multiparous sows. *Veterinary Medicine International*. Vol. 6, pp. 6. doi: 10.461.

Costa, E.P.; Vilela, C.G.; Carvalho, F.F.; Costa, A. H.P.; Podda, M.C.A.; Pinheiro, R. W. (1999). Oxitocina no sêmen diluído de varrões II - Influência na taxa de repetição de estro e número de leitões nascidos. *Proceedings of IX Congresso Brasileiro de Veterinários Especialistas em Suínos (ABRAVES)*, Belo Horizonte/MG, outubro, 2005.

Costa, E.P.; Amaral Filha, W.S.; Costa, A.H.A.; Carvalho, F.F.; Santos, A.K.; Silva, A.F. (2004). Influence of the lactation length in the subsequent litter size of sows. *Animal Reproduction*, Vol.1, No.1, (October/December 2004), pp. 111-114, ISSN 1806-9614

Dallanora, D.; Mezalira, A.; Katzer, L. H.; Bernardi, M. L.; Bortolozzo, F. P.; Wentz, I. (2004). Desempenho reprodutivo de fêmeas suínas inseminadas pela técnica intrauterina ou tradicional. *Pesquisa Agropecuária Brasileira*. v. 39, n.8, p. 815 - 819.

Dias, C.P., Uemoto, D.A., Marchetti, A. N., Pozzobon, M.C., Bortolozzo, F.P., Wentz, I., Borchardt Neto, G., Brant, G. (1999). Caracterização do reflexo de tolerância ao homem em fêmeas suínas. *Proceedings of Congresso Brasileiro de Veterinários Especialistas em Suínos (ABRAVES)*, Belo Horizonte/MG, outubro, 1999.

Diehl, G.N.; Amaral Filha, W.S.; Kummer, R.; Koller, F.; Bernardi, M.L.; Wentz, I. & Bortolozzo, F.P. (2006). Nova pipeta para inseminação intra-uterina em suínos. *Ciência Rural*, Vol.36, No.1, 2006, pp.179-185, ISSN 0103-8478.

Fantinati, P.; Zannoni, A.; Bernardini, C.; Webster, N.; Lavitrano, M.; Forni, M.; Seren, E.; Bacci, M.L. (2005). Laparoscopic insemination technique with low numbers of spermatozoa in superovulated prepuberal gilts for biotechnological application. *Theriogenology* v.63 pp. 806–817.

Feitsma, R. Artificial insemination in pigs, research and developments in The Netherlands, a review. (2009). *Acta Scientiae Veterinariae*, Vol. 37, No. 1, pp. 61-71, ISSN 1678-0345.

Foxcroft G, Aherne F. (2000). Manejo de marrãs e fêmeas de primeiro parto: Parte VI. Fatores que afetam a fertilidade de fêmeas primíparas desmamadas. *Proceedings of Simpósio Internacional de Reprodução e Inseminação Artificial em Suínos*, pp.186-198, Foz do Iguaçu, Paraná, Brasil, 2000.

Gerrits, R.J.; Lunney, J.K.; Johnson, L.A.; Pursel, V.G.; Kraeling, R.R.; Rohrer, G.A.; Dobrinsky, J.R. (2005). Perspectives for artificial insemination and genomics to improve global swine populations. *Theriogenology*. V.63, p.283 - 299.

Grunert E, Birgel EH. 1982. *Obstetrícia veterinária* (3ª edição). Editora Sulina, Porto Alegre, RS, Brasil.

Guérin, B.; Pozzi N. (2005). Viruses in boar semen: detection and clinical as well as epidemiological consequences regarding disease transmission by artificial insemination. *Theriogenology*. V.63: p.556-572.

Hafez, E.S.E.; Hafez, B. (2000). *Reproduction in farm animals* (7.ed.), Blackwell Publishing, ISBN 978-0-6833-0577-7, Maryland, USA.

Hansen, D. (2004). Resultados práticos da inseminação pós ou trans-cervical em suínos. *Proceedings of 2° Congresso Latino Americano de Suinocultura e 4° Congresso de Suinocultura do Mercosul*. Foz do Iguaçu, Paraná, 2004.

Ivanow, E. I. (1907). De la fe´condation artificielle chez lês mammife`res. *Arch. Sci. Biol.* Vol, 12, (1907), pp. 377–511.

Koketsu Y, Dial GD, King VL. (1997a). Influence of various factors on farrowing rate on farms using early weaning. *Journal of Animal Science.*, vol.75, (1997),pp. 2580-2587.

Koketsu Y, Dial GD, Pettigrew JE, King VL. (1997b). Influence of feed intake during individual weeks of lactation on reproductive performance of sows on commercial farms. *Livestock Production Science*, Vol. 49, (1997), pp. 217-225.

Langendijk, P.; Soede, N.M.; Kemp, B. (2005). Uterine activity, sperm transport, and the role of boar stimuli around insemination in sows. *Theriogenology*. Vol.63, p. 500–513.

Machado GS, Machado JV, Mayrink RR. 2000. Experiência com desmame precoce em granjas brasileiras-1 Aspectos reprodutivos. *Proceedings of Simpósio Internacional de Reprodução e Inseminação Artificial em Suínos*, pp.114-130, Foz do Iguaçu, Paraná, Brasil, 2000.

Maes D, Nauwynck H, Rijsselaere T, Mateusen B, Vyt P, de Kruif A, Van Soom A. (2008). Diseases in swine transmitted by artificial insemination: an overview. Theriogenology. Vol. 70, No. 8, (November 2008), pp. 1337-1345.

Martín Rillo, S.; de Alba Romero, C.; Romero Rodrigues, A.; Cidoncha R.; Ziecik A.J. (2001). Litter Size and Vagina-Cervix Catheter Penetration Lenght in Gilts. *Reproduction Domestic Animals*. Vol. 36, No. 6, pp. 297-300. DOI: 10.1046

Martínez, E.A.; Vazquez, J.M.; Roca, J. et al. (2001). Deep intrauterine insemination and embryo transfer in pigs. *Reproduction*, vol. 58(Suppl), pp.301-311.

Martínez, E.A.; Vazquez, J.M.; Roca, J. et al. (2002). Minimum number of spermatozoa required for normal fertility after intrauterine insemination in non-sedated sows. *Reproduction*, vol. 123, pp.163-170.

Martínez, E.A.; Vazquez, J.M.; Roca, J.; Cuello C.; Gil, M.A.; Parrilla I.; Vazquez, J.L. (2005a). An update on reproductive technologies with potential short-term application in pig production. *Reproduction Domestic Animals*, vol. 40, No.4, (August 2005), pp.300-309, ISSN 0936-6768

Martínez, E.A.; Vazquez, J.M.; Parrilla I.; Cuello C.; Gil, M.A.; Tornel, J.A.; Roca, J.; Vazquez, J.L. (2005b). Low-dose deep intrauterine insemination in sows under conditions: Incidence of unilateral fertilizations. *Reproduction Fertility and Development*, vol. 17, No.1 & 2 (Abstract 19 - *Proceedings of the Annual Conference of the International Embryo Transfer Society, Copenhagen, Denmark, January 2005)*, (January 2005), pp.159-160, DOI: 10.1071/RDv17n2Ab19

Martínez, E.A.; Vazquez, J.M.; Parrilla I.; Cuello C.; Gil, M.A.; Rodriguez-Martinez, H.; Roca, J.; Vazquez, J.L. (2006). Incidence of unilateral fertilizations after low dose deep intrauterine insemination in spontaneously ovulating sows under field conditions. *Reproduction Domestic Animals*, vol. 41, No.1, (February 2006), pp.41-47, DOI: 10.1111.

Mezalira, A.; Dallanora, D.; Bernardi, M. L.; Wentz, I.; Bortolozzo, F. P.(2005). Influence of sperm cell dose and post-insemination backflow on reproductive performance of intrauterine inseminated sows. *Reproduction in Domestic Animals*, v.40, p.1-5.

Mburu, J.N.; Einarsson, S.; Lundeheim, N.; Rodriguez-Martinez, H. (1996). Distribution, number and membrane integrity of spermatozoa in the pig oviduct in relation to spontaneous ovulation. *Animal Reproduction Science*. vol. 45, No.1, (December 1996), pp.109-121.

Nääs, I.A. Influência do ambiente na resposta reprodutiva de fêmeas. *Proceedings of Simpósio Internacional de Reprodução e Inseminação Artificial em Suínos*, pp.253-262, Foz do Iguaçu, Paraná, Brasil, 2000.

Nishikawa, Y. (1964). History and development of artificial insemination in the world. In: *Proceedings of 5th International Congress Animal Reproduction Artificial Insemination*, Trento, Italy. 1964.

Pinheiro, R.W. Avaliação de parâmetros reprodutivos, com auxílio de ultra-sonografia, em fêmeas suínas na região de Ponte Nova-MG. Viçosa, MG: UFV, Impresso Universidade Federal de Viçosa, 2000. 46 f. Dissertação (Mestrado em Medicina Veterinária) - Universidade Federal de Viçosa, Viçosa.

Podda, M. C. A.; Costa, E.P.; Pinheiro, R.W.; Vilela, C.G.; Paiva, F.P.; Carvalho, F.F.; Costa, A.H.A. Oxitocina no sêmen diluído de varrões. I – Influência nos aspectos físicos do sêmen e morfológicos dos espermatozóides *Proceedings of Congresso Brasileiro de Veterinários Especialistas em Suínos (ABRAVES)*. pp. 343-344. Belo Horizonte, Minas Gerais, Brasil, outubro, 1999.

Rath, D. Low dose insemination in the sow - A Review. (2002). *Reproduction of Domestic Animals.* v.37, pp. 201 - 205.

Roppa, L. (September/October 2006). Perspectivas da produção mundial de carnes, 2006 a 2030. *Revista Pork World,* Editora Paulínia, n. 34, pp. 16 - 27 , São Paulo, SP.

Soede, N.M., Kemp, B. (1996). Timing of AI and ovulation in sows. *Proceedings of International Conference On Boar Semen Preservation,*1996

Spencer, K.W.; Purdy, P.H.; Blackburn, H.D.; Spiller, S.F.; Stewart, T.S.; Knox, R.V. (2010). Effect of number of motile, frozen-twawed boar sperm and number of fixed-time inseminations on fertility in estrous-synchronized gilts. *Animal Reproduction Science,* Vol. 121, (July 2010), pp.259-266, doi:10.1016/j.anireprosci.2010.07.002.

Steverink, D.W.; Soede, N.M., Bouwman, E.G. (1998). Semen backflow after insemination and its effect on fertilization in sows. *Journal of Reproduction and Fertility,* v.111, p.165-171, 1998.

Sumransap, P.; Tummaruck P.; Kunavongkrit, A. (2007). Sperm distribution in the reproductive tract of sows after intrauterine insemination. *Reproduction Domestic Animals,* vol. 42, No.2, (2007), pp.113-117, ISSN 0936-6768.

Tummaruk, P.; Sumransap, P.; Techakumphu, M.; Kunavongkrit, A. (2007). Distribution of Spermatozoa and Embryos in the Female Reproductive Tract after Unilateral Deep Intra Uterine Insemination in the Pig. *Reproduction Domestic Animals,* vol. 42, No.6, (December 2007), pp.603-609, ISSN 0936-6768.

Vazquez, J. L.; Martínez, E. A.; Vazquez, J. M.; Lucas, X.; Gil, M. A.; Parrilla, I.; Roca, J. (2000). Development of a non-surgical deep intrauterine insemination technique. *Proceedings of International Conference on Sêmen Preservation,* Beltsville, 2000.

Vazquez, J.M.; Martinez, E.A.; Roca, J.; Gil, M.A.; Parilla, I.; Cuello, C.; Carvajal, G.; Lucas, X.; Vazquez, J.L. (2005). Improving the efficiency os sperm Technologies in pigs: the value of deep intrauterine insemination. *Theriogenology.* Vol. 63, No.2 (January 2005), pp.563-547. doi:10.1016

Vazquez, J.M., Martinez, E.A., Roca, J., Gil, M.A., Parrilla, I., Cuello, C., Carvajal, G., Lucas, X., Vazquez, J.L., (2005). Improving the efficiency of sperm technologies in pigs: the value of deep intrauterine insemination. *Theriogenology,* Vol. 63, pp. 536–547.

Vazquez, J.M.; Roca, J.; Gil, M.A.; Cuello, C.; Parrilla, I.; Vazquez, J.L.; Martínez, E.A. (2008). New developments in low-dose insemination technology. Theriogenology. Vol. 70, No. 8, (November 2008), pp. 1216-1224, DOI: 10.1016.

Viring, S.; Einarsson, S. (1981) Sperm distribuition within the genital tract of naturally inseminated gilts. *Nordisch Veterinarian Medicine,* v.33, p.145-149.

Waberski D, Petrunkina AM, Töpfer-Petersen E. (2008). Can external quality control improve pig AI efficiency? Theriogenology. Vol. 70, No. 8, November, pp. 1346-51.

Watson, P. F. & Behan, J. R. (2002). Intrauterine insemination of sow with reduced sperm numbers: results of a commercially based field trial. *Theriogenology.* Vol. 57, pp. 1683 - 1693.

Weber, D.; Bennemann, P.E.; Wentz, I.; Bortolozzo, F.P. (2003). Avaliação do Custo de Doses Inseminantes Produzidas em Centrais de Inseminação Artificial de Suínos em Sistema Fechado. *Proceedings of XI Congresso Brasileiro de Veterinários Especialistas em Suínos (ABRAVES),* Goiânia - GO, outubro, 2003.

7

Sperm Preparation Techniques for Artificial Insemination - Comparison of Sperm Washing, Swim Up, and Density Gradient Centrifugation Methods

Ilaria Natali
Sterility Center, Gynecology and Obstetrics Unit,
S.S. Cosma and Damiano Hospital, Pistoia
Italy

1. Introduction

The Artificial Insemination (AI) is the first option treatment for infertile couples with cervical factor subfertility, mild-moderate male subfertility and unexplained infertility. With the exception of cases in which the use of in vitro fertilization (IVF or ICSI) is strictly due as a consequence of a severe male or female factor, the artificial insemination must be part of a gradual approach to the techniques of artificial insemination. This is particularly the case since the AI is a valid low-cost method, minimally invasive and easily acceptable for the female's hormone treatment (Aribarg & Sukcharoen, 1995).

The AI, as other assisted reproductive techniques, needs a selection of the ejaculated spermatozoa before the performance of the treatment. In fact, some components of the seminal fluid may become an obstacle to the fertilization when the in vitro fertilization or the intrauterine insemination are performed (Bjorndahl et al., 2005). Spermatozoa and leukocytes produce many oxygen radicals that alter the possibility of the sperm-oocyte fusion after repeated centrifugations. So, the selection of the sperms from the other components with methods like the swim up technique or the gradient density centrifugation must be preferred (Aitken & Clarkson, 1988).

Some different techniques are used to prepare the spermatozoa for the AI, but the choice strongly depend on the quality of the semen, that is on the concentration, motility and morphology, in order to obtain the higher number of good spermatozoa, even from the poorest semens.

The principle techniques of sperm preparation consist of migration, density gradient centrifugation and filtration techniques. While for the migration the method is based on movement of the spermatozoa, for density gradient centrifugation and filtration techniques the method is based on a combination of the motility and the retention at phase borders and adherence to filtration matrices, respectively (Henkel & Schill, 2003).

The main techniques used for the AI are the sperm washing, the swim-up technique, and the density gradient centrifugation and they will be described as follow. The aim of the present chapter is to shed light on the key principles and the best method for sperm selection in order to obtain higher pregnancy rate.

2. Sperm preparation techniques

2.1 Semen collection

The semen consists of a suspension of spermatozoa stored in the epididymes that, at the moment of the ejaculation, is mixed with the secretions of the accessory glands. These glands are mainly the prostate and the seminal vesicles, while the bulbourethral glands and the epididymes represent only the minor contribution of the ejaculate.
Two main fractions are present in the seminal fluid; the first one is prostatic, rich in spermatozoa. The last fraction of the semen consists of vesicular fraction, less rich in spermatozoa (Bjorndahl & Kvist, 2003).
During ejaculation, it is very important to collect the entire volume of the sample: if the first fraction (rich in spermatozoa) is lost, the assessment of the semen features will be more difficult. In case of the AI, the semen sample will not contain the best portion of the spermatozoa.
For these reasons, the first step throughout the sperm preparation, is the correct sperm collection.
The semen collection is strongly recommended after an abstinence period of 2-3 days (Jurema et al., 2005; Marshburn et al., 2010) to maximize the conception rate. A sterile container (non-toxic for the spermatozoa) will be used and the collection of the semen will occur in a private room very close to the laboratory. All of these elements are mandatory for the therapeutic use. After the collection, the name of the couple should be clearly written on the container.

2.2 Choice of the technique

The techniques for the selection of the most efficient spermatozoa are very important for clinical practice. The choice of the best technique for semen preparation, before the AI, strictly depends on the quality of the sample (Canale et al., 1994). So, if we have a sample with normal count, motility and morphology of sperms we choose a sperm washing or a swim up method. By contrast, with a suboptimal quality sample we usually prefer a density gradient centrifugation. With the first methods, we obtain good quality sperms; while the density gradient centrifugation is usually preferred for the greater number of mobile spermatozoa selected from poor characteristics samples (low number, motility and morphology samples). Each technique can be changed or improved with simple changes, in order to optimize the recovery of the sperms.
The efficiency of the sperm selection is expressed as the concentration of spermatozoa with normal motility (that is progressively motile spermatozoa, according to the definition of the World Health Organization Manual of 2010) (WHO Manual, 2010).
Glass-wool columns are reported to be as effective as density gradient for the separation of spermatozoa also with intact acrosome from semen with suboptimal characteristics (Rhemrev et al., 1989; Sterzik et al., 1998), but this technique is less used.
The swim up method and the density gradient centrifugation produce different levels of contamination in the sample in the final preparation. In fact, the swim-up technique produces an higher level of non-sperm components (e.g. debris, bacteria) and the diffusion of other substances (e.g. the prostatic zinc) from the semen into the overlaying medium respect of the density-gradient centrifugation (Bjorndahl et al., 2005). Some differences also exist in the presence and the production of the Reactive Oxygen Species (ROS) and the

sperm DNA damage, associated with high levels of ROS, after the application of the two main techniques (Irvine et al, 2000; Zini et al, 1993, 2009).
The final volume of the preparation depends on the technique performed. If the IntraUterine Insemination (IUI) is performed, 0,3-0,4 milliliters (ml) of spermatozoa resuspended in sterile medium is required. If the case of the Fallopian Tube Sperm Perfusion (FSP), the volume of the suspension must be 4 ml, because it must perfuse the uterus and the both tubes. Because of its simplicity the first technique is the most used, even if some authors, comparing the IUI versus the FSP, demonstrate the superiority of the FSP technique about the pregnancy rate in stimulated cycles (Fanchin, 1995).

3. The sperm count

Before and after the treatment of the seminal fluid, the following parameters must be evaluated in line with the WHO Manual 2010.

- Volume (ml)
- Concentration (millions/ml)
- Motility (Progressive motility)
- Morphology (%normal sperms)

In addition, it is very important to establish the concentration of spermatozoa with progressive motility in the final preparation. The concentration of the progressive spermatozoa is calculated by multiplying the percentage (%) of the progressive sperms for the concentration of the sperms in the final preparation.

$$[PS] = \%PS \text{ X } [S]_f \quad (1)$$

The total number of the progressive spermatozoa is calculated by multiplying the concentration of the progressive sperms for the final volume of the suspension.

$$TPS = [PS] \text{ X } V_f \quad (2)$$

The total number of the progressive sperms in the preparation before the AI may be defined as a threshold value in predicting outcome in AI. This threshold is not absolute and may vary from study to study, even if some authors have identified this value in 10 million sperms (Miller et al., 2002; Van Voorhis et al., 2001).

4. Sperm washing

For the best quality samples (number and motility of sperms) the sperm washing is often performed (Boomsma et al., 2004) for the AI. The procedure simply consists in the washing of the semen with a sterile medium added with human albumin. After the fluidification of the sample, the entire volume is divided in fractions of not more than 2 ml into centrifuge tubes. The sterile medium of the equal volume (e.g. for the volume of the sample of 2 ml the medium added is 2 ml) is added in each tube and gently mix with a sterile pipette. After

---

[1] P=Progressive; S=Spermatozoa; [PS]=Concentration of Progressive Spermatozoa; $[S]_f$=Concentration of the sperms of the final preparation.

[2] TPS=Total Number of the Progressive Spermatozoa; [PS]=Concentration of Progressive Spermatozoa; V_f =Final volume of the preparation.

that, the samples are centrifuged at 300g (the rpm must be calculated for the centrifuge in each laboratory) for 10 min and than the supernatant is very carefully removed with a sterile pipette. The pellet is resuspended in 1 ml of the medium, gently mixed and centrifuged again for 5 min at 300g. The supernatant is removed again and the final pellet is resuspended in sterile medium for the AI.
It is very important to determine the count and the motility of the final preparation before the insemination.
In spite of the simplicity and velocity of the method, it must be reminded that the repeated centrifugations without the separation of the good sperms from leukocytes and dead sperms can produce many oxidative species and the damage of the sperms function (Aitken & Clarkson, 1988).

5. Swim up method

The swim up is the most common technique used in IVF laboratories and is preferred if the semen sample has a normal number of good sperms (normozoospermia). By this technique, the sperms are selected on their motility and the capability to swim out of the seminal plasma.
If the "direct swim up" is performed, after the fluidification of the sample, the entire volume (well mixed) is divided in fractions of 1 ml into centrifuge tubes (round bottom is preferred). 1,3 ml of culture medium is placed over the semen with extreme attention in each tube. The tubes must be put in the incubator, inclined at an angle around 45° and incubated at 37°C for 30-60 min. By inclining the tubes at 45°, we increase the surface between the medium and the semen and we improve the capability of the sperms to swim out of the semen and to reach the medium. After that, the tube must be returned in the vertical position and 1 ml of the supernatant of each tube can be gently removed, aspirating the sperms from the upper meniscus downwards with a sterile pipette (Henkel et al., 2003).
In alternative, the culture medium can be placed in each tubes and the semen can be stratified under the medium, in order to obtain a much cleaner surface between the semen and the medium. In addition, the recovery of the sperms can be optimized by increasing the number of the tubes and decreasing the volume of the semen in each tube. 2 ml of medium are added to the supernatant of each tubes and than centrifugated at 300g for 10 minutes. The supernatant is removed again and the pellet is resuspended in the sterile medium for the AI.
The "not direct" swim up from pellet is performed with the centrifugation of the semen followed by the stratification of the medium over the resuspended pellet. The liquefied semen is divided in fractions of 1 ml into each tubes, the medium is added (1:1) and after the centrifugation the supernatant is gently removed. Over the resuspended pellet, 1,3 ml of medium is replaced with caution and the tubes is put into the incubator from 30 to 60 min at 37°C (inclined at 45°); after the migration of the sperms, the volume of the semen for the AI is removed and the sperm count and motility are assessed.
The centrifugation for the direct swim up occurs after the migration of the sperms, that is, after the separation of the good sperms from the leukocytes and dead sperms. These species, usually produce the reactive oxygen species after the centrifugation (Irvine et al, 2000; Zini et al, 1993, 2009) so the direct swim up is the preferred method respect to the "not direct" swim up to select sperms for the AI.

6. Density gradient centrifugation

This is the preferred technique to select the greater number of motile spermatozoa in cases of severe oligozoospermia, teratozoospermia or asthenozoospermia. In this method, good quality sperms can be separated from dead sperms, leukocytes and the other components of the seminal plasma by a density discontinuous gradient. Cells with different density and motility can be selected during the centrifugation by the colloidal silica coated with silane of the gradient; the sperms with high motility and good morphology are at the bottom of the tube, finally free from dead spermatozoa, leukocytes, bacteria and debris.

The most applied discontinuous density-gradient is a two layers density-gradient, formed by a top layer of 40% (v/v) and a lower layer of 80% (v/v). Density gradient media are available in commerce ready to use or ready to make the different density layers; the top layer phase (40%) is prepared by adding 4 ml of density gradient medium to 6 ml isotonic sterile medium (BWW, Earle, Ham F-10 or HTF) supplemented with HAS (Human Serum Albumin); the lower layer phase (80%) is prepared by adding 8 ml of density gradient medium to 2 ml of isotonic sterile medium. The density gradient is prepared by layering 1 ml of 40% medium over the 80% medium, or by layering the 80% medium under the 40% medium in a conical centrifuge tube (not the round bottom tube!). The number of the tubes depends on the volume of the semen sample, but the total volume could be divided in not more of 1 ml of semen per tube.

After the fluidification, 1 ml of the semen is layered over the upper layer (40%) and centrifuged at 300g for 15 minutes. If the volume of each layer is reduced (<1ml) the spermatozoa have to migrate for a less distance between the layers and so the greater number of motile spermatozoa can be recovered. The centrifugation time and force can be varied depending on the quality of the sample: for example, the centrifugation time can be increased for specimens with high viscosity. After the centrifugation, most of the supernatant must be gently removed and the pellet is placed into a new, clean tube; here, the pellet is well resuspended in 5 ml of medium to remove the density gradient medium. It is centrifuged at 200g for 10 minutes. At the end of the centrifugation, the supernatant is removed and 5 ml of new medium are added. The centrifugation is repeated again and the final pellet is resuspended in the sterile medium for the AI.

The concentration and the motility after the preparation can be determined. It must be stressed that the sterile conditions and materials are essential when we perform the technique for therapeutic applications.

Nevertheless, the two main techniques produce different levels of contamination in the sample and of the production of ROS (see above). In addition, the swim-up technique produces an higher level of non-sperm components respect of the density-gradient centrifugation. The density gradient centrifugation recovers spermatozoa with improved motility but lower DNA integrity instead of the swim up technique, as the literature suggests (Zini et al., 1999, 2000). Several studies demonstrate that sperm DNA damage is associated with lower natural pregnancy rates (Loft et al., 2003; Spano et al., 2000) and lower IUI pregnancy rates (Evenson et al., 2008).

7. Conclusions

The AI is the still most used reproductive technique as it is relatively simple and low-cost. It is essential to select the most motile and normal morphological spermatozoa from the ejaculate as soon as possible, first because some components of the ejaculate contrast with the fertilizing capability of the spermatozoa (Bjorndahl et al., 2005; Mortimer et al., 1998). Then, because spermatozoa and leukocytes produce many oxygen radicals that can negatively influence the fertilizing sperm function (Agarwal & Sekhon, 2010; Aitken et al., 1998; De Jonge, 2002; Shamsi et al., 2008; Sharma & Agarwal, 1996; Zini & Sigman, 2009). So, the methods who separates the functional sperms from the other cells must be preferred (Aitken & Clarkson, 1988). The choice of the best method to select the functionally competent sperms depends on the features of the samples.

The swim up technique and the density gradient centrifugation have different efficiency in separating the sperms: the sperms isolated with the swim up are clean and motile, but damaged by the ROS and with higher DNA integrity; the sperms isolated with the density gradient centrifugation are not damaged by the ROS but with low DNA integrity.

When we compare the pregnancy rate after artificial insemination obtained with the sperm washing, the advanced sperm preparation methods (swim up and density gradient centrifugation) offer the higher rate of pregnancies (Carrell et al., 1998). These data indicate that the correct choice of the method of sperm selection can represent a good chance of pregnancy, after ovarian stimulation, in the artificial insemination.

Finally, the threshold value of 10 million sperms in the final preparation for the IUI has a predictive value for the pregnancy rate in IUI. Some authors demonstrate that when the total count of the progressive sperms is less than 10 millions the pregnancy rate decreased, even if, in practice, a pregnancy is also possible with an inferior total sperm count (Miller et al., 2002; van Weert et al., 2004; Van Voorhis et al., 2001).

If the total sperm count is very low, and in presence of a severe male factor, other alternative must be considered, like the In Vitro Fertilization (IVF).

8. Acknowledgments

I want to thank the book editor Milad Manafi for comments and support.

9. References

Agarwal, A. & Sekhon, L.H. (2010). The role of antioxidant therapy in the treatment of male infertility. *Human Fertility*, Vol.13, No.4, (December 2010), pp.217–225, ISSN 1464-7273

Aitken, R.J. & Clarkson, J.S. (1988). Significance of Reactive Oxygen Species and Antioxidants in Defining the Efficacy of Sperm Preparation Techniques. *J of Androl*, Vol.9, No.6, (November/December 1988), pp.367-76

Aitken, J.R.; Gordon, E., Harkiss, D., Twigg, J.P., Milne, P., Jennings, Z. & Irvine, D.S. (1998). Relative Impact of Oxidative Stress on the Functional Competence and Genomic Integrity of Human Spermatozoa. *Biol of Reprod*, Vol.59, (1998), pp.1037–1046

Aribarg, A. & Sukcharoen, N. (1995). Intrauterine insemination of washed spermatozoa for treatment of oligozoospermia. *Int J Androl*, Vol. 18, No. 1, (1995), pp.62-6

Bjorndahl, L. & Kvist, U. (2003). Sequence of ejaculation affects the spermatozoon as a carrier and its message. *Reprod Biomed Online*, Vol.7, No. 4, (October/November 2003), pp.440-8

Bjorndahl, L.; Mohammadieh, M., Pourian, M., Soderlund, I. & Kvist, U. (2005). Contamination by seminal plasma factors during sperm selection. *J of Androl*, Vol.2, (December 2005), pp.170-73

Boomsma, C.M.; Heineman, M.J., Cohlen, B.J. & Farquhar, C. (2004). Semen preparation techniques for intrauterine insemination. Cochrane Database of Systematic Reviews 2004; (3):CD004507

Canale, D.; Giorgi, P.M., Gasperini, M., Pucci, E., Barletta, D., Gasperi, M. & Martino, E. (1994). Inter and intra-individual variability of sperm morphology after selection with three different techniques: layering, swim up from pellet and percoll. *J Endocrinol Invest*, Vol. 17, No. 9, (October 1994), pp.729-32

Carrell, D.T.; Kuneck, P.H., Peterson, C.M., Hatasaka, H.H., Jones, K.P. & Campbell, B.F. (1998). A randomized, prospective analysis five sperm preparation techniques before intrauterine insemination of husband sperm. *Fertil Steril*, Vol. 69, No. 1, (January 1998), pp. 122-26

De Jonge, C. (2002). The clinical value of sperm nuclear DNA assessment. *Hum Fertil*, Vol. 5, No. 2, (May 2002), pp.51-3

Evenson, D.P. & Wixon, R. Data analysis of two in vivo fertility studies using Sperm Chromatine Structure Assay-derived DNA fragmentation index vs. pregnancy outcome. *Fertil Steril*, Vol. 90, No. 2, (October 2008), pp.1229-31

Fanchin, R.; Olivennes, F., Righini, C., Hazout, A., Schwab, B. & Frydman, R. (1995). A new system for fallopian tube sperm perfusion leads to pregnancy rates as high as standard intrauterine insemination. *Fertil Steril*, Vol. 64, No. 3, (September 1995), pp. 505-510

Henkel, R.R. & Schill, W-B. (2003). Sperm preparation for ART. *Reproductive Biology and Endocrinology*, Vol. 1, (2003), p.108

Irvine, D.S.; Twigg, J.P., Gordon, E.L., Fulton, N., Milne, P.A. & Aitken, R.J. (2000). DNA integrity in human spermatozoa: relationships with semen quality. *J Androl*, Vol. 21, No. 1, (January/February 2000), pp.33-44

Jurema, M.W.; Vieira, A.D., Bankowski, B., Petrella, C., Zhao,Y., Wallach, E. & Zacur, H. (2005). Effect of ejaculatory abstinence period on the pregnancy rate after intrauterine insemination. *Fertil Steril*, Vol. 84, No. 3, (September 2005), pp.678-81

Loft, S.; Kold-Jensen, T., Hjollund, N.H., Giwercman, A., Guyllemborg, J., Ernest, E., Olsen, J., Scheike, T., Poulsen, H.E. & Bonde, J.P. (2003). Oxidative DNA damage in human sperm influences time to pregnancy. *Hum Reprod*, Vol. 18, (2003), pp.1265-72

Marshburn, P.B.; Alanis, M., Matthews, M.L., Usadi, R., Papadakis, M.H., Kullstam, S. & Hurst, B.S. (2010). A short period of ejaculatory abstinence before intrauterine insemination is associated with higher pregnancy rates. *Fertil Steril*, Vol. 93, No. 1, (January 2010), pp. 286-88

Miller, D.C.; Hollenbeck, B. K., Smith, G.D., Randolph, J.R., Christman, G.M., Smith, Y.R., Lebovic, D.I. & Ohl, D.A. (2002). Processed total motile sperm count correlates with pregnancy out come after intrauterine insemination. *Urology*, Vol. 60, (2002), pp. 497–501

Mortimer, S.T.; Swan, M.A. & Mortimer, D. (1998). Effect of seminal plasma on capacitation and hyperactivation in human spermatozoa. *Hum Reprod*, Vol. 13, No. 8, (1998), pp.2139–2146

Rhemrev, J.; Yejendran, R.S., Vermeiden, J.P. & Zaneveld, L.J. (1989). Human sperm selection by glass wool filtration and two-layer, discontinuous Percoll gradient centrifugation. *Fertil Steril,* Vol. 51, No. 4, (April 1989), pp.685-90

Shamsi, M.B.; Kumar, R. & Dada, R. (2008). Evaluation of nuclear DNA damage in human spermatozoa in men opting for assisted reproduction. *Indian J Med Res,* Vol. 127, (2008), pp.115-123

Sharma, R.K. & Agarwal, A. (1996). Role of reactive oxygen species in male infertility. *Urology,* Vol. 48, No. 6, (December 1996), pp.835-50

Spano, M.; Bonde, J.P., Hjollund, H.I., Kolstad, H.A., Cordeli, E. & Leter, G. (2000). Sperm chromatine damage impairs human fertility. *Fertil Steril,* Vol. 73, (2000), pp.43-50

Sterzik, K.; De Santo, M., Uhlich, S., Gagsteiger, F. & Strehler, E. (1998). Glass wool filtration leads to a higher percentage of spermatozoa with intact acrosomes: an ultrastructural analysis. *Hum Reprod,* Vol. 13, No. 9, (September 1998), pp.2506-11

Van Voorhis, B.J.; Barnett, M., Sparks, A.E.T., Syrop, C.H., Rosenthal, G., Dawson, J. (2001). Effect of the total motile sperm count on the efficacy and cost-effectiveness of intrauterine insemination and in vitro fertilization. *Fertil Steril,* Vol. 75, No. 4, (April 2001), pp. 661-8

van Weert, J-M; Repping, S, Van Voorhis, van der Veen, F, Bossuyt, P.M.M. & Mol, B.W.J. (2004). Performance of the postwash total motile sperm count as a predictor of pregnancy at the time of intrauterine insemination: a meta-analysis. *Fertil Steril,* Vol. 82, No. 3, (September 2004), pp.612-20

World Health Organization. (2010). WHO laboratory manual for the examination and processing of human semen. Fifth edition. 2010, Geneva

Zini, A.; de Lamirande, E. & Gagnon, C. (1993). Reactive oxygen species in semen of infertile patients: levels of superoxide dismutase- and catalase-like activities in seminal plasma and spermatozoa. *Int J Androl,* Vol. 16, No. 3, (June 1993), pp.183-8

Zini, A.; Mark, V., Phang, D. & Jarvi, K. (1999). Potential adverse effect of semen processing on human sperm deoxyribonucleic acid integrity. *Fertil Steril,* Vol. 72, No. 3, (September 1999), pp.496-9

Zini, A.; Finelli, A., Phang, D. & Jarvi, K. (2000). Influence of semen processing technique on human sperm integrity. *Urology,* Vol. 56, No. 6, (December 2000), pp.1081-4

Zini, A. & Sigman, M. (2009). Are tests of sperm DNA damage clinically useful? *J of Androl,* Vol. 30, No. 3, (May/June 2009), pp.219-29

8

Effect of Vitamin E on the Development of Testis in Sheep

Hailing Luo, Suyun Ge, Dubing Yue, Leyan Yan, Xu Xu, Kun Liu and Fei Yuan
State Key Laboratory of Animal Nutrition, College of Animal Science and Technology, China Agricultural University, Beijing, PR China

1. Introduction

Vitamin E (VE) is a term that encompasses a group of potent, lipid-soluble, chain-breaking antioxidants. Structural analyses have revealed that molecules having VE antioxidant activity include four tocopherols (α-, β-, γ-, and δ-tocopherols) and four tocotrienols (α-, β-, γ-, and δ-tocotrienols). One form, a-tocopherol, is the most abundant form in nature , has the highest biological activity. As a naturally occurring antioxidant, VE is located in biological membranes where it acts to protect the membrane PUFA—polyunsaturated fatty acid (PUFA) from oxidation and attenuate oxidative damage to the cellular membranes (Sugiyama, 1992). Tappel (1962), Burton and Ingold (1986) and Esterbauer et al. (1991) found VE was effective in preventing lipid peroxidation and other radical-driven oxidative events. VE was first isolated from green leafy vegetables by Herbert Evans and Katherine Bishop, two prominent researchers from Berkeley and described as a fertility factor in 1922, then was named tocopherol in 1924 and synthesized in 1938 (Sen et al., 2007). The role of VE in reproductive performance was shown up that supplementing VE increased total sperm output and sperm concentration in boars (Brzezinska-Slebodzinska et al., 1995), rabbits (Yousef et al., 2003) and rams (Luo et al., 2004; Yue et al., 2010).

Impairment of mammalian fertility has also been attributed to VE deficiency. The crucial role of VE in animal reproduction has been recognized since 1922 (Evans and Bishop, 1922). To date, there are approximately 100 publications on this topic, which highlight the beneficial effects of this antioxidant on viability, membrane integrity and motility of spermatozoa of different species. The protective effects of VE against oxidative damage of sperm cells become even more significant when hygienic conditions are poorly controlled, as they frequently occur in field. Such conditions are associated with increased incidence of infections/inflammations of reproductive apparatus. During inflammation, the antioxidant defence of reproductive system downplays and generates an oxidative stress (Potts and Pasqualotto, 2003), which may impair testis function and affect negatively semen characteristics (O'Bryan et al., 2000). Because of high content of polyunsaturated membrane lipids, testicular tissue becomes one of the targets for oxidative stress (Mishra and Acharya, 2004).

VE supplementation in diet can protect the cell membrane from oxidation and improve the survival rates of cells. Adding VE in diet also increased activity of total anti-oxidation competence (T-AOC), superoxide dismutase (SOD) and glutathione peroxidase (GSH-PX), decreased content of nitric oxide (NO), malondialdehyde (MDA) and activity of nitric oxide synthase (NOS) in testis in Boer goat (Zhu et al., 2010). In Aohan fine-wool sheep, supplementing VE have a positive role in reducing MDA level and improving the activities of SOD and GSH-PX in testicular cell membrane and mitochondria (Yue et al, 2010) and improving testicular marker enzyme, such as ATPase, lactate dehydrogenase (LDH), sorbitol dehydrogenase (SDH), and alkaline phosphatase (ALP) activity (Yan et al, 2010).

Some reports proved that VE had effects on reproductive organs. Marin-Guzman et al. (1997) found the length and width of testis in boar were larger in group of VE supplementation at 220 IU/kg in diet than in group without VE supplementation ($P>0.05$). Soleimani et al. (2009) found testis volume of rat in VE treated group (100 mg/kg per day) was bigger than in Control ($P>0.05$), the thickness of germinal epithelium and diameter of seminiferous tubules in VE treated group was increased compared with Control ($P<0.05$). VE deficiencies caused testicular degeneration in poultry (Todorovic et al., 2002), rat and hamster (Sidney et al., 1975) and resulted in a lower number of germ cells and a reduction in sperm production (Cooper et al., 1987). Wu et al. (1973) and Wilson et al. (2003) found deficiency of VE may lead to reproductive organ damage, such as degenerative spermatogonium, testicular damage and degeneration of the seminiferous tubules.

In view of the above, VE can reduce the oxidative damage on reproductive organs and the effects of VE on reproductive efficiency have been described in several species. But for growing fine-wool sheep, the evidence of effects on the development of reproductive organs has been scant. Therefore, the objective of the present study was conducted to determine the effect of VE on the development of the testis of Aohan fine-wool sheep.

2. Material and methods

2.1 Animals and management

Thirty male growing Aohan fine-wool sheep (local breed, 5 months old) weighing an average of 24.58±3.12 kg were purchased from the Aohan fine-wool sheep breeding farm of Inner Mongolia Autonomous Region, China. A basic ration was fed with a forage/concentrate ratio of 6/4. The formulation is shown in Table 1 and was made according to the NRC feeding standard (1985). The sheep were divided randomly into five groups, one control and four treatments. Each group was supplemented VE with 0, 20, 200, 1000 or 2400 IU $sheep^{-1}$ d^{-1} for 12 months, which are 0, 1, 10, 50, 120 times of NRC feeding standard. These levels were based on previous research (Luo et al., 2004; Liu et al., 2005; Zhu et al., 2009, 2010). The Control received 4.3 IU $sheep^{-1} \cdot d^{-1}$ VE which existed in basal diet. VE powder consisting of VE acetate (1 mg contains 1 IU VE) was bought from the Zhejiang Guobang Pharmaceutical Co., Ltd (China). In this study, all procedures involving animals were conducted under the approval of China Agricultural University Animal Care and Use Committee.

2.2 Methods

Three Aohan fine-wool sheep in each group were randomly chosen for slaughter at the age of 17 months to collect the testis. Ipsilateral testis were dissected from their surrounding connective tissues and put into phosphate buffer to prepare for biopsy. H&E stained slides were used according to the system described by Karl et al. (2005) and the Motic Image Manipulation system was used to measure sample indexes.

Ingredients	%	Nutrient contents of DM	
Forage	60	CP (%)	4.86
Concentrate	40	EE (%)	8.97
		NDF (%)	31.23
		ADF (%)	22.33
		Vitamin E (IU/Kg)	3.42
The composition and nutrient level of the concentrate			
Ingredients	%	Nutrient content of DM	
Corn	62	CP (%)	18.68
Soybean meal	26	EE (%)	14.41
Wheat bran	8	NDF (%)	10.14
$CaHPO_4$	2	ADF (%)	6.52
Salt	1	Vitamin E (IU/Kg)	7.56
Additives	1		

CP: crude protein; EE: ether extract; NDF: neutral detergent fiber; ADF: acid detergent fiber

Table 1. The composition and nutrient level of the diet

2.3 Statistical analyses

Data were subjected to one-way analysis of variance (ANOVA) followed by Duncan's new multiple range tests with the SAS 9.1 software program to determine the level of significance among mean values. Results were expressed as a mean and standard error. Values of $P<0.05$ were considered significant.

3. Results

Table 2 showed the effect of different levels of VE in diet on testis indexes. The width, length, transverse girth, vertical girth and testis volume in treatments were larger than Control respectively ($P>0.05$), the order was Group 2>Group 3>Group 1>Group 4>Control.

Item	Control	Group 1	Group 2	Group 3	Group 4
Width (cm)	5.59±0.65	5.90±1.35	6.69±0.40	6.23±0.78	5.89±1.12
Length (cm)	8.64±0.82	9.56±2.09	10.51±0.63	10.14±1.60	9.32±1.48
Transverse girth (cm)	13.42±1.85	14.85±2.77	16.90±0.28	15.58±1.52	14.63±2.79
Vertical girth (cm)	19.63±2.01	21.03±3.54	24.22±1.71	22.67±3.04	20.93±3.96
Volume (cm^3)	289.63±98.12	383.85±255.42	495.17±81.67	426.81±156.44	358.20±172.70

Values in same row with same superscript differ insignificantly ($P>0.05$), with different superscripts differ significantly ($P<0.05$).

Table 2. Effect of Vitamin E on testis indexes

The effect of VE supplementation in diet on histological indexes of testicle was presented in Table 3 and Fig.1. VE supplementation in diet increased the thickness of germinal epithelium, that in Group 2 (143.72 μm), Group 4 (141.28 μm) was significantly larger ($P<0.05$) than in Control (75.05 μm) respectively, but Groups 1 (91.31 μm) and 3 (116.02 μm) did not significantly differ with Control ($P>0.05$).

Item	Control	Group 1	Group 2	Group 3	Group 4
Density of sertoli cell (number per seminiferous tubule)	10.03 ± 2.08^{b}	11.20 ± 2.13^{ab}	13.57 ± 0.56^{a}	13.40 ± 1.13^{a}	13.33 ± 1.27^{a}
Density of spermatogenic cell (number per seminiferous tubule)	60.13 ± 25.18^{b}	93.03 ± 44.90^{ab}	145.10 ± 52.79^{a}	137.35 ± 19.59^{ab}	113.80 ± 36.05^{ab}
Density of leydig cell (number/mm2)	285.14±14.82	299.74±18.30	325.87±15.69	320.49±6.52	313.57±38.10
Thickness of germinal epithelium (μm)	75.05 ± 17.21^{b}	91.31 ± 36.23^{ab}	143.72 ± 28.17^{a}	116.02 ± 15.24^{ab}	141.28 ± 29.48^{a}
Diameter of seminiferous tubule (μm)	303.93 ± 51.41^{c}	334.02 ± 57.55^{bc}	465.78 ± 56.16^{a}	374.32 ± 16.73^{abc}	443.66 ± 64.45^{ab}

Values in same row with same superscript differ insignificantly (P>0.05), with different superscripts differ significantly (P<0.05).

Table 3. Effect of Vitamin E on histological indexes of testicle

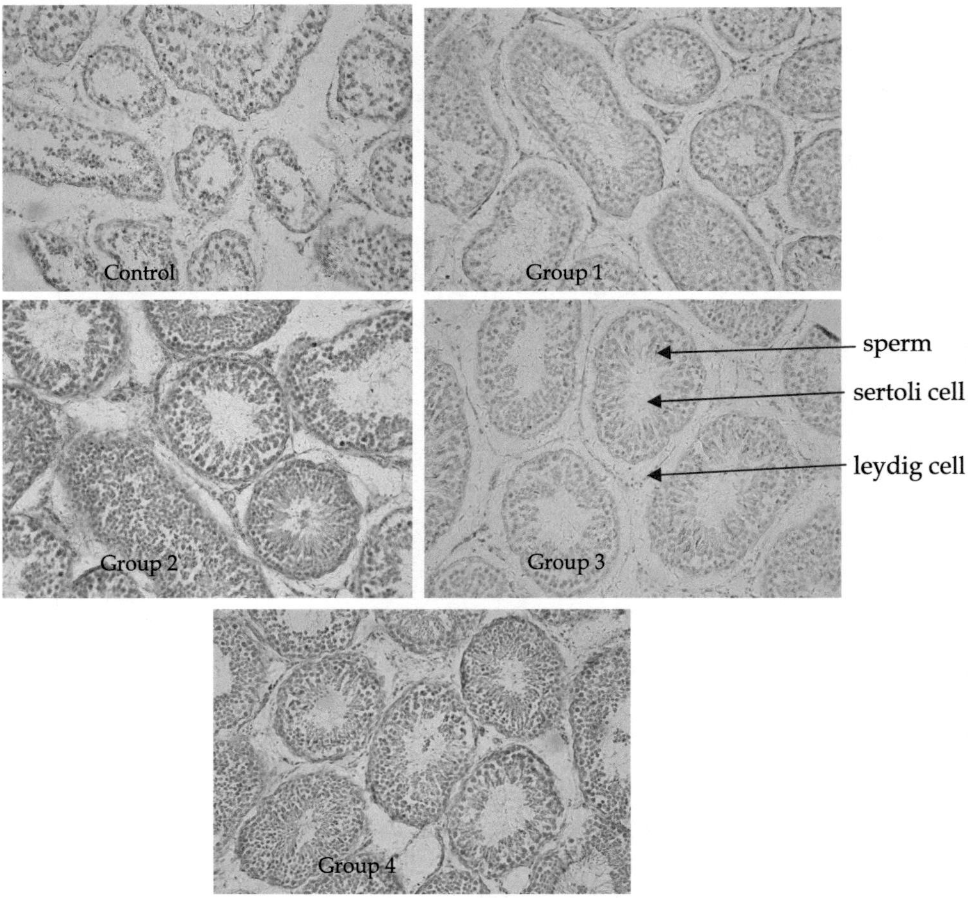

Fig. 1. Effect of Vitamin E level in diet on histological structure of testis (400×)

Compared with the Control, supplementing VE in diets increased the diameter of seminiferous tubule, it was significantly wider in Group 2 (at the level of 200 IU $sheep^{-1}$ d^{-1}) than in Control and Group 1 (P<0.05). Furthermore, the diameter of seminiferous tubule in Group 4 was also significantly wider than in Control (P<0.05). No significant differences were observed between Control and Group 1, or Group 3 (P>0.05).

Although the density of leydig cell in treatment groups was larger than in Control, no significant differences were observed among Control and treatment groups (P>0.05). Feeding with dietary VE tended to have a higher density of sertoli cell, it was significantly increased in Group 2, Group 3 and Group 4 compared with Control (P<0.05).VE supplementation improved the density of spermatogenic cell, that was significantly higher in Group 2 than in Control (P<0.05) and no significant differences were observed between Control and other treatment groups (P>0.05).

4. Discussion

Marin-Guzman et al. (1997) presented the length and width of testis in boar were larger in group of VE supplementation at 220 IU·kg^{-1} in diet than in group without VE supplementation, testis volume of rat in VE treated group (100 mg·kg^{-1}·d^{-1}) was bigger than in Control (Soleimani Mehranjani et al., 2009, P>0.05). Similar results were observed in the present study, the width, length, transverse girth, vertical girth and volume of testis in VE treated groups were higher than Control, but no significant differences were observed between Control and treatment groups (P>0.05).

This study proved that for Aohan fine-wool sheep, the thickness of germinal epithelium, diameter of seminiferous tubule and the density of spermatogenic cell, sertoli cell and leydig cell in VE treatment groups were larger than in Control. Similar results have been proved in Boer goats in our previous research (Zhu et al., 2009), which showed that diameters of seminiferous tubules and numeric density of spermatogenic cells tended to be larger in 80 IU kid^{-1} d^{-1} VE supplemented group compared to the control group ($P<0.05$). However, no significant effects were observed on thickness of germinal epithelium and numeric density of leydig cells ($P>0.05$).

Sertoli cells are the nurse cells for the spermatogonium in the seminiferous tubules and can thus influence the development of the sperm precursor cells and the subsequent number of spermatids. This effect may be accomplished through their production of various factors such as plasminogen activator, transferrin, and sertoli cell growth factor (Lacroix et al., 1977; Feig et al., 1980; Skinner and Griswold, 1980). Besides, sertoli cells can maintain high concentrations of androgens in seminiferous tubules and epididymis (Lacroix et al., 1977), they can also transport testosterone from the testis into epididymis (Krishnamoorthy et al., 2005). Our research showed supplementing VE in diet increased the density of sertoli cell, which in Group 2, Group 3 and Group 4 was significantly higher than in Control respectively ($P<0.05$) and Group 2 was the highest. The results indicated that VE supplementation can promote the growth of sertoli cells.

The spermatogenic cell is the sum of spermatogenous cell, spermatocyte, spermatoblast and sperm male germ cells may be susceptible to oxidative stress because of high concentrations of PUFAs and low antioxidant capacity (Vernet et al., 2004). It is reported that dietary deficiencies of VE in growing males causes degenerative spermatogonium, resulting in a lower sperm concentration (Cooper et al., 1987; Lin et al., 2005). In this study, the density of spermatogenic cell in VE supplemented groups increased, that in Group 2 (200 IU $sheep^{-1}$ d^{-1}) was significantly higher than in Control ($P<0.05$).

Testosterone secretion is critical for male secondary sexual differentiation and leydig cells are the principal source of testosterone production in the males (Ren-Shan et al., 2007). ROS can be produced in leydig cells through mitochondrial respiration (Chen et al., 2001) as well as through the cytochrome P450 enzymes of the steroidogenic pathway (Hornsby, 1989; Peltola et al., 1996). VE's function as an antioxidant, can quench lipid peroxidation and eliminate the ROS to protect the leydig cells from damage. Mather et al. (1983) reported that VE could prolong the survival and function of porcine leydig cells cultured in vitro. In our study, the density of leydig cell in treatment groups was larger than in Control, but no significant differences were observed among Control and treatment groups (P>0.05).

VE supplementation in diet increased the thickness of germinal epithelium. Significant differences were observed between Group 2, Group 4 and Control (P<0.05). The seminiferous epitheliums contained three different germ cell generations: spermatogonia, spermatocytes and spermatids and one kind of sertoli cell, which suggests the thickness of germinal epitheliumwas determined by the numbers of the spermatogenic cells and sertoli cells (Garcia-Gil et al., 2002). The spermatogenic cells and sertoli cells in VE supplemented groups increased in our research. This is in agreement with the findings of Soleimani Mehranjani et al. (2009), who found the thickness of germinal epithelium in VE treated rat increased compared with Control (P<0.05). Zhu et al. (2009) also presented the thickness of germinal epitheliums in Boer kids were higher with VE than in Control, but differences between the Control and treatment groups were not significant (P>0.05).

In our study, compared with the Control, supplementing VE in diets increased the diameter of seminiferous tubule. At the level of 200 IU sheep^{-1} d^{-1}, the diameter of seminiferous tubule was significantly wider than Control and Group 1 (P<0.05), the result was similar to the research of Zhu et al.(2009), who reported that when Boer kids were supplemented with 0, 80, 320 and 880 IU kid^{-1} d^{-1} VE for 5 months, the diameter of seminiferous tubule of the testis in Group 2 (80 IU kid^{-1} d^{-1}) increased significantly compared to other groups (P<0.01). The diameter increased to maximum level at a different supplementation dose for different breeds (80 IU kid^{-1} d^{-1} in Boer goat, Zhu et al., 2009 and 200 IU sheep-1 d^{-1} in Aohan fine-wool sheep in this study). The differences could be attributed to differences species or supplementation practices.

5. Conclusion

This study shows VE supplemented in diet can improve density of spermatogenic cell, sertoli cell, diameter of seminiferous tubule and thickness of germinal epithelium, especially at 200 IU sheep^{-1} d^{-1} VE supplement concentration. These results indicate that VE has a positive role in improving the development of testis in Aohan fine-wool sheep.

6. Acknowledgements

The present study is supported by the project from the China Agricultural Ministry (200903060) and the earmarked fund for China Agriculture Research System-39.

7. References

Brzezinska-Slebodzinska, E.; Slebodzinski, AB.; Pietras, B.; Wieczorek, G. (1995). Antioxidant effect of Vitamin E and glutathione on lipid peroxidation in boar semen plasma. *Biol. Trace Elem. Res*, 47: 69-74

Burton, GW.; Ingold KU. (1986). Vitamin E: application of the principles of physical organic chemistry to the exploration of its structure and function. *Acc. Chem. Res,* 19: 194-201

Chen, H.; Cangello, D.; Benson, S.; Folmer, J.; Zhu, H.; Trush, MA.; Zirkin, BR. (2001). Age-related increase in mitochondrial superoxide generation in the testosterone-producing cells of Brown Norway rat testes: relationship to reduced steroidogenic function. *Exp. Gerontol,* 36 (8): 1361-1373

Cooper, DR.; King, OR.; Carpenter, MP. (1987). Effect of Vitamin E deficiency on serum concentrations of follicle stimulating hormone and testosterone during testicular maturation and degeneration. *Endocrinology,* 120: 83-90

Esterbauer, H.; Dieber-Rotheneder, M.; Striegl, G.; Waeg, G. (1991). Role of Vitamin E in preventing the oxidation of low density lipoprotein. *Am. J. Clin. Nutr,* 53: 314-321

Evans, HM.; Bishop, KS. (1922). On the existence of a hitherto unrecognized dietary factor essential for reproduction. *Science,* 56: 650-651

Feig, LA.; Bellve, AR.; Erickson, NH.; Klagsburn, M. (1980). Sertoli cells contain a mitogenic polypeptide. *Proc. Natl. Acad. Sci. USA,* 77: 4774-4778

Garcia-Gil, N.; Pinart, E.; Sancho, S.; Badia, E.; Bassols, J.; Kádár, E.; Briz, M.; Bonet S. (2002). The cycle of the seminiferous epithelium in Landrace boars. *Anim. Reprod. Sci,* 73 (3-4): 211-225

Ge, RS.; Chen, GR.; Cigdem T.; Matthew, PH. (2007). Phthalate ester toxicity in leydig cells:developmental timing and dosage considerations. *Reprod. Toxicol,* 23 (3): 366-373

Hornsby PJ. (1989). Steroid and xenobiotic effects on the adrenal cortex: mediation by oxidative and other mechanisms. *Free Radic. Biol. Med,* 6 (1): 103-115

Karl, L.; Patrick, K.; Fredrik, H.; Andrzej, M.; Leif, N.; Stig, EH.; Rodriguez, M. (2005). Delayed effects on plasma concentration of testosterone and testicular morphology by intramuscular low-dose di (2-ethylhexyl) phthalate or estradiol benzoate in the prepubertal boar. *Theriogenology,* 64 (5): 1170-1184

Krishnamoorthy, G.; Murugesan, P.; Muthuvel, R.; Gunadharini, DN.; Vijayababu, MR.; Arunkumar, A.; Venkataraman, P.; Aruldhas, MM.; Arunakaran, J. (2005). Effect of Aroclor 1254 on Sertoli cellular antioxidant system, androgen binding protein and lactate in adult rat in vitro. *Toxicology,* 212 (2-3): 195-205

Lacroix, M.; Smith, FE.; Fritz, IB. (1977). Secretion of plasminogen activator by Sertoli cell enriched cultures. *Mol. Cell. Endocrinol,* 9: 227-236

Lacroix M, Smith FE, Fritz IB. 1977. Secretion of plasminogen activator by Sertoli cell enriched cultures. Mol. Cell Endocrinol. 9 (2): 227-236

Lin, YF.; Chang, SJ.; Yang, JR.; Lee, YP.; Hsu, AL. (2005). Effects of supplemental Vitamin E during the mature period on the reproduction performance of Taiwan native chicken cockerels. *Br. Poultry Sci,* 46 (3): 366-373

Liu, HB.; Luo, HL.; Liu, ZH.; Shi, ZH.; Zhao, HB. (2005). Effect of dietary Vitamin E concentration on semen quality of goat. *Chin. J. Anim. Sci,* 10: 12-14 (in Chinese)

Luo, HL.; Jia, ZH.; Zhu, SE.; Ding, JZ. (2004). Effect of Vitamin E on the qualities of fresh and frozen thawed ram semen. *China Herbivores* 24: 14-16 (in Chinese)

Marin-Guzman, J.; Mahan, DC.; Chung, YK.; Pate, JL.; Pope, WF. (1997). Effects of dietary selenium and Vitamin E on boar performance and tissue responses, semen quality, and subsequent fertilization rates in mature gilts. *J. Anim. Sci,* 75: 2994-3003

Mather, JP.; Saez, JM.; Dray, F.; Haour, F. (1983). Vitamin E prolongs survival and function of porcine Leydig cells in culture. *Acta Endocrinol. (Copenh.),* 102 (3): 470-475

Mishra, M.; Acharya, UR. (2004). Protective action of vitamins on the spermatogenesis in lead-treated Swiss mice. *J. Trace Elem. Med. Biol,* 18 (2): 173-178

O'Bryan, MK.; Schlatt, S.; Phillips, DJ.; De Kretser, DM.; Hedger, MP. (2000). Bacterial lipopolysaccharide-induced inflammation compromises testicular function at multiple levels in vivo. *Endocrinology,* 141: 238-246

Peltola, V.; Huhtaniemi, I.; Metsa-Ketela, T.; Ahotupa, M. (1996). Induction of lipid peroxidation during steroidogenesis in the rat testis. *Endocrinology,* 137 (1): 105-112

Potts, JM.; Pasqualotto, FF. (2003). Semilal oxidative stress in patients with chronic prostatitis. *Andrologia,* 35: 304-308.

Regina BF.; Maret, GT. (1999). Vitamin E: function and metabolism. *FASEB J,* 13: 1145-1155

Sen, CK.; Khanna, S.; Rink, C.; Roy, S. (2007). Tocotrienols: the emerging face of natural vitamin E. *Vitam Horm,* 76: 203-61

Sidney, I.; Mauey, KE.; Mason. (1975). Antisterility Activity of d-a-Tocopheryl Hydroquinone in the Vitamin E-deficient Male Hamster and Rat. *J. Nut,* 105: 491-494

Skinner, MK.; Griswold, MD. (1980). Sertoli cells synthesize and secrete transferrin-like protein. *J. Biol. Chem,* 225: 9523-9525

Soleimani, MM.; Noorafshan, A.; Momeni, HR.; Abnosi, MH.; Mahmoodi, M.; Anvari, M.; Hoseini, SM. (2009). Stereological study of the effects of Vitamin E on testis structure in rats treated with para-nonylphenol. *Asian J. Androl,* 11: 508-516

Sugiyama, M. (1992). Role of physiological antioxidants in chromium (VI)-induced cellular injury. *Free Radical Biol. Med,* 12: 397-407

Tappel, AL. (1962). Vitamin E as the biological lipid antioxidant. *Vitam. Horm,* 20: 493-510

Todorovic, M.; Jokic, Z.; Davidovic, V. (2002). The influence of selenium and Vitamin E in poultry nutrition. *Biotech. Anim. Husb,* 18: 231-238

Vernet, P.; Aitken, RJ.; Drevet, JR. (2004). Antioxidant strategies in the epididymis. *Mol. Cell. Endocrinol,* 216 (1-2): 31-39

Wilson, MJ. Kaye, D.; Edward, SW.; Quach, HT.; Sinha, AA.; Vatassery, GT. (2003). Effect of Vitamin E deficiency on the growth and secretory function of the rat prostatic complex. *Exp. Mol. Pathol,* 74: 267-275

Wu, SH., Oldfield, JE.; Whanger, PD.; Weswig, PH. (1973). Effect of selenium, Vitamin E and antioxidants on testicular function in rats. *Biol. Reprod,* 8 (5): 625-629

Yan, LY.; Yue, DB.; Luo, HL.; Jin, XX.; Xu, X. (2010). Effect of Vitamin E supplementation on the enzymatic activity of selected markers in Aohan fine-wool sheep testis. *Anim. Reprod. Sci,* 122: 264-269

Yousef, MI.; Abdallah, GA.; Kamel, KI. (2003). Effect of ascorbic acid and Vitamin E supplementation on semen quality and biochemical parameters of male rabbits. *Anim. Reprod. Sci,* 76: 99-111

Yue, DB.; Yan, LY.; Luo, HL.; Jin, XX.; Xu, X. (2010). Effect of Vitamin E supplementation on semen quality and the testicular cell membranal and mitochondrial antioxidant abilities in Aohan fine-wool sheep. *Anim. Reprod. Sci,* 118: 217-222

Zhu, H.; Luo, HL.; Meng, H.; Zhang, GJ.; Yan, LY.; Yue, DB. (2010). Effect of Vitamin E supplement in diet on antioxidant ability of testis in Boer Goat. *Anim. Reprod. Sci,* 117: 90-94

Zhu, H.; Luo, HL.; Meng, H.; Zhang, GJ. (2009). Effect of Vitamin E supplementation on development of reproductive organs in Boer goat. *Anim. Reprod. Sci,* 113: 93-101

9

Evaluation of a New Method and Diagnostic Test in Semen Analysis

Petra Zrimšek
*Clinic for Reproduction and Horses,
Veterinary Faculty,
University of Ljubljana,
Slovenia*

1. Introduction

Sperm concentration is an important parameter affecting fertility. Animal species of agricultural interest are mainly produced by artificial insemination (AI) which contributes highly to the development of worldwide swine production, making the impact of the male in reproductive efficiency of the pig herds more crucial (Jounala et al., 1998).

The efficiency of AI (fertility rate and prolificacy) is directly dependent on the quality of semen doses and on the number of spermatozoa used for insemination (Camus et al., 2011). In commercial farms, routine examination of boar semen is performed aiming to predict the male's fertility. Evaluation of concentration is crucial to adapt dilution rate and to optimize sperm concentration which will directly impact fertility performance. In the first part of a present chapter we address the basic concepts of a method comparison study and present an example of a method comparison experiment concerning determination of sperm concentration.

Various laboratory methods techniques are used to evaluate sperm quality, such as sperm concentration, motility, viability, and morphology. However, there is no single semen assay that provides complete information about semen quality (Holt & Medrano, 1997; Johnson et al., 2000; Liu & Baker, 2002). Studies in domestic animals showed that these semen characteristics were often not significantly correlated to fertility, while the most valid assessment of boar semen quality is to obtain viable pregnancies and normal offspring following AI (Tsakmakidis et al., 2010). Since fertilization is a complex process involving a huge number of events, fertility research must not only device more predictive laboratory tests, but also properly combine different assays aiming to predict male fertilizing ability, as spermatozoa should satisfy many requirements for successful fertilization (Quintero-Moreno et al., 2004). Assessment of metabolic status of spermatozoa could provide a useful tool for evaluation of semen quality, because sufficient metabolism for energy production is one of the several attributes that a sperm must posses to fertilize an oocyte. In the second part of this chapter developing and diagnostic evaluation of a spectrophotometric application of the resazurin reduction assay will be presented.

Learning objectives of a chapter are to:

- Investigate repeatability in continuous data

- Perform method agreement
- Construct Bland-Altman plots
- Explain limits of agreement between two methods
- Chose an appropriate regression analysis used in the interpretation of comparing data
- Define the diagnostic parameters: specificity, sensitivity, accuracy, predictive values of a test
- Recognize the validity and usefulness of the test
- Evaluate the performance of a diagnostic test using ROC (receiver operating characteristic) analysis
- Construct and compare ROC curves
- Determine optimal cut-off point for a test
- Explain the developing of a new method in semen evaluation

2. Method agreement for determining sperm concentration

Semen samples, which often contain a variety of cells (immature germ cells, blood cells, epithelial cells, and cellular debris) in addition to spermatozoa, differ markedly from blood samples because of their heterogeneity. There is also no specific standard available for sperm cells of each species. It is therefore important to compare a new, more appropriate or additional method to a conventional one. The counting chamber technique for estimating sperm count appears to be adequate because of its simplicity, low cost and reproducibility. However, photometers are widely used routinely for determining sperm concentration by many AI organisations, for bulls and boars as well as other species (Woelders, 1991). They need to be evaluated before use, because accurate concentration measurement is the first and crucial step of the semen preparation process for production of semen doses (Camus et al., 2011). Correct assessment of sperm concentration is essential to ensure that the number of sperm per insemination dose meets requirements and that the maximal number of doses can be produced per ejaculate.

The increasing use of AI in swine emphasizes the need for the distribution of good quality sperm by the AI centres (Vyt et al., 2004). Boar sperm quality is routinely assessed by measuring concentration, morphology and motility of spermatozoa (Johnson et al., 2000). Determination of sperm concentration is essential in evaluating fertility, whether *in vivo* or *in vitro*. However, there is no agreed method for use as a standard. Knuth et al. (1989) showed that introduction of an unevaluated laboratory method, without appropriate quality control, can cause a bias in semen analysis. However, the methodology of semen evaluation is complex, and standardization is difficult (Brazil et al., 2004). For example, the first large scale, nation-wide proficiency testing program for clinical andrology laboratories in the United States reported that the inter-laboratory coefficient of variation for manual sperm concentration determination was 80%, with a range for a single semen specimen of 3 – 492 x 10^6 /ml (Keel et al., 2000). The accuracy, reliability and repeatability of different instruments that evaluate sperm concentration of raw semen have already been compared in several previous studies (Christensen et al., 2004; Hansen et al., 2006; Prathalingam et al., 2006; Anzar et al., 2009; Camus et al., 2011). Variation in the results from different laboratories could be due to the lack of standardisation of methods between laboratories (Maatson, 1995).

The reason for comparing methods is often that a quicker, more convenient and more economical adaptation has been made to an existing method. Studies comparing a new method with an established method are performed to assess whether the new measurements are comparable with existing ones (Jensen & Kjelgaard-Hansen, 2006).

2.1 Precision of the evaluated methods

It is necessary to establish that a method is repeatable before comparing two measurements for reproducibility (Petrie & Watson, 1999). Repeatability of boar semen concentration assessment depends on instruments and procedures, for example CV for instruments FACS, HEMO, Photo C254, SpermVision, UltiMate and SP-100 were 2.7, 7.1, 10.4, 8.1, 5.4 and 3.1%, respectively (Hansen et al., 2006). Imade et al. (1993) reported similar overall precision (5.9%) for the Makler chamber, whereas CV for sperm counts in sperm suspensions can be higher, for example 18.6% (Christensen et al., 2005) or even 26.3% (Mahmoud et al, 1997). It is generally admitted that intra-observer CVs are often greater than 10%. Although guidelines for standardizing the procedure have been proposed, relatively important degrees of intra- and inter- technician or inter-laboratory variability have been reported. In the external quality assessment (EQA) reported by Neuwinger and coworkers (1990), which involved 10 experienced German laboratories in the evaluation of 8 sperm samples, the mean CV was 37.5%. From the data of the external quality control obtained under the British Fertility Society and reported by Matson (1995), the calculated inter-individual CV for sperm concentration was 64.7% for 24 semen samples collected by technicians from 20 laboratories.

2.2 Method agreement

According to the literature, a very common way of investigating method agreement is to perform a paired t-test or to calculate a correlation coefficient to provide a measure of agreement. However, in this instance, neither method is appropriate for the following reasons (Petrie & Watson, 1999). The paired t-test tests the null hypothesis that the difference is zero. If the differences between pairs are large - indicating that the methods do not agree - but are evenly scattered around zero, then the result is non-significant. We can only conclude that there is no bias, not that the methods agree. Correlation is a statistical method used to quantify any association between two continuous variables (Ma & Smith, 2003). The correlation coefficient provides a measure of the linear association between the measurements obtained by the two methods. It provides an indication of how close the observations in the scatter diagram are to a straight line. R measures the strength of a relation between two variables, not the agreement between them (Bland and Altman, 1999). For example, the Pearson correlation coefficient gives no information of value in method comparison studies, because R can be highly significant even when there is an obvious bias between the two methods. It measures the strength of association, rather than agreement, although in the literature it has been used in many studies, such as comparison between different methods to determine sperm concentration (Prathalingam et al., 2006). R was also used to evaluate agreement between assessments within lab technician in sperm analysis (Christensen et al., 2005). In order to assess agreement, it is necessary to know how close the points are to the line of equality, i.e. the 45° line (Petrie & Watson, 1999). Therefore, in the study of Sokol et al. (2000), comparison of two methods for measuring sperm concentration using only Wilcoxon signed rank test and F-test, appears to be insufficient.

Scatter plots and absolute and relative bias plots give the best overview of comparisons of data (Twormey, 2004; Twormey, 2005). Absolute bias plots are also called Bland and Altman plots, usually used for method comparison (Bland and Altman, 1999). In absolute bias plots, the biases are plotted against their average value for each sample. The mean of these differences ($\bar{d}$) is an estimate of the average bias of one method relative to that of the other. If this value is zero, then the two measurements agree on average. However, this does not imply that they agree for each individual measurement.

In order to assess how well the paired measurements agreed with each other, limits of agreement have to be determined. The upper and lower limits of agreement are calculated as

$$\bar{d} \pm 2s_{difff} \quad (1)$$

where $\bar{d}$ is the mean of differences for all the samples (average bias) and s_{diff} is the standard deviation of the differences; $2s_{diff}$ is also referred to as the British Standard Institution repeatability (or, reproducibility, as appropriate) coefficient and indicates the maximum difference likely to occur between two measurements. This coefficient is the value below which the bias between paired results may be expected to lie (Petrie & Watson, 1999).

We performed method agreement between two clinical laboratory methods for determining boar sperm concentration using the statistical programme Analyse-it, General + Clinical Laboratory statistics, version 1.71, where linear regression, Deming regression and Passing Bablok regression can be applied in the evaluation. We chose Deming regression, because it is appropriate for describing the relationship between two variables, both measured with error. In the case of observed increasing imprecision, i.e. where a proportional bias between methods is detected, the Passing Bablock regression procedure is more accurate than Deming's method. When the assumption that the independent variable is determined without error is satisfied, linear regression should be used to describe the agreement between two methods (Jones & Payne, 1997). The intercept is calculated, as in conventional least squares regression, as the mean of y minus the product of the slope and the mean of x. The standard error (SE) of the intercept defines how much the line might vary in the y direction, and SE of the slope defines how much the line might pivot about the central point through the means of x and y. Thus, SEs allow calculation of the confidence intervals of the slope and the intercept (Jones & Payne, 1997).

2.3 Experiment: Agreement between two methods of sperm concentration measurement

In the present study we compared two clinical laboratory methods for determining boar sperm concentration, the Makler chamber and the photometer (Photometer SDM5, Minitüb, Germany) (Mrkun et al., 2007). Prior to method comparison, precision of each method was assessed. Scatter plots with fitted regression line, and absolute and relative bias plots were used to get the best overview of comparative data (Twormey, 2004; Twormey, 2005). Deming regression was applied to describe the relationship between variables both measured with error by proposing that the sum of the squares of the deviations from a line should be minimised in both the x and the y directions at the same time, thus taking account of the analytical imprecision of each method (Jones & Payne, 1997). The purpose of this study was to compare the two methods and to assess method agreement together with the appropriate regression analysis used in the interpretation of the data.

2.3.1 Semen samples

Twenty-three semen samples were obtained from eight 12 to 24 month old boars of various breeds. Each semen sample was collected with gloved hand using a clean semen collecting flask that filters out gel, dust and bristles, while the boar mounted a dummy sow. Semen samples were diluted 1:2 with BTS semen extender (Beltsville Thawing Solution, Truadeco, Netherlands) and delivered to the laboratory.

2.3.2 Counting with the Makler chamber

Immediately before each semen aliquot was analysed, the entire semen specimen was vortexed. To render the spermatozoa immotile and to prepare the semen samples for the Makler chamber (Sefi Medical Instruments, Israel), semen samples were diluted 1:2 with distilled water. 6 parallel dilutions of each semen sample were prepared and the average of the measurements on each used as the representative value.

Following dilution, sperm suspensions were again vortexed and an aliquot of 5 µl was loaded into the Makler chamber. The next step was to assess whether sperm were evenly distributed or whether there were movements in the fluid in the counting chamber. If either of these problems was observed; the chamber was cleaned and refilled. The fields were chosen according to a prescribed pattern: 10 fields spaced left to right and 10 fields spaced top to bottom. Chosen fields formed a plus sign centred in the middle of the chamber, excluding the areas 2-3 mm from the chamber edges. Only recognizable spermatozoa, including lost heads, were counted, while other cells and lost tails were ignored. The concentration in the original semen sample was calculated from the total number of sperm in the counting area.

2.3.3 Counting with a photometer

Sperm concentration was determined by measuring the sample opacity, as the percentage transmittance of light through a sample, using a photometer (Photometer SDM5, MiniTüb, Germany). Boar ejaculates are normally too opaque, so a small semen sample was diluted with an isotonic solution before measuring. A blank tube was loaded with 3.5 ml 0.9% NaCl and a sample tube with 70 µl semen sample added to 0.9% NaCl. Sperm concentration was determined from a previous calibration of the spectrophotometer, performed by the manufacturer (Photometer SDM5, MiniTüb, Germany). Six measurements were made for each semen dilution.

2.3.4 Precision of the evaluated methods

The precision of each method was determined by making 6 measurements of each of 23 semen samples. Coefficients of variation (CV) were calculated for each method and scatter graphs of CV versus average sperm count for each semen sample were constructed. In our study CVs were calculated to be 6.6 ± 3.5 % and 1.6 ± 0.6 % for Makler chamber and photometer, respectively. Both methods yielded acceptable precision (Christensen et al., 2005), although the precision of the Makler chamber was significantly poorer.

In a diagram of the CV plotted against the average for each sperm concentration, the scatter of the points is random for the photometer (Fig.1). In contrast, for the Makler chamber, the size of CV is related to the size of the sperm concentration, shown by the higher CVs for lower sperm counts (Fig.2).

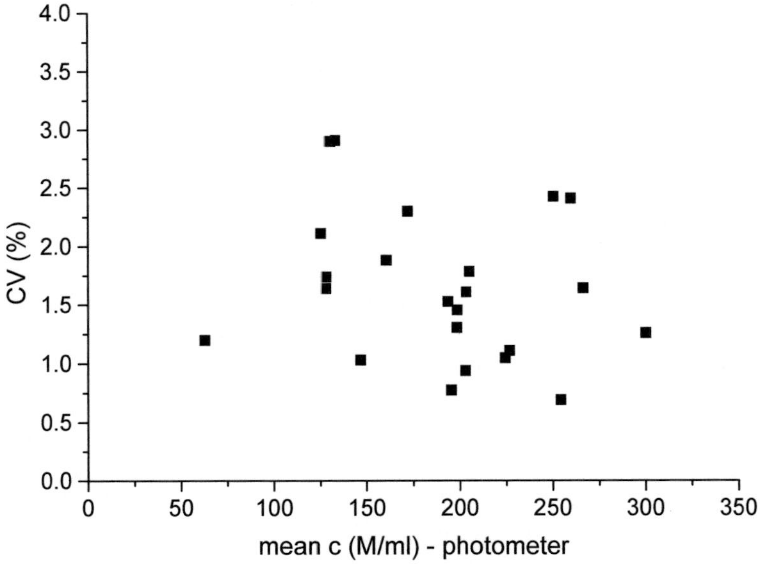

Fig. 1. Coefficient of variation (CV) versus mean sperm count for the photometer method
Mean counts were calculated as the average of six parallel counts for each sample

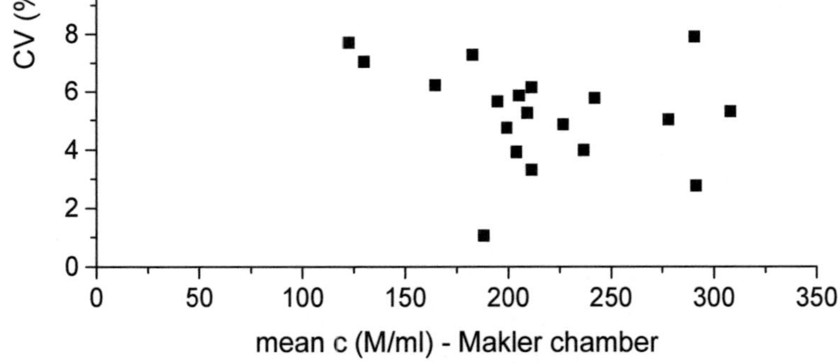

Fig. 2. Coefficient of variation (CV) versus mean sperm count determined by the Makler chamber method
Mean counts were calculated as the average of six parallel counts for each sample

2.3.5 Method agreement between Mackler chamber and photometer

We were interested in assessing the similarity between sperm counts measured with Makler chamber and photometer, so we compared pairs of measurements. For this purpose, we calculated the differences between pairs of measurements of sperm counts - by Makler chamber and photometer - obtained by each method for each sperm sample.

The mean percentage bias between methods was - 0.6 ± 6.9 %. The scatter of the points lies in the interval -15 to 15 % (Fig. 3), which is in the range of satisfactory between-run reproducibility of the assay. From the absolute bias plot (Fig. 4) it is also evident that the scatter is random, indicating that the size of the difference between sperm counts obtained by two methods is not related to the size of the counts. Thus, no proportional bias has been detected. Average absolute bias was close to zero (-1.092 ± 15.237 M/ml). Sperm counts obtained with Makler chamber and photometer agree; 90% of the differences lie within the limits of agreement (Fig. 4), confirming that the level of agreement between the methods was satisfactory. Therefore, measurements of sperm concentration with photometer and counting chamber techniques are equally appropriate for estimating sperm counts.

Using scatter diagrams with regression lines fitted, we established that the paired measurements, sperm counts obtained with Makler chamber and with photometer, were close to the line of equality. Deming regression was used to solve the problem of describing the relationship between sperm counting with methods, both measured with error. Deming's method gives only a single regression line, whether x or y is used as the "independent variable" (Fig. 5).

The estimated intercept for the regression line, 4.7069 M/ml, does not differ much from zero. The estimated regression equation indicates that the points are close to the line of equality, i.e. the 45 ° line and SE of the slope (0.0600) indicates that there is almost no pivoting of the line about central point through the means of x and y.

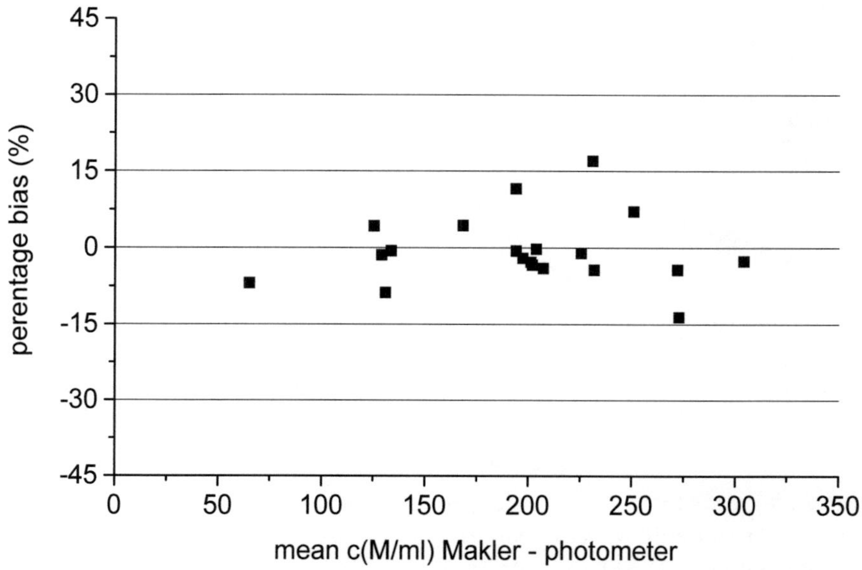

Fig. 3. Relative bias plot of sperm concentration obtained by Makler chamber versus concentration obtained by photometer

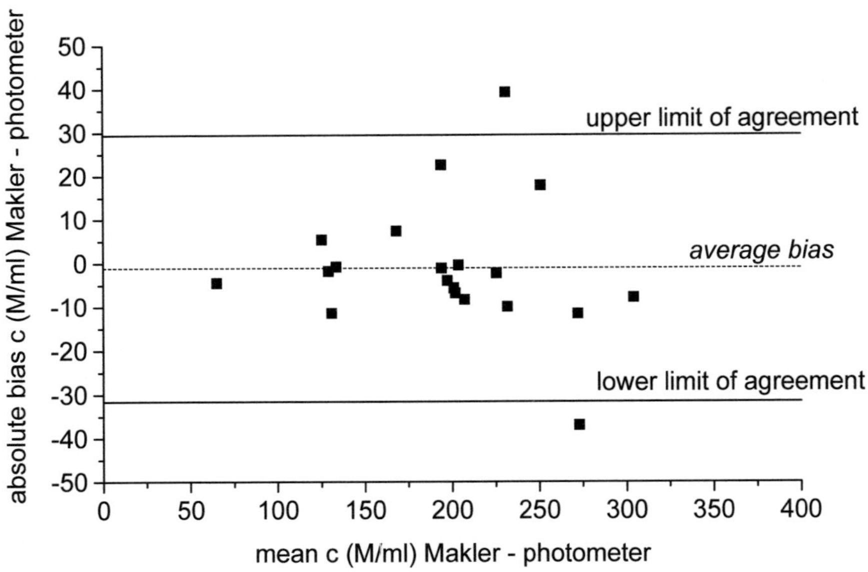

Fig. 4. Absolute bias plot of sperm concentrations obtained by Makler chamber versus concentrations obtained by photometer showing average bias and limits of agreement

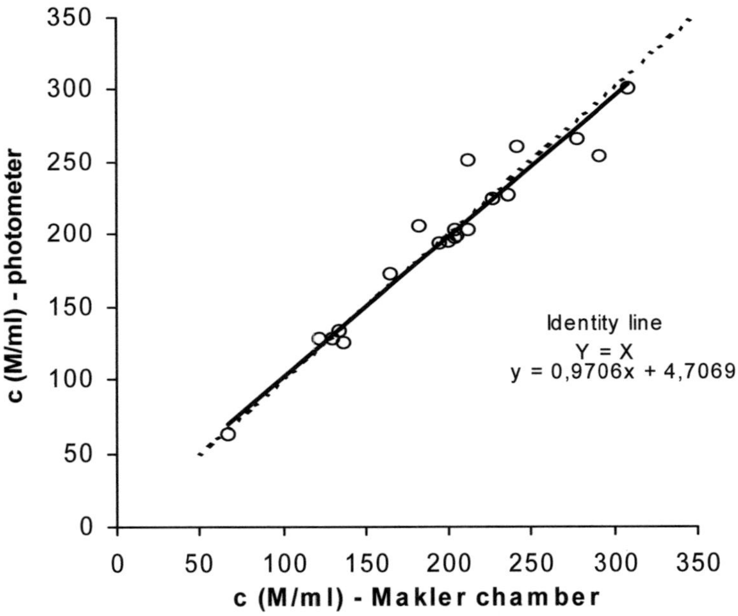

Fig. 5. Scatter diagram of sperm concentration obtained by photometer versus sperm concentration obtained with Makler chamber, with Deming regression line fitted

- - - - - : line of equality (Y=X)

______ : Deming regression line:

c (photometer) = 4.7069 + 0.9706 x c (Makler chamber)

3. Development and diagnostic evaluation of spectrophotometric application of the resazurin reduction assay to evaluate boar sperm quality

There are several attributes that a sperm must posses to fertilize an oocyte, including motility, normal morphology, sufficient metabolism for energy production, and membrane integrity. Although various analytical techniques have been developed to evaluate sperm quality, including sperm concentration, motility, viability and morphology, there is no single method that provides complete information about semen quality (Holt & Medrano, 1997; Johnson et al., 2000). Due to the complexity of the fertilization process, single tests are not able to predict fertility. Instead, a set of semen tests has to be selected with high relevance for important sperm traits and low redundancy of assay results (Petrunkina et al., 2007). Moreover, particularly in pig industry, the choice of semen test has considered cost effectiveness. Routine testing of fresh boar sperm predominantly aims to identify subfertile boar ejaculates. In number of countries, liquid preserved boar semen is used after several days of *in vitro* storage. It's well known that boars differ in their capacity to maintain sperm function during preservation *in vitro*. These differences can only be partially visualized by standard sperm parameters, such as loss of motility and membrane integrity (Waberski et al., 2011). However, the battery of diagnostic methods used by the industry is as yet restricted (Tejerina et al., 2008). A reliable, simple, cost effective and rapid method of assessing the quality of boar spermatozoa would be of benefit to livestock producers and veterinary practitioners (Dart et al., 1994). Reproductive performance depends on metabolic processes; therefore assessment of metabolic status of spermatozoa could provide valuable information for predicting sperm fertilizing capacity. The resazurin reduction assay, one of the methods for evaluating the metabolic status of spermatozoa, depends on the ability of metabolically active spermatozoa to reduce the resazurin redox dye to resorufin. Dehydrogenase activity of spermatozoa is manifested as a visual colour change from blue (resazurin) to pink (resorufin) and further to white (dihydroresorufin) (Glass et al., 1991; Fuse et al., 1993; Reddy Venkata Rami et al., 1997). The resazurin reduction assay using visual detection of colour change is quite subjective and varies between evaluators (Wang et al., 1998). The colour change of resazurin is usually matched with a colour chart, consisting of a spectrum of colours from blue to pink, varying between investigators. The possibility of human error therefore, has led to the spectrophotometric modification of the resazurin reduction test. It has been mostly used for the evaluation of human semen (Mahmoud et al., 1994, Rahman & Kula, 1997; Zalata et al., 1998; Reddy Venkata Rami & Bordekar; 1999) but, to our knowledge, in veterinary medicine only for evaluating ram (Wang et al., 1998) and boar semen quality (Zrimšek et al., 2004). The visual assay has been used for evaluating stallion (Carter & Ericsson, 1998), bull (Dart et al., 1994), sheep (Cooper et al., 1996; Martin et al., 1999) and boar (Mesta et al., 1995) semen. Spectrophotometric measurement of resazurin reduction provides a quantitative and objective method.

The aim of the present study was to develop and evaluate diagnostically the spectrophotometric application of the resazurin reduction test for evaluating boar sperm quality (Zrimšek et al, 2004; Zrimšek et al., 2006). Following Zalata et al. (1998), who developed a spectrophotometric method of resazurin reduction to evaluate human semen we extracted the developed colour after the assay with boar semen with butanol and measured the absorbance in the clear upper layer of butanol, eliminating the problem of sample turbidity. The optimisation and developing of the test included several steps as follows:

- determination of specific absorbance wavelength, used for analysis on the basis of absorbance spectra of resazurin and resorufin

- optimisation of the test procedure
- determination of repeatability of the assay
- correlations between resazurin reduction assay and various semen parameters; Spearman rank correlation analysis
- relationship between resazurin reduction and concentration of motile spermatozoa and sperm index; linear regression analysis
- statistical comparison of the results obtained between the groups of satisfactory and unsatisfactory semen; Mann-Whitney U-test
- diagnostic evaluation of the assay; ROC analysis
- stability of butanol extracts in terms of A_{610}; measuring agreement

In this study, receiver operating characteristics (ROC) was used to determine the optimal cut-off value and diagnostic accuracy of the resazurin reduction assay. A complete picture of test accuracy is presented by the ROC plot, which provides a view of the whole spectrum of sensitivities and specificities as functions of selected cut-off values (Greiner et al., 2000). A global summary statistic of the diagnostic accuracy of the assay was quantified by the area under the ROC curve. Likelihood ratios were used to revise the probability of the semen status in individual samples (Greiner et al., 1995).

3.1 Development of resazurin reduction assay

3.1.1 Semen samples and analysis

Forty-one semen samples from eight 12-24-month-old boars of various breeds were included in the study. Semen was collected with a glove hand using a clean semen collecting flask that filters out gel, dust and bristles, while the boar mounted a dummy sow. Semen was kept at the temperature collected and analyzed within 1 h. Sperm concentration and motility characteristics were determined by computer-assisted semen analysis (Hamilton Thorne IVOS 10.2; Hamilton Thorne Research, MA, USA) with a Makler counting chamber (Sefi Medical Instruments, Haifa, Israel). Sperm morphology was examined on Giemsa-stained samples (Hafez, 1993). Sperm index (SI) was calculated by multiplying sperm concentration by the square root of percentage sperm motility multiplied by the percentage of normal sperm morphology (Mahmoud et al., 1994). Combining concentration, motility and morphology in sperm index allows the concentration of active spermatozoa to be determined, and may provide a better means of evaluating semen quality than assessing the characteristics, mentioned above, independently.

3.1.2 Determination of specific absorbance wavelengths of resazurin and resorufin

Before developing the assay, specific absorbance wavelengths of resazurin and resorufin were determined. Ten µl 1.8 mM resazurin (Sigma, Steinheim, Germany) in physiological saline was added to 1 ml of 1:2 dilution of semen sample in BTS and incubated at 37°C in a water bath. After the semen sample completely turned to pink, the developed dye (resorufin) was extracted from the solution by adding n-butyl alcohol (Sigma, Germany) and fast vortexing. The control sample (blue colour solution) was prepared by adding butanol immediately after the resazurin. After centrifugation, the blue (resazurin) and pink (resorufin) solutions were separated from the clear upper layers of butyl alcohol and were scanned in the range from 400 to 850 nm, using a scanning spectrophotometer (UV/VIS Spectrometer Lambda 12, Perkin Elmer). Resazurin exhibits an absorption peak at 610 nm, while that of resorufin is at 575 nm (Fig. 6). There was minimal overlapping between absorption peaks of resazurin and resorufin at 610 nm; therefore the absorbance at 610 nm was used in further analysis.

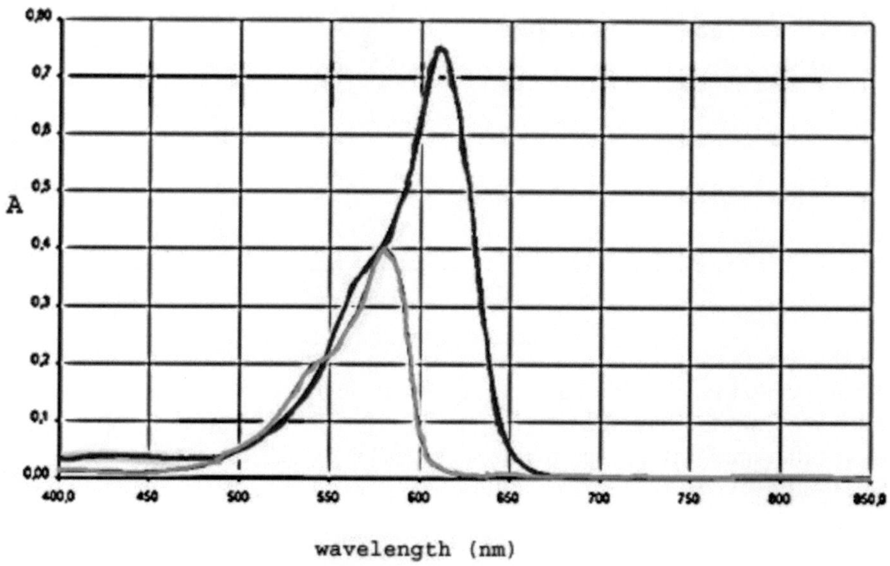

Fig. 6. Specific absorbance wavelengths of resazurin (–) and resorufin (–)

3.1.3 Resazurin reduction assay and correlation with semen parameters

The resazurin reduction assay was performed within 1 h after semen collection. Briefly, 30μL of 1.8mmol/L resazurin (Sigma, Steinheim, Germany) diluted in physiological saline was added to 3mL of semen sample diluted 1: 2 with Beltsville thawing solution semen extender (Beltsville Thawing Solution, Truadeco, the Netherlands) and incubated at 37°C in a water bath for 10min. After incubation, two sub-samples of 1mL were added to 1.5 mL of butanol (Merc, Germany). After rapid vortexing, samples were centrifuged at 3 000×g for 10min. Absorbance in the clear upper layer of butanol was measured at 610mm (UV/VIS Spectrometer Lambda 12; Perkin Elmer Corp., Analytical Instruments, Norwalk, CT, USA). The within-run coefficient of variation, calculated as 7.79±4.06 %, confirmed satisfactory repeatability of the assay. Spearman rank correlation analysis was used to determine the correlation between resazurin reduction assay and semen parameters such as sperm density, morphology, motile sperm concentration, viable sperm concentration and sperm index. We observed the highest correlations of resazurin reduction with sperm concentration followed by motile sperm concentration and viable sperm concentration. Inverse correlations indicate that better values of seminal parameters are correlated with a lower level of absorbance, indicating a stronger reducing capacity of the dye (resazurin). There were correlations ($P<0.001$) between the reduction of resazurin and motile sperm concentration ($r=0.81$) and SI ($r=0.82$), therefore resazurin reduction assaay was further diagnostically evaluated according to motile sperm concentration and sperm index. Scatter-plots and linear regression equations are shown in Figures 7 and 8.

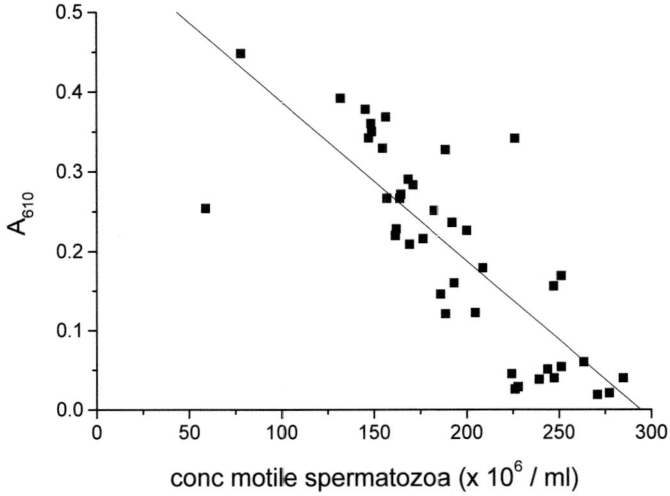

Fig. 7. Relationship between the reductions of resazurin expressed as absorbance and the concentration of motile spermatozoa
Regression equation: C (motile spermatozoa) = 258.345 – 0.325 x A_{610}

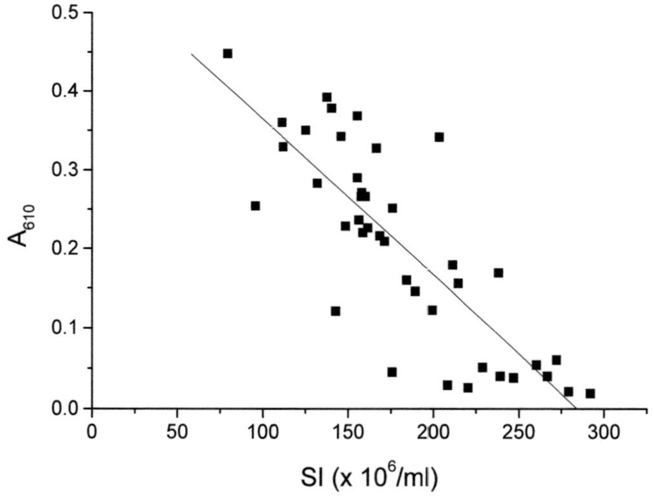

Fig. 8. Relationship between the reductions of resazurin expressed as absorbance and sperm index
Regression equation: SI = 250.546 – 0.339 x A_{610}

3.2 Diagnostic evaluation of resazurin reduction assay

Semen samples were divided into satisfactory (SAT) and unsatisfactory (UNSAT) according to various criteria. Criteria considering the concentration of motile sperm included pre-selected minimums of 160, 200 and 240×10^6 sperm/mL. Criteria considering the concentration of motile, normal sperm (SI) included pre-selected minimums of 140, 180 and 220×10^6sperm/mL. There was a significant difference between the absorbance values in groups of satisfactory and unsatisfactory semen samples (P<0.001) based on motile spermatozoa/mL and sperm index. Box plot in Fig.9 represents the values of A_{610} in both groups divided according to motile sperm concentration and sperm index.

The performance of diagnostic tests is usually described in terms of sensitivity and specificity (Jones & Payne, 1997). In the present study, receiver operating characteristics (ROC) analysis was used to determine the optimal cut-off value and diagnostic accuracy of the resazurin reduction assay by using boar semen. A complete picture of test accuracy is presented by the ROC plot, which provides a view of the whole spectrum of sensitivities (true positive rate) against one minus specificities (false positive rate) as functions of selected cut-off values (Greiner et al., 2000). A"good" test is one which has a high true positive rate and a low false positive rate and whose value, therefore, lies close to the top left-hand corner of the ROC curve (Petrie & Watson, 1999). A global summary statistic of the diagnostic accuracy of the assay is quantified by the areas under ROC curves (AUC). Likelihood ratios (LR) are used to revise the probability of the semen status in individual samples (Greiner et al., 1995). However, a complete ROC analysis, including AUC, provides an index of accuracy by demonstrating the limits of a test's ability to discriminate between different semen status values (Zwieg et al., 1993).

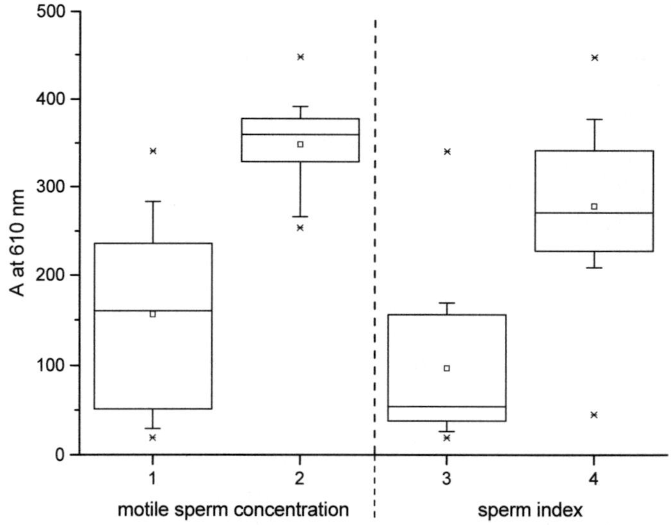

Fig. 9. Values of A_{610} in groups of satisfactory (group 1, group 3) and unsatisfactory (group 2, group 4) semen samples based on the motile sperm concentration (160x10^6 sperm/ml) and sperm index (180x10^6 sperm/ml)

ROC curves (Analyse-it, General + Clinical Laboratory statistics, version 1.71; Analyse-it Software Ltd., Leeds, UK) were applied to identify optimal test cut-off values. A positive test result (T+) was recorded when spermatozoa in a sample reduced resazurin from blue to pink, resulting in A_{610} below the cut-off value. A negative test result (T-) was recorded when spermatozoa in a sample did not reduce resazurin from blue to pink, resulting in A_{610} above the cut-off value. Sensitivity (Se) and specificity (Sp) for each cut-off value were calculated as the proportion of positive test results (T+) for SAT samples and negative test results (T-) for UNSAT samples according to complete 2x2 table (Table 1).

$$Se = TP/(TP+FN) \quad (2)$$

$$Sp = (TN)/(TN + FP) \quad (3)$$

Test result	Semen samples status		Total
	Satisfactory (SAT)	Unsatisfactory (UNSAT)	
Positive (T+)	True positive (TP)	False positive (FP)	TP + FP
Negative (T-)	False negative (FN)	True negative (TN)	FN + TN
Total	TP + FN	FP + TN	

Table 1. Complete 2x2 table

ROC curves plotted all sensitivity versus 1-specificity for the complete range of cut-off points (Greiner et al., 2000; Yuan et al., 2004). Sensitivity and specificity were estimated at 39 cut-off values. A diagonal line in a plot corresponds to a test that is positive or negative just by chance.

All possible combinations of sensitivity and specificity that can be achieved by changing the test's cut-off value were summarized by a single parameter; that is, AUC (Greiner et al., 2000). The slope of the ROC curve represents the LR for a diagnostic test, and the tangent at a point on the ROC curve corresponds to the LR for a single test value represented by that point (Choi et al., 1998).

$$LR=Se/(1-Sp) \quad (4)$$

The optimal cut-off values were selected based on the best balance of sensitivity, specificity and Youden index (J) along with larger increases in LR for each criterion value (Weiss et al., 2003-2004).

$$J = Se+Sp-1 \quad (5)$$

The diagnostic potential of resazurin reduction assay according to motile sperm concentration and SI was not different on the basis of AUC. The AUC was the same for criteria of 200×10^6 motile sperm/mL and 180×10^6 motile, normal sperm/mL (AUC=0.92; standard error for ROC curve (SE)=0.047 and 0.048, respectively; $P<0.0001$; Figure 10). On the basis of LR, absorbance lower than or equal to the optimal cut-off point were 11.3 and 7.1 times as likely to be found in satisfactory as in unsatisfactory semen samples according to SI and motile sperm concentration, respectively.

A plot of sensitivity, specificity and Youden index as a function of the cut-off value provides a useful visualisation and is helpful in selecting optimal cut-off values of the assay (Greiner, 2000). The selection of cut-off values of absorbance at 610nm according to different criteria for motile sperm concentration and SI are presented in Figures 11 and 12, respecitvely.

Values of Youden index peaked at a cut-off point of A_{610} at 0.209 for pre-selected minimum concentration of motile sperm concentration of 200×10^6sperm/mL (Figure 12B) and SI of 180×10^6 sperm/mL (Figure 12B). The optimal cut-off value at A_{610} of 0.209 therefore provided the best discrimination power according to both motile sperm concentration and SI. At this point, maximum overall accuracy was achieved for both cases. This cut-off value yielded estimates of sensitivity of 88.2% and 94.1% with corresponding specificities of 87.5% and 91.7% for motile sperm concentration and SI, respectively.

A

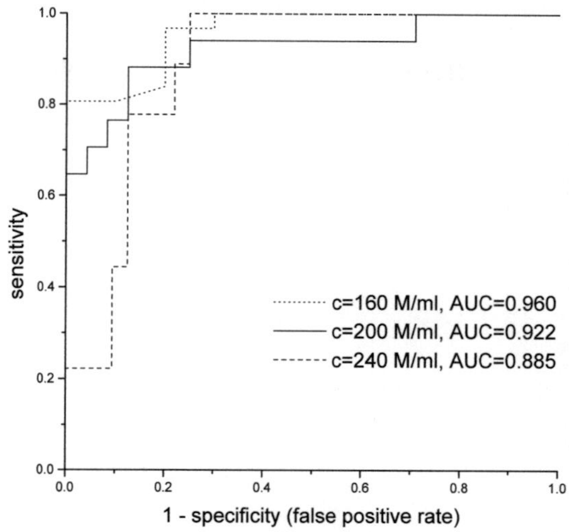

B

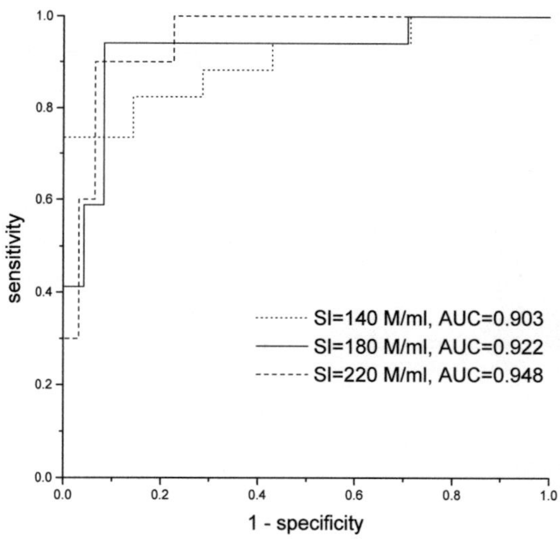

Fig. 10 (A, B). ROC plots of resazurin reduction assay for identifying semen samples with pre-selected minimum concentration of motile sperm concentration (A) and motile and normal sperm (B).

However, in clinical use of the test, it is often important to 100% correctly identify satisfactory or unsatisfactory samples. Therefore, a cut-off value of A_{610} at 0.342 was selected to enable 100% correct identification of unsatisfactory semen samples. For both criteria, the test is 100% sensitive at A_{610} of 0.342. A cut-off value at A_{610} of 0.121 gives 100% specificity for motile sperm concentration and 95.8% specificity for SI. For pre-selected minimum concentration of motile sperm concentration of 160×10^6 sperm/mL and SI of 140×10^6sperm/mL, 100% specificity was obtained at the optimal cut-off value of A_{610} at 0.254, whereas only moderate levels of sensitivity were observed (80.6% and 73.5%, respectively; Figures 11A and 12A). In contrast, at the highest criteria values 100% sensitivity corresponded to only moderate levels of specificity (Figures 11C and 12C). In contrast, semen samples with A_{610} below 0.121 in the resazurin reduction assay were 100%

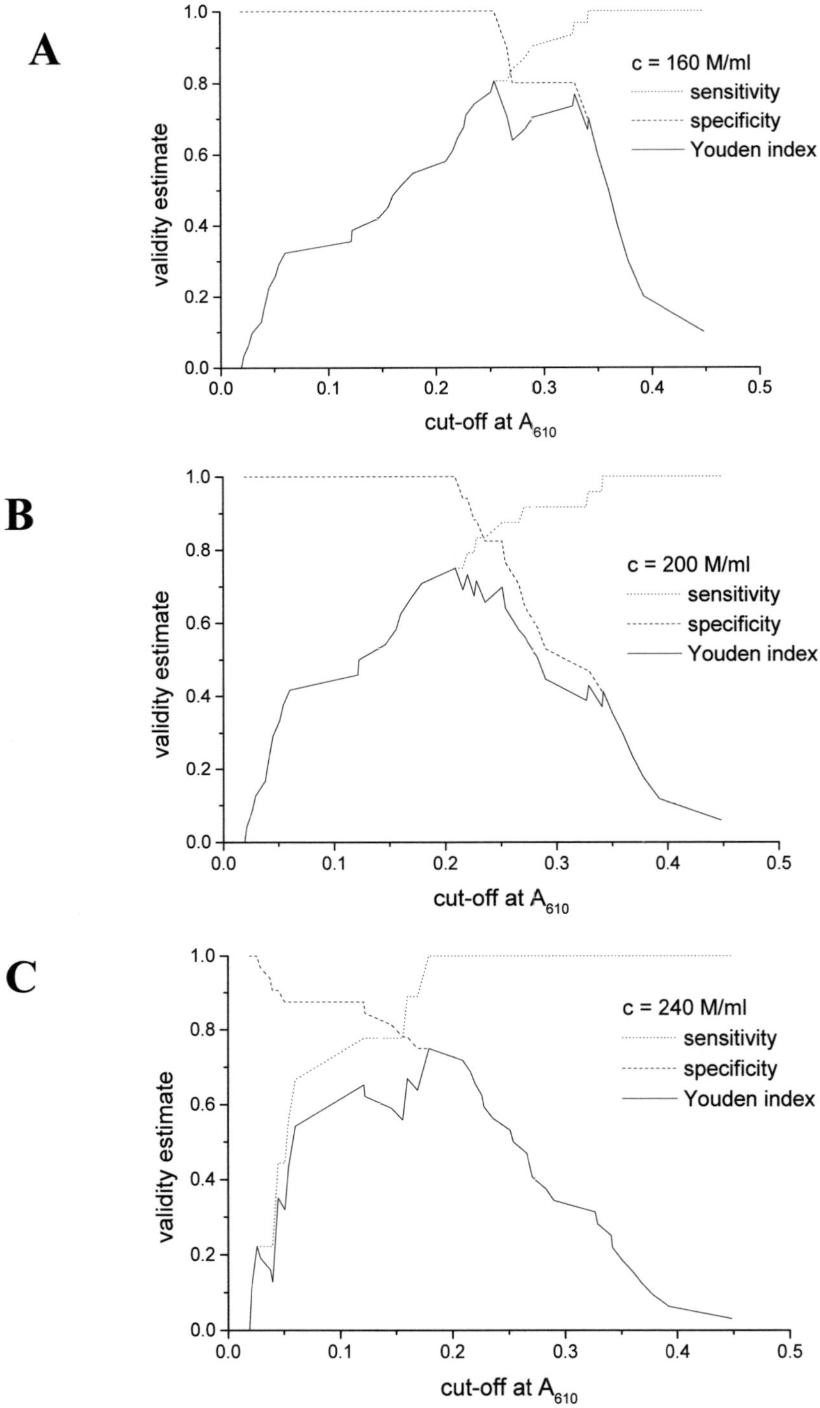

Fig. 11 (A, B, C). Plot of the diagnostic specificity, sensitivity and Youden index of resazurin reduction assay according to motile sperm concentration as a function of the cut-off value at 610nm.

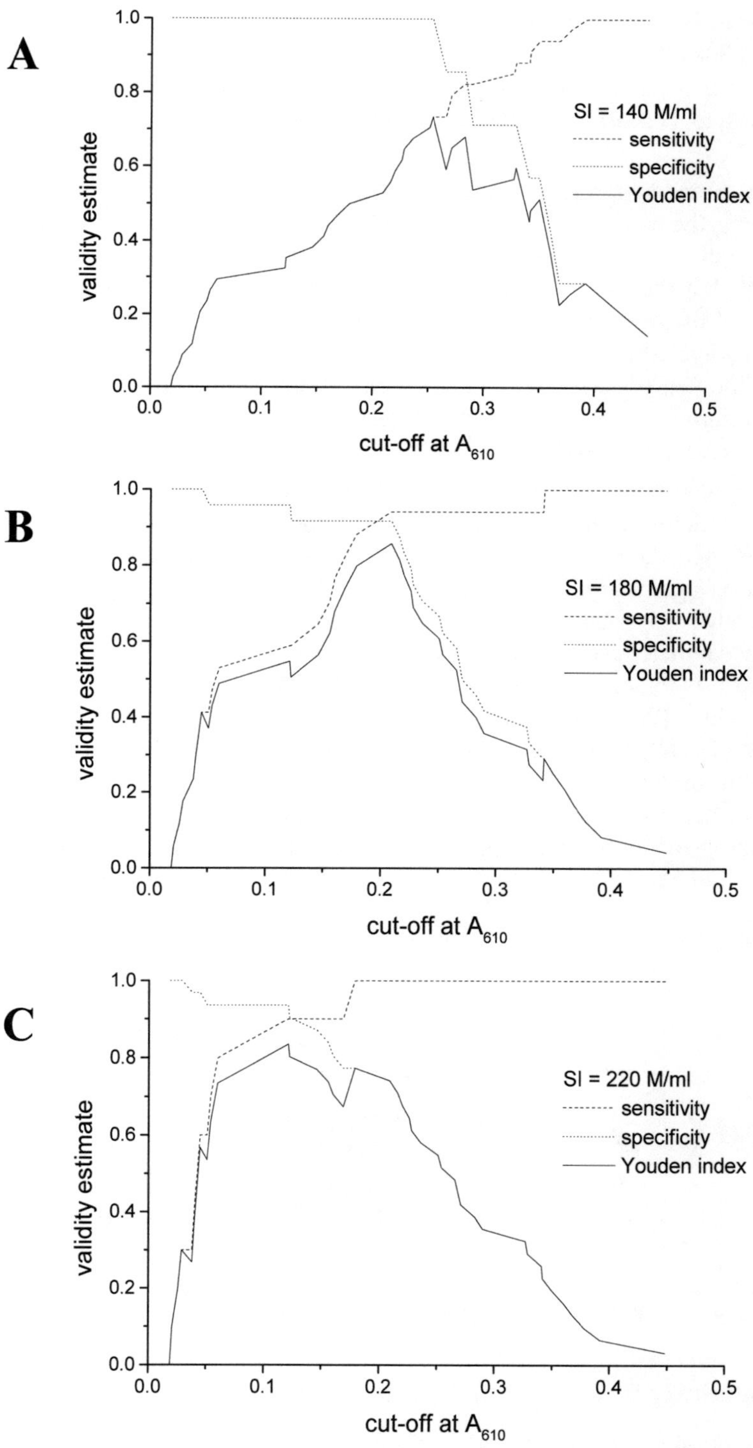

Fig. 12 (A, B, C). Plot of the diagnostic specificity, sensitivity and Youden index of resazurin reduction assay according to sperm index as a function of the cut-off value at 610nm.

and 95.8% correctly identified as satisfactory according to the criteria of 200×10^6 motile sperm/mL or 180×10^6 motile, normal sperm/mL, respectively. In our quantitative test, the maximum overall accuracy of 92.9% confirmed the high discrimination power for boar semen according to a criterion value of SI at 180×10^6sperm/mL.

3.3 Stability of butanol extracts in terms of A610

After developing the assay, we wondered if it was possible to measure the absorbance at a later date, i.e. within a day or even a week of the assay. A satisfactory level of agreement would indicate that the modification was successful, which in turn would greatly enhance the usefulness of the assay as it could then be performed even if a spectrophotometer was not immediately available.

We measured the A_{610} of each butanol extract of 112 samples on days 0, 1 and 7 after storage at 4°C. The differences were obtained between A_{610} at day 0 (A0) and day 1 (A1) and between days 0 (A0) and 7 (A7).

The limits of agreement were calculated as follows: limits = $\bar{d} \pm 2sdiff$, where $\bar{d}$ is the mean of differences for all the samples, and sdiff is the standard deviation of the differences. 2sdiff is also named the reproducibility coefficient. Differences between absorbances (A1 - A0) were plotted against their average value ((A1 + A0)/2) for each sample. Satisfactory agreement is achieved when minimum 95% of the absolute differences are less than the reproducibility coefficients (Petrie & Watson, 1999).

It is necessary to establish that a method is repeatable before comparing two measurements for reproducibility (Petrie & Watson, 1999). The within-run coefficient of variation, calculated as 7.79 ± 4.06 %, confirmed satisfactory repeatability of the method, therefore the pairs of measurement of A610 were allowed to compare. The differences between measurements (A_{610}) immediately after centrifugation (day 0) and after 7 days were plotted against the average of these values. 95.54 % of differences lie within the limits of agreement (Fig. 13).

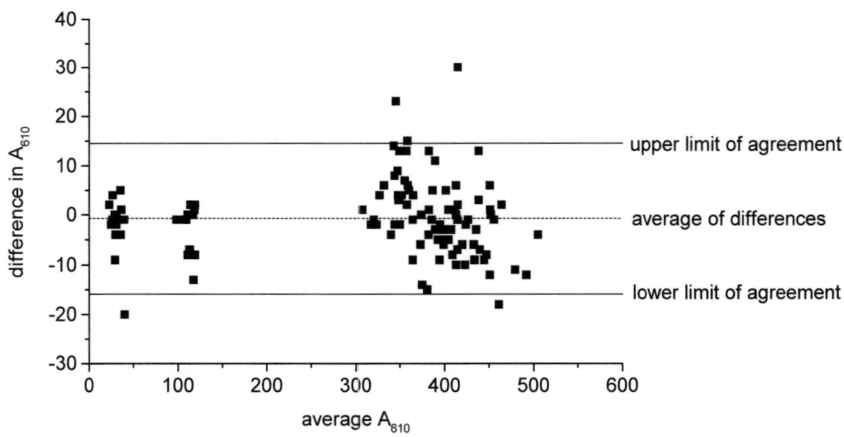

Fig. 13. A_{610} values as a function of time of measurement

Measurements obtained on the day of performing the test and the measurements after 24 hours also agree; 99.1 % of the differences lie within the limits of agreement (data not shown). The results obtained leading to the conclusion that we can measure A_{610} of butanol

extracts within 7 days from the day of test performing, confirming a great practical value of the method.
In a diagram of the differences between absorbances plotted against their average, the scatter of the points is random (Fig. 13) indicating, that the size of the discrepancy between the two absorbance is not related to the size of the absorbance. More than 95 % of absolute differences were less than the reproducibility coefficients in both cases of testing the stability of butanol extracts. This is a satisfactory agreement, therefore we can measure the absorbance immediately after performing the test or within 7 days of that time. Therefore the test is useful even if spectrophotometer is not available at the location of semen evaluation. The results obtained leading to the conclusion that we can measure A_{610} of butanol extracts within 7 days from the day of test performing, confirming a great practical value of the method.

4. Conclusions

The usefulness of sperm counting is greatly enhanced by the simplicity of determination by photometer (Photometer SDM5, MiniTüb, Germany) in on-farm AI laboratories. The use of photometer for determining sperm concentration would, therefore, be of benefit also to livestock producers in evaluating the quality of boar semen.
The resazurin reduction assay was shown to be a reliable, easy-to-perform test that requires no sophisticated equipment. It was demonstrated that the results of the assay can be used to select semen samples with minimum requirements of sperm concentration, motility and normal morphology, which are all combined in sperm index. Because reproductive performance depends on metabolic processes, the assessment of metabolic rates of spermatozoa could provide even better or more complete information about semen quality than other tests. It allows the concentration of active spermatozoa to be determined, and may provide a better means of evaluating semen quality than assessing the characteristics, mentioned above, independently. Expressing the latter in semen evaluation is complex, although fertility results from insemination with evaluated semen could provide a gold standard of fertilizing capacity. Additional research is required for relevant and valid information about replacing or updating the methodology of semen evaluation.

5. Acknowledgements

This work was supported by the Slovenian Ministry of Higher Education, Science and Technology, programme group "Endocrine, immune, nervous and enzyme responses in healthy and sick animals" (P4-0053).
Special thanks go to author's collegues who contributed to the research work, presented in this chapter: Janko Mrkun, DVM, PhD, Marjan Kosec, DVM, PhD, Janez Kunc, DVM, MSc, Maja Zakošek Pipan, DVM.

6. References

Anzar, M., Kroetsch, T., Buhr, M.M. (2009). Comparison of different method for assessment of sperm concentration and membrane integrity with bull semen. *J Androl*, 30, 6, pp. (661-668)

Bland J.M. & Altman D.G. (1999). Measuring agreement in method comparision studies. Stat Methods Med Res 8, pp. (135-160)

Brazil, C., Swan, S.H., Tollner, C.R., Treece, C., Drobnis, E.Z., Wang, C., Redmon, J.B. & Overstreet, J.W. (2004). Quality control of laboratory methods for semen evaluaion in a multicenter research study. *J. Androl.*, 25, pp. (645 - 656)

Carter, R.A., Ericsson, S.A., Corn, C.D., Weyerts, P.R., Dart, M.G., Escue, S.G. & Mesta J. (1998). Assessing the fertility potential of equine semen samples using the reducible dyes methylene green and resazurin. *Arch Andro*, 40, 1, pp. (59-66)

Camus, A., Camugli, S., Leveque, C., Schmitt, E. & Staub, C. (2011). Is photomertry an accurate and reliable method to assess boar semen concentration? *Theriogenology*, 75, pp. (577-583)

Choi, B.C. (1998). Slopes of a Receiver Operating Characteristic Curve and Likelihood Ratios for a Diagnostic Test. *Am J Epidemiol*, 148, pp. (1127-1132)

Christensen, P., Stenvang, J. & Godfrey, W. (2004) A flow cytometric method for rapid determination of sperm concentration and viability in mammalian and avian semen. *J Androl*, 25, 2, pp. (255-264)

Christensen, P., Stryhn, H. & Hansen, C. (2005). Discrepancies in the determination of sperm concentration using Bürker-Türk, Thoma and Makler counting chambers. *Theriogenology*, 63, 4, pp. (992-1003)

Cooper, T.A., Wang, S., Liu, Y., Bunch, T.D. & Holyoak, G.R. (1996). A new method to evaluate the viability of cryopreserved ram semen using a resazurin reduction assay. *Theriogenology*, 45, 1, pp. 313.

Dart, M.G., Mesta, J., Creshaw, C. & Ericsson, S.A. (1994). Modified resazurin reduction test for determining the fertility potential of bovine spermatozoa. *Arch Androl*, 33, pp. (71-75)

Fuse, H., Okumura, M., Kazama, T. & Katayama T. (1993). Comparison of resazurin test results with various sperm parameters. *Andrologia*, 25, pp, (153-157)

Glass, R.H., Drouin, M.T., Ericsson, S.A., Marcoux, L.J., Ericsson, R.J. & Sullivan H. (1991). The resazurin reduction test provides an assessment of sperm activity. *Fertil Steril*, 56, pp. (43-46)

Greiner, M., Sohr, D.& Göbel, P. (1995). A modified ROC analysis for the selection of cut-off values and the definition of intermediate results of serodiagnostic tests. *J Immunol Methods*, 185, pp. (123-132)

Greiner, M., Pfeiffer, D. & Smith, R.D. (2000). Principles and practical application of the receiver-operating characteristic analysis for diagnostic tests. *Prev Vet Med*, 54, pp. (23-41)

Hafez, E.S.E. (1993). Semen evaluation. In: *Reproduction in Farm animals (6th ed.)*. Hafez, E.S.E., pp. (405-423), Philadelphia, PA

Hansen, C., Vermeiden, T., Vermeiden, J.P.W., Simmet, C., Day, B.C. & Feitsma, H. (2006). Comparision of FACSCount AF system, improved Neubauer hemacytometer, Corning 254 photometer, SpermVision, UltiMate and NucleoCounter SP-100 for determination of sperm concentration of boar semen. *Theriogenology*, 66, pp. (2188-2194)

Holt, W.V. & Medrano A. (1997). Assessment of boar sperm function in relation to freezing and storage. *J Reprod Fertil*, Suppl., 52, pp. (213-222)

Imade, G.E., Towobola, O.A., Sagay, A.S. & Otubu, J.A. (1993). Discrepancies in sperm count using improved Neubauer, Makler, and Horwells counting chambers *Arch Androl*, 31, 1, pp. (17-22)

Jensen, A.L. & Kjelgaard-Hansen, M. (2006). Method comparison in the clinical laboratory, *Vet Clin Pathol.*, 35, pp. (276-286)

Johnson, L.A., Weitze, K.F., Fiser, P. & Maxwell, W.M. (2000). Storage of boar semen. *Anim Reprod Sci*, 62, pp. (143-172)

Jones, R.G. & Payne, R.B., (1997). Analytical methods: control and comparison. In: *Clinical Investigation and Statistics in Laboratory Medicine*, Jones, R.G. & Payne, R.B., pp. (27-65), ACB Venture Publications, London

Juonala, T., Lintukangas, S., Nurttila, T. & Andresson, M. (1998). Relationship between semen quality and fertility in 106 AI-Boars, *Reprod Domest Anim*, 33, pp. (155-158)

Keel, B., Quinn, P., Schmidt, C., Serafy, N, Jr, Serafy, N. Sr. & Schalue, T. (2000). Results of the American association of Bioanalysts national proficiency testing programme in andrology, *Hum Reprod*, 15, pp (680-686)

Knuth, U.A., Neuwinger, J. & Nieschlag, E. (1989). Bias to routine semen analysis by uncontrolled changes in laboratory environment - detection by long-term sampling of monthly means for quality control, *Int J Androl*, 12, pp. (375-383)

Liu, D.Y. & Baker, H.W.G. (2002). Evaluation and assessment of semen for IVF/ICSI, *Asian J Androl*, 4, pp. (281-285)

Ma, D. & Smith, F.G. (2003). Correlation and regression. In: *Key topics in Clinical Research*, Smith, F.G. & Smith, J.R., pp. (147-151), BIOS Scientific Publishers Limited, Oxford

Maatson, P. (1995). External quality assessment for semen analysis and sperm antibody detection: results of a pilot scheme, *Hum Reprod*, 10, pp. (620-625).

Mahmoud, A.M., Comhaire, F.H., Vermeulen, L. & Andreou, E. (1994). Comparison of the resazurin test, adenosine triphosphate in semen, and various sperm parameters, *Hum Reprod*, 9, pp. (1688-1693)

Mahmoud, A.M.A., Depoorter, B., Piens, N. & Comhaire, F.H., (1997). The performance of 10 different methods for the estimation of sperm concentration, *Fertil and Steril*, 68, 2, pp. (340-345)

Martin, L.M., Crenshaw, C.C., Dean, J.A. Jr., Dart, M.G., Purdy, P.H. & Ericsson, S.A. (1999). Determination of the number of motile sperm within an ovine semen sample using resazurin, *Small Rumin Res*, 32, pp. (161-165)

Mesta, J., Ericsson, S.A., Dart, M.G., Wansley, R.G. & Weyerts, P.R. (1995) Assesment of fertility potential of porcine spermatozoa using the reducible dyes methylene green and resazurin. *Journal of Animal Science*, 73, (Suppl. 1), pp. (26)

Mrkun, J., Kosec, M., Zakošek, M., Zrimšek, P. (2007). Method agreement between measuring of boar sperm concentration using makler chamber and photometer. *Acta vet (Beogr.)*, 57, 5/6, pp. (563-572)

Neuwinger, J., Behre, H.M. & Nieschlag, E. (1990). External quality control in the andrology laboratory: an experimental multicenter trial, *Fertil Steril*, 54, pp. (308-314)

Petrunkina, A.M., Waberski, D., Günzel-Apel, A.R. & Töpfer-Petersen, E. (2007). Determinants of sperm quality and fertility in domestic species. *Reproduction*, 134, pp. (3-17)

Petrie, A. & Watson, P. (1999). Additional Topics. In: *Statistics for veterinary and animal science*, Petrie, A., Watson, P., pp. (168-181), Blackwell Science, Oxford

Prathalingam, N., Holt, W., Revell, S., Jones, S. & Watson, P. (2006). The precision and accuracy of six different methods to determine sperm concentration. *J Androl*, 27, 2, pp. (257-262)

Quintero-Moreno, A., Rigau, T. & Rodriguez-Gil, J.E. (2004). Regression analysis and motile sperm subpopulation structure study as improving tools in boar semen quality analysis, *Theriogenology*, 61, pp. (673-690)

Rahman, N.A. & Kula, K. (1997). Enlarged spectrum of seminological diagnoses using the resazurin colour reaction, a spectrophotometric application, *Int J Andro,* 20, pp. (17-22)

Reddy Venkata Rami, K., Meherji, P.K., Gokral, J.S. & Shahani, S.K. (1997). Resazurin reduction test to evaluate semen quality. *Indian Journal of Experimental Biology,* 35, pp. (369-373)

Reddy Venkata Rami & K., Bordekar, A.D. (1999). Spectrophotometric analysis of resazurin reduction test and semen quality in men. *Indian J Exp Biol,* 37, pp. (782-786)

Sokol, R.Z., Shulman, P. & Paulson, R.J. (2000). Comparison of two methods for the measurement of sperm concentration. *Fertil Steril,* 73, 3, pp. (591-594)

Tejerina, F., Buranaamnuay, K., Saravia, F,, Wallgren, M. & Rodriguez-Martinez, H. (2008). Assessment of motility ejaculated, liquid-stored boar spermatozoa using computerized instruments, *Theriogenology,* 69, pp. (1129-1138)

Tsakmakidis, I.A., Lymberopoulos, A.G. & Khalifa, T.A.A. (2010). Relationship between sperm quality traits and filed-fertility of porcine semen. *J Vet Sci,* 11, 2, pp. (151-154)

Twormey, P. (2004). Plasma glucose measurement with the Yellow Springs Glucose 2300 STAT and the Olympus AU640. *J Clin Pathol,* 57, pp. (752-754).

Twormey, P. (2005). How do we really compare methods in the clinical laboratory? *Proceedings of Statistics Workshop & Clinics, EuroMedLab,* Glasgow, May 2005

Vyt, P., Maes, D., Rijsselaere, T., Dejonckheere, E., Castryck, F. & Van Soom, A. (2004). Motility Assessment of Porcine Spermatozoa: a Comparison of Methods. *Reprod Dom Anim,* 30, pp. (447–453)

Yuan, Y.M., Xin, Z.C., Jiang, H., Guo, Y.J., Liu, W.J., Tian, L. & Zhu, J.C. (2004). Sexual function of premature ejaculation patients assayed with Chinese Index of Premature Ejaculation, *Asian J Androl,* 6, pp. (121-126)

Waberski, D., Schapmann, E., Henning, H., Reisenbeck, A. & Brandt, H. (2011). Sperm chromatin structural integrity in normospermic boars is not related to semen storage and fertility after routine AI, *Theriogenology,* 75, pp. (337-345)

Wang, S., Holyoak G.R., Panter, K.E., Liu, G., Evans, R.C., Bunch, T.D. (1998) Resazurin reduction assay for ram sperm metabolic activity measured by spectrophotometry. Proc Soc Exp Biol Med, 217, pp. (197-202)

Weiss, H.L., Niwas, S., Grizzle, W.E. & Piyathilake, C. (2003-2004). Receiver operating characteritic (ROC) to determine cut-off points of biomarkers in lung cancer patients. *Dis Markers,* 19, pp. (273-278)

Woelders, H. (1991). Overview of in vitro methods for evaluation of semen quality, *Reprod Domest Anim Suppl,* pp. (145-164)

Zalata, A.A., Lammertijn, N., Christoper, A. & Comhaire, F.H. (1998). The correlates and alleged biochemical background of the resazurin reduction test in semen. *Int J Androl,* 21, pp. (289-294)

Zwieg, M.H. & Campbell, G. (1993). Receiver-Operating Characteristic (ROC) Plots: A Fundamental Evaluation Tool in Clinical Medicine, *Clin. Chem.,* 39/40, pp. (561-577)

Zrimšek, P., Kunc, J., Kosec, M., Mrkun, J. (2004). Spectrophotometric application of resazurin reduction assay to evaluate boar semen quality. *Int J Androl,* 27, 1, pp. (57-62)

Zrimšek, P., Kosec, M., Kunc, J., Mrkun, J. (2006). Determination of the diagnostic value of the resazurin reduction assay for evaluating boar semen by receiver operating characteristic analysis. *Asian J Androl,* 8, 3, pp. (343-348)

10

Particularities of Bovine Artificial Insemination

Antônio Nelson Lima da Costa, Airton Alencar de Araujo
and José Valmir Feitosa
Federal University of Ceara
Brazil

1. Introduction

In beef production systems a good reproductive performance is essential for the efficient management and production. The production of cattle can be divided into two sectors: dairy and meat production. In many European countries and developing countries, even the cattle is used as a source of meat and milk and are called dual fitness. Unlike in countries such as Australia, Brazil and the United States, the functions of production of meat and milk were separated and the creation of selective breeding is directed to a single feature.

The productive and reproductive performance of cattle herd is directly related to the service period, calving interval, number of service per conception and number of calves weaned. Artificial insemination (AI) has been proven worldwide and has proven to be a viable technical and economical to increase the genetic gain and increase efficiency, especially in production systems for meat and milk.

In cattle, AI despite presenting a series of known proven advantages, gradually being replaced by fixed-time artificial insemination (FTAI) because of lack of skilled labor, logistical problems in large AI programs, in failures detection of estrus; costs for implementing the program, no optimization of herd reproductive efficiency, and the difficulty of practical application in field conditions.

In this chapter discuss techniques to improve conception rates using artificial insemination, such as: improved detection of estrus, a reduction in calving interval, implementation of FTAI; calving and breeding seasons, care with the semen, body condition score of females, the female gynecological evaluation, diagnosis of pregnancy, parturition rate.

After the reading of these topics, many barriers bovine artificial insemination will be elucidated, and the artificial insemination technique is best applied in various conditions of management of cattle herds worldwide.

2. Improvement in detection of estrus

Worldwide there are reports that indicate low rates of service in artificially inseminated cattle, mainly due to problems in the detection of estrus. While few cows are detected in heat losses occur in significant herd reproductive efficiency, and commitment of the artificial insemination program. This commitment is even higher in *Bos indicus* cattle, whose breeding behavior has special features - heat of short duration with a high percentage of expression during the night (Galina et al., 1996, Pinheiro et al., 1998). This feature was confirmed with the radiotelemetry system (Heat-watch) in Nelore, Angus x Nelore and Angus to the terrain under the same management (Mizuta, 2003). The results are indicative that the heat of Nelore (*Bos indicus*) and Nellore x Angus is about 4 hours less than the duration of estrus Angus cows (*Bos taurus*).

The secretion of estrogen, a manifestation of oestrus LH surge and ovulation are closely related and well known. With follicular growth, the amount of estrogen secreted increases to a peak serum concentration, triggering a preovulatory LH surge, follicular maturation and ovulation, lasting 27 hours. The goal of increased concentrations of estrogen is triggering hormonal cascade of events that includes the LH surge and a series of changes that promote follicular ovulation, and sexual behaviors associated with acceptance of mounts.

The main characteristic of estrus is the posture of immobility assumed by acceptance of the cows and ride. High producing cows milk manifest estrus of shorter duration than cows with lower production (Lopez et al., 2004). Females of childbearing age are pregnant or in the luteal phase of the cycle (under the domain of progesterone) are less likely to mount other females are in estrus. Almost 86% of females who ride other females are in estrus and proestrous (under the domain of the estrogen). Consequently, it should be kept open or barren females with other similarly to occur as much sexual behavioral interactions (Helmer and Britt, 1985). The type of flooring is essential for the expression of mounts and immobility. When you can choose, cows in estrus spend 73% of time on the ground and not on the concrete and assemble increases by 15 times in paddocks of land in relation to the concrete. Moreover, the duration of estrus and immobility also increases on gravel (Vail & Britt, 1990).

Over the years various devices have been developed to detect estrus and they were effective as an aid in visual identification, as Bos indicus tend to present turnover night (Baruselli et al., 2004). These devices range from the tail to paint the most sophisticated pedometers (figure 1) and tags that track electronic activity detectors and electronic pressure "HeatWatch. The pedometers have been used to measure activity or movement of the cow through a microprocessor chip and miniature device is fixed to a collar or bracelet. A cow in estrus walks about 4 times more than another that is not in estrus. These devices can be accessed manually or automatically when the cow enters the milking parlor or through receiving antennas mounted in the stalls. The information is sent to a computer and compared with individual basal activity of the same cow over a similar time interval of 2 or 3 days earlier. If the activity has increased significantly this cow, this cow is identified by a warning light that flashes on the ankle or on the computer, generating a warning report to the responsible to verify whether it is in heat and should be inseminated (Stevenson, 2001).

Using these devices in heifers, it was found that they are effective in identifying animals with short periods of estrus and few events of immobility. When compared the accuracy of heat identification of 49 heifers with synchronized estrus, with pedestrian detection by the farm, it failed to comply with estrus in 13 of 49 heifers (26%), while the electronic device identified all foodstuffs (Stevenson et al., 1999). Remembering that the aids can be used to increase the efficiency of our detection of estrus, but not to replace it.

Intensive detection of estrus was defined as 2 h of heat detection in the mornings and afternoons and one additional hour of estrus detection around noon. The detection was defined as a casual observation of the cows in the mornings and afternoons for 30 minutes. In the same herd, cows of both groups underwent intensive observation and casual, were

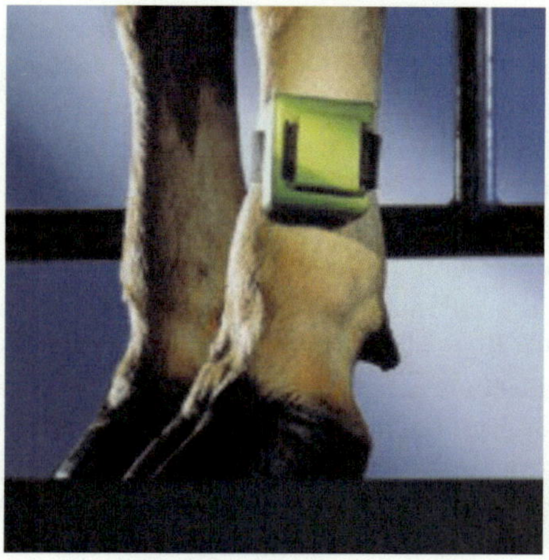

Fig. 1. Cow with pedometer in previous member

synchronized with the same protocol and inseminated by the same technician. In animals with the intensive detection of estrus, the percentage of cows observed in estrus increased in 30% conception rate in 20% and pregnancy rate doubled in this group. The highest conception rates among cows intensively observed may have been the result of a more appropriate time of artificial insemination relative to ovulation (Geary et al., 2000).

Whenever is observed a cow in heat, it should be removed from the herd as soon as possible because it diverts attention from other cows are in heat in two ways. First, when are making the detection of estrus, each time a cow is in a position to accept mounts noted his number. If the cow is being mounted, has been identified previously, then get distracted and fail to see other cows. Second, there is always regarded as timid cows to avoid the pushing of estrous behavior and estrous pass through undetected. These cows may show signs of estrus when the cow in estrus ruling was removed. The only time when one considers the possibility of letting the cows are in heat in the pasture to help identify other cows in heat is when you do not make use of estrus synchronization and when it is expected that less than 5% of cows in the herd come into estrus per day (Geary et al., 2005).

All of estrus detection devices should be used cautiously and their results interpreted by trained people, since people are the most important component in any program of estrus detection and artificial insemination. The ability to detect estrus in the interpretation and common sense are key to the success of an accurate detection of estrus and this increases the rate of submission to artificial insemination.

3. Reducing the gap between births

Calving interval (CI) covers the period between two consecutive deliveries from a cow and a yearly calving interval is a common goal for both beef producers and for the milk. Long intervals are uneconomical because cows with extended intervals produce little milk and fewer calves per year. It is one of the main parameters to measure the reproductive efficiency of cattle.

The CI can be divided into two components: the interval from calving to conception and during pregnancy. The first covers the period from calving to the establishment of a new pregnancy and is the main determinant of CI being the parameter usually manipulated to

achieve a desirable CI. The second component comprises an average of 285 days, varying only according to the genetics of both the matrix and the player and can only be reduced by inducing premature parturition.
To get an CI for 365 days, the interval between delivery and conception should not be longer than 80-85 days. A key factor for achieving these goals is good nutrition. A study conducted in Florida stressed the importance of dry matter intake for cows in early cyclicity. Cows with higher dry matter intake returned to cycle faster and lost less weight postpartum (Staples et al., 1998). Care of the dry matter intake and body condition is essential and should begin well before birth in the last 100 days of lactation. So there will be enough time to adjust body condition and prepare all the cows in their dry period and lactation next breeding season.
The relationship between energy balance and ovulation is directly related to the pattern of LH secretion, which is the gonadotropin responsible for follicular maturation and ovulation. After delivery, there is limited secretion of LH, but as approach the time of first ovulation, the basal concentration of LH secretion increases and the pattern becomes more pulsatile. The LH pulse frequency should occur at hourly to support follicular maturation and ovulation. The first ovulation occurs two weeks after the increased frequency of LH pulses. Thus, it should provide a well balanced diet and palatable to cows to meet their metabolic needs as soon as possible after birth, stimulating consumption fractionated into four meals a day until the cows to produce milk and ovulate early, reducing the CI (Butler and Smith, 1989).
Another factor that must be considered is the diagnosis of pregnancy, IE this should be done up to 30 days after artificial insemination, and the empty livestock referred for procedures such as fixed-time artificial insemination. Resynchronization of repeat breeder cows is also an alternative to reduce the CI, because prior to the diagnosis of pregnancy can identify animals that are empty and reinseminated them, improving conception rates and shortening the CI (Chebel et al., 2006). Furthermore can mention other factors that influence the duration of the CI as appropriate handling and deposition of semen, the ability of artificial insemination, animal care not to subject him to stress management, such as abuse, also contribute a good mineralization for the appearance of fertile estrus, improvement in the design and decrease the CI.

4. Application of fixed-time artificial insemination

The fixed-time artificial insemination (FTAI) has become very popular because of reduced manpower and independence of estrus detection, since there are many difficulties to detect cows in heat, especially at night. The rates of detection of estrus and submission to artificial insemination are limiting factors due to the type of installation, which limit the expression of estrus, or lack of skilled labor for estrus detection. For artificial insemination programs are successful in herds not using hormonal intervention, the rate of estrus detection should exceed 70%. Most programs result in FTAI pregnancy rates similar to those obtained following the detection of natural estrus.
The inefficiency of reproductive cows causes great frustration and losses for farmers. Even under ideal conditions, the reproductive process is far from perfect, considering the myriad factors involved in producing a live calf. The reproductive efficiency involves not only proper management of cows, but also management of carers and inseminate. The conception rates of lactating dairy cows declined from the 50's in the USA, while the annual yield per cow increased 3.3 times (Lucy, 2001). Given the inverse relationship of milk yield

and fertility, there is a genetic antagonism between milk yield and reproductive traits manifested primarily in first lactation cows, but good management practices such as use of FTAI, can overcome this inverse correlation and allowed its acceptable levels of reproductive efficiency.

The programmed insemination is a method that plans and manages a program of artificial insemination of a herd. This lineup of estrous cycles has some advantages such as convenience of scheduling tasks and use of manpower, control the occurrence of estrus, ovulation, or both, and knowledge of the estrous cycle and reproductive status of females in the herd. The categories of reproductive status are scheduled to open cows at first artificial insemination, cows inseminated to be subjected to pregnancy diagnosis, cows scheduled to open re-insemination; open cows destined for disposal (will not be inseminated) and cows confirmed pregnant. Thus, the programmed insemination can be applied in two distinct groups: cows that are scheduled for their first insemination and cows confirmed to be opened after diagnosis of pregnancy and scheduled for re-insemination. The programmed insemination involves hormonal timing of estrus, ovulation, or both. In the USA, FTAI programs are used in 90% of herds, with 86% of synchronizing first services, 77% of re-synchronization of repeaters and 59% of treatments for cystic cows in anovulatory or anestrus (Caraviello et al., 2006).

The best program is the simplest and easiest to apply, varying with the level of training of officials of the farm. In this case, simplicity means lower number of manipulations in cows during the implementation of a protocol. Employees should be trained to take a disciplined approach and comprehensive programs work, i.e., the implementation of the protocols should be approximately 100% to achieve a greater number of pregnant cows and fewer discharges of pregnant cows.

Some studies have evaluated the cost-effectiveness of fixed-time artificial insemination protocols. One study estimated the value of a pregnancy in a flock where half of the cows were inseminated only after the detection of natural estrus, compared to the application of FTAI the other half of the cows. In herds with low estrus detection, the cost of pregnancy was significantly reduced with the use of FTAI compared detection only. In herds with high rates of detection of estrus, the cost of pregnancy was higher with the use of FTAI, but there was a better reproductive performance of cows treated. The highest costs of pregnancy were associated with damage resulting from longer periods opened and account for up to 83% of total costs (Tenhagen et al., 2004). Thus, the use of a system of FTAI is considered a profitable alternative for large commercial flocks in the estrus detection rates are low.

5. Breeding seasons and calving

The breeding season or insemination consists of a period of the year in which breeding females are exposed to males or are inseminated, and calving season is closely correlated, because the births are concentrated in a pre-determined by the breeding season or insemination. It is a strategy for increasing productivity in terms of number of weaned calves, zero cost, rationalizing the reproductive activity of animals with the concentration of deliveries, facilitating and regulating the management of livestock.

The most widely used method of breeding in central Brazil is one where the bull stays with the herd throughout the year. As a result, births are distributed throughout the year, despite a higher concentration during the months from July to September. The occurrence of births at times inappropriate affect the calves, due to higher incidence of diseases and parasites, or the lower availability of pasture for sows during the lactation period. The biggest drawback, however, that limits the use of rides throughout the year, concerns the difficulty of controlling the health of livestock and livestock due to lack of uniformity (age and weight) of animals. These factors ultimately affect the selection of cattle for increased reproductive potential, rather than female fertility (Embrapa, 2011).

The advantages in adopting the breeding season are many and are related to the calves, the matrices and the production system. With regard to calves, they will be born in more favorable time of year with a lower incidence of ectoparasites and endoparasites, with proper nutrition will have a greater supply of fodder, assist in the formation of more uniformity, reduced mortality, increased weaning weight and easy of recreating. Concerning the matrices, the mating season coincides with the increased availability of forage providing suitable conditions for the restoration of reproductive activity with higher pregnancy rates, select arrays to better reproductive efficiency after the breeding season and diagnosis gestation selecting the best females, and lactating occurring over a period of good supply of food. The advantages to the production system is characterized in rationalization of manpower, purchase of inputs less frequently, and much lower price, and ease of adoption of other practices such as early weaning, supplementation of calves, estrous synchronization and artificial insemination of matrices (Santos, 2003).

The choice of the breeding season depends on several factors such as climatic conditions, availability of pasture land, labor, adequate time for the birth of calves and purpose of production, i.e., commercial or purebred animals. Based on these facts, it is much easier to work towards the establishment of a nature to breeding season in the property, aiming to streamline the reproductive activity in both the biological and practical.

When the producer chooses to adopt the breeding season of short duration (2-3 months), replacing the system where there insemination of cows throughout the year, we recommend a gradual reduction in the period of insemination, eliminating every year one to two months to reach the optimal duration, so there is no reduction in fertility. For heifers, it is recommended to advance the breeding season in 30 days than cows, so they have more time to restore their reproductive activity when they become primiparous. Adequate protein supplementation of females during the breeding and supply of mineral throughout the year contribute to elevation of the reproduction of the herd.

6. Care of semen

The canister is an insulated container with vacuum insulation, for the preservation of semen, and for that he should receive liquid nitrogen, which preserves the doses of semen frozen at a temperature of -196°C (one hundred ninety-six degrees Celsius) indefinitely, provided they maintain a certain level, supplying them periodically. It should be handled with the utmost care to avoid damage that may result in losses. To lessen the risks to the canister, it is advisable to build a wooden box for packaging, avoiding shocks, movements are too fast, and overturn spilling its entire contents.

The liquid nitrogen evaporates constantly, and the inseminator is alert to prevent loss of semen due to lack of nitrogen. To do so, you should always measure your level with appropriate meter; never letting the level below 15 cm. High consumption of nitrogen can indicate problems with the canister as well as the formation of frost or condensate on any external surface may also indicate defects.

The thawing of semen at appropriate temperatures, according to the recommendations of the supplier is required to maximize post-thaw survival and motility of sperm. The cold shock can be avoided by maintaining the temperature, because when the blade is exposed for 30 seconds at room temperature, the temperature drops to 35°C to 23°C. Heating the artificial insemination pipette and maintenance of the temperature of the semen to its insertion into the vagina prevents thermal shock. Only straws should be thawed enough to inseminate cows in 10 minutes. All equipment must be kept artificial insemination extremely clean.

The deposition of semen in inadequate reproductive tract may be a limiting factor when the coach is not sure of the location of the pipette tip. Surveys show that less motile sperm reaching the oviduct when the semen is deposited in the cervix. Insemination, the goal is to reach the body of the uterus. When in doubt, it is better to deposit the semen in one or both uterine horns and fertility will be less compromised than if the semen is deposited only in the cervix. As 85 to 90% of the semen is expelled from the female reproductive tract by retrograde flow, it is essential that the total dose is deposited in the uterus.

The use of sexed semen has become common, but it is important to remember that it is different from the conventional. To achieve 90% purity of a specific sex, sperm are treated with fluorescent dyes and X and Y chromosome sperm are separated by a cell separator (flow cytometry) based on fluorescence intensity after exposure to the laser beam. There are many data Dairy Heifers, describing a design with sexed average, around 70% to 80% of the design of conventional semen used in the first service. The specific reason for this drop in fertility in artificial insemination with sexed semen, as compared to conventional, is still unknown. Nevertheless, given the potentially negative effects of the procedures for sexing, of course it is very important to the careful handling of sexed semen to optimize fertility.

Sexed semen for commercial use, is currently stored in straws thin (0.25 mL), containing 2.1 million sperm. Although 0.25 mL straws were handled similarly to 0.5 mL, the smaller diameter makes them more sensitive to errors in handling semen. The deposition of sexed semen in the uterus of the heifer must be as fast as possible, not exceeding 5 minutes. Fertility variations found after the use of sexed semen are quite large and are determined by several factors, including error handling and storage of semen. Handle carefully sexed and consider the ongoing evaluation of procedures, because every successful artificial insemination program starts with good handling practices Semen.

7. Body condition score of females

The estimate of the nutritional status of ruminant livestock of interest by assessing body condition (BC) is a subjective measure based on the classification of animals with the coverage of the muscle and fat mass. Therefore, the body condition score (BCS) estimates the nutritional status of animals by means of visual assessment and / or tactile and represents an important tool of management. The method is fast, convenient and cheap; it reflects the energy reserves of the animals and serves as an aid in the identification of practices to be adopted in the nutritional management of the herd.

The assessment of body condition or its variation to estimate body reserves is more appropriate than the measurements of body weight, for its analysis independent of the size and physiological status of the animal. The importance of body assessment scores stems from the knowledge about the partition of nutrients according to the priority needs of the animal. The premise is to maintain life and then to preserve the species. Thus, Adams and Short (1988) proposed the following order of partition of energy nutrients: 1. basal metabolism, 2. mechanical activities, 3. growth, 4. set of basic bodily reserves of energy, 5.

ongoing maintenance of pregnancy, 6. lactation, 7. extra reserves of energy, 8. estrous cyclicity, ovulation and early pregnancy, and 9. excess reserves. Therefore, the reproductive functions, in terms of partition of nutrients, are not priorities for the animal economy (Wright & Russel, 1984).

Knowledge of body condition score herd contributes to decisions on measures of impact on production and costs of livestock development. In fact, you can set times to wean the calves or to define when and how to supplement the diet of breeders, aiming to reduce the period of postpartum anestrus (Moraes et al., 2007). Furthermore, knowing the body condition score is useful even in the prediction of productive performance (Short et al., 1996) and reproductive performance (Dunn & Moss, 1992).

The score is obtained by the visual and tactile (palpation) of the animal by a trained professional. There are scores of different scales, which vary in concept, the topology of the points of observation and animal species for which they are applied. The notes are given to animals in accordance with the amount of tissue reserves, especially fat and muscle in certain areas of the body, often associated with specific anatomic landmarks, such as certain bony protrusions, ribs, spinous processes of the spine, processes transverse spine, flank, tip of the ileum, above the tail, sacrum and lumbar vertebrae. Extreme scores 1 and 5 (obese and cachectic) are undesirable in any scale and in any animal species studied (figure 2).

The monitoring of changes in the body condition score and body weight provides information on the reproductive potential of the cows (Dunn & Moss, 1992), which is

Score 1

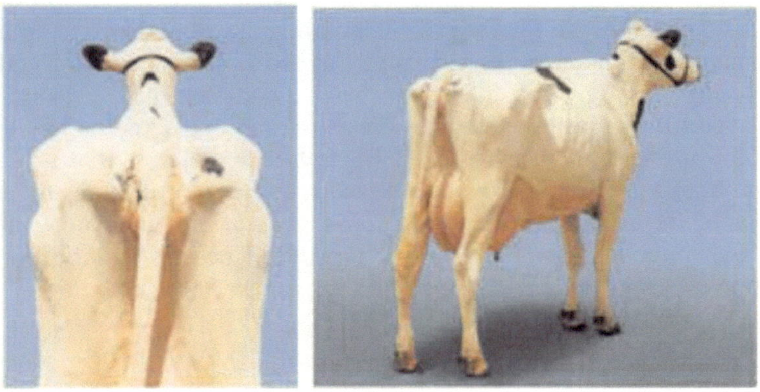

Score 2

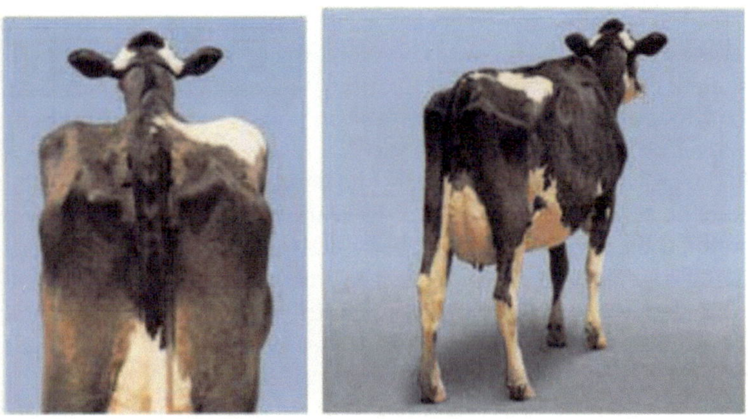

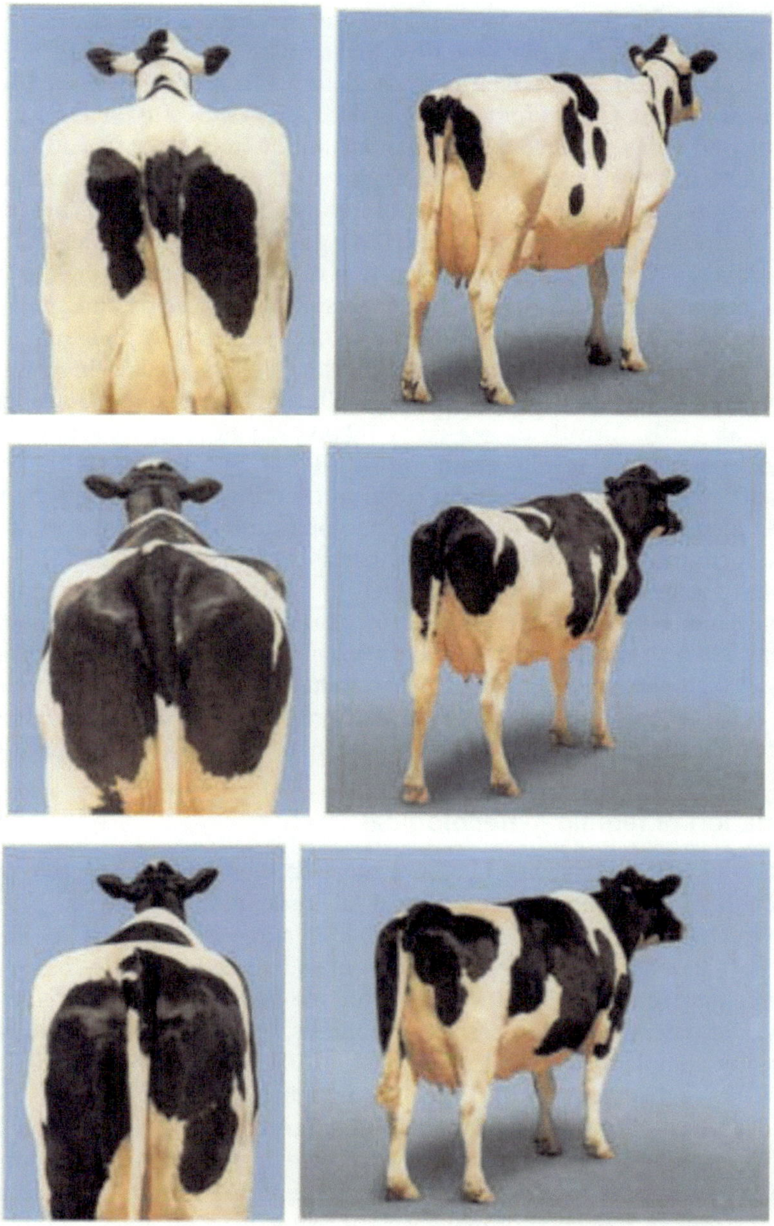

Score 3

Score 4

Score 5

Fig. 2. Body condition score of dairy cows.

directly related to nutrition in the pre-delivery and postpartum period. Kunkle et al. (1994) found that body condition score at calving and during breeding season is closely related to the interval between births, the proportion of cows not pregnant at the end of the breeding season, milk production and cow weight at weaning. Cows with body condition at calving cycle more rapidly than those with body condition score.

In cows of high milk production is expected high demand for nutrients and thus mobilization of reserves in the first three to five weeks postpartum. This phenomenon is accompanied by rapid weight loss and BCS, which submits the ovarian follicles to large metabolic changes. Such variations affect the normal development of follicles and lower levels of progesterone. This scenario is associated with reduced fertility (Butler and Smith, 1989). Indeed, Walters (2000) found that the decrease in BCS after delivery decreased by 42% the quality of oocytes collected by follicular aspiration from Holstein cows.

Vizcarra et al. (1998) inferred that the nutritional status influence postpartum luteal activity and concentrations of glucose, insulin and saturated fatty acids, which are high in cows with high body condition score at calving. According to Walters (2000), this framework explains why the delay of first ovulation in postpartum cows with negative energy balances. In fact, low plasma levels of glucose, insulin, non-esterified fatty acids and growth factor type 1 insulin are associated with inhibition of pulse frequency of luteinizing hormone and estradiol production by the dominant follicle (Walters, 2000). In cows that consume adequate dry matter during this period, follicular development is apparently normal (Staples et al., 1991). Already decreased by 1.0 point in the body condition score in these first five weeks postpartum resulted in lower fertility at first service (Britt, 1992). In contrast, over-conditioning, ie very high body condition score cows at the end of the pre-delivery caused an increase in service period and embryonic mortality (Flipot et al., 1988).

The productivity and profitability of farms are closely related to achieving high reproductive rates, which are only achieved through the adoption of certain management practices. Among these, science-based nutrition should provide the matrix of metabolic conditions ideal to meet certain strategic moments of the production cycle, such as the breeding season, the season of birth and lactation season. In this context, the body condition score is a useful tool in assessing the nutritional status of the animal and therefore has strategic application in reproductive management of herds that are artificially inseminated.

8. Evaluation of female gynecological

All females of reproductive age in a herd must be submitted to gynecological examination for selection of suitable animals for artificial insemination program. This is an internal examination by rectal palpation, ultrasound and vaginoscopy and can be complemented by laparoscopy and biopsy. On rectal palpation and ultrasonography are checked the size, consistency and contraction of the uterus, uterine horns and symmetry. In the ovaries are observed consistent form and size of follicles, cysts and persistent corpus luteum. Vaginoscopy complements rectal palpation and ultrasonography, because it turns out the shape of the vaginal portion of cervix, the opening degree of the cervical canal, mucosa color, moisture content and characteristic vaginal and cervical mucus.

The pelvic examination should be thorough, seeking to know and understand the best possible animal's reproductive status, either for a simple confirmation of pregnancy or to identify diseases or reflection of management that is harming their reproductive efficiency. Gynecological examination involves a complete evaluation of all components of the external and internal genitalia, with emphasis on the ovaries, combining the findings of the examination with a score of animal body, with its history and with the herd.

For purposes of gynecological evaluation should consider the following groups of animals: from 20 to 30 days postpartum, postpartum with abnormal vaginal discharge, irregular estrous cycles, not seen in estrus 60 days postpartum; covered or inseminated by two or more times, and that return to estrus 45 days after artificial insemination. In the historical survey of the animal should always consider the age, number of childbirths and their conditions and cyclicality observed, as these factors may reflect the ovarian function and

reproductive efficiency. Are essential, too, about the coverage, treatment for retained placenta and uterine infection, drugs and dosages, treatment outcome, nutritional program for the animals used in pre-natal and post partum, body condition at calving, stage lactation, milk production and herd health program.
It is crucial at the end of gynecological examination, classify the animals examined according to their reproductive status in pregnant and not pregnant, the latest being identified as normal or with any individual or reproductive problems reflecting a management problem. The results of gynecological examination of different groups of animals held in a coherent and detailed by a veterinarian, provides a satisfactory understanding of the breeding herd during the exam, allowing them to be defined and adopted measures to keep the reproductive efficiency of flock.

9. Diagnosis of pregnancy

Pregnancy diagnosis is an important tool for the management of rural property. This must be done by a veterinarian trained at around 28-30 days after artificial insemination by rectal palpation and / or ultrasonography. There are other methods that can be used for diagnosis of pregnancy such as: no return to service, measurement of progesterone, pregnancy-specific proteins, estrone sulfate, breast enlargement and abdominal distension. The accurate diagnosis of pregnancy is important in establishing and maintaining optimal reproductive performance. The producer should know as early as possible if the female is covered or not pregnant for it to be inseminated again.
A cow is diagnosed not pregnant if she has been observed in estrus approximately 21 days after artificial insemination. The percentage of cows not observed in estrus around this period is known as the rate of no return and is not a method to estimate pregnancy rates. As the percentage of cows ovulating truly seen in estrus is often low, the rate of return not overestimate the rates of pregnancy. If a cow is in estrus detected three weeks after artificial insemination, it can still be pregnant and her artificial insemination can cause miscarriage. One must be careful to confirm that it is true and not in heat pregnant through other methods of pregnancy diagnosis.
The detection of pregnancy by measurement of hormones, especially if they occur in milk has advantages when interference is minimal with the cow and risk-free pregnancy. The measurement of progesterone to verify pregnancy also offers the possibility of diagnosing the twenty-first day. In pregnant cows, progesterone concentrations in milk and blood remain high between the twenty-first and twenty-fourth day after ovulation, when they would be basal in the animal not pregnant. The simplest procedure is to obtain a sample of milk from the cow 21 days after artificial insemination. If the progesterone level is low, the cow is not pregnant. If the progesterone level is high, the cow may be pregnant.
The factor of early pregnancy is a gestation dependent protein complex that has been detected in the serum of various species. It is detected using an immunological technique, the rosette inhibition test. It is expected that this substance appear in the serum soon after conception and disappear very quickly after embryonic death. Two additional proteins, protein B pregnancy specific bovine and bovine pregnancy associated glycoprotein, can also be measured during early pregnancy in the cow.
The availability of ultrasound has been a major advance in the diagnosis and monitoring of pregnancy reproductive taking the advantage of not being invasive. The baby begins to fill the uterine horn near the seventeenth day of gestation and can be seen as an non-echogenic area. In the nineteenth day, the amniotic sac has expanded considerably and the lumen of

the uterus can be observed. In the twenty-second day you can hear the heartbeat with the thirtieth day embryo and fetus is very visible.
Rectal palpation of the fetus relies on the ability to detect the presence of a fetus growing in one of the uterine horns by inserting the arm into the rectum of the cow. This can be a dangerous procedure, since trauma can be generated in both the cow and the fetus and must therefore be done by a trained examiner. In non pregnant animal and the animal in early pregnancy, the uterine horns can be felt in size and approximately equal diameters. It is possible to detect a difference in the size of the two uterine horns from 35-40 days of gestation forward.
The identification of components produced by the fetus, rather than the mother, has advantages in the diagnosis of pregnancy. Estrogens are produced by the bovine fetus and the concentrations of estrone sulfate in maternal plasma increases from the seventeenth day of gestation. The content of estrone sulfate in milk reflects the plasma and estrone sulfate test positive at 15 weeks of gestation provides 100% effective diagnosis of pregnancy. In most cases, detection of non-pregnancy at this late stage is of little value in reproductive management, but can be used as a confirmatory test after diagnosis of early pregnancy.
The mammogensis or mammary gland development as a result of pregnancy can be detected in heifers as early as four months of pregnancy. Promoters like growth steroids can stimulate similar changes which may be a confounding factor. It is only during the last days of gestation, when the udder is distended with colostrum, the breast development may be regarded as accurate diagnosis of pregnancy.
The abdomen of the pregnant animal is getting distended around the seventh month of pregnancy. If a hand is pushed firmly against the right side of the abdomen, the fetus can sometimes be felt rebounding against the hand. It is not a reliable indicator of pregnancy.
Pregnancy diagnosis is a vital aid for reproductive management and must be sought the best combination of earliness and accuracy.

10. Calving rate

Cows get pregnant has always been and will remain the major challenge of cattle. Over the years many methods evaluation were developed, but, unfortunately, with the interval between data calving, days in milk at first AI, percentage of pregnant cows on visit the veterinarian and the first AI conception do not tell the whole story, that is, do not reflect reality.
Averages can leave much to be desired, especially when analyzing calving interval. Two herds may have intervals of 13 months births, but in the herd A the cows were pregnant in the early part and the remaining lactation and late lactation and few between. While in herd B pregnancies are distributed during lactation, and the vast majority of cows becomes pregnant at the beginning of lactation and the rest evenly distributed during lactation. Herd B has a performance reproductive better, but the average interval between births of the two herds is equal. The most reliable measure that reflects what is happening in the herd and has resulted in the birth of calves is the calving rate.
The calving rate is the percentage of cows calved in the total of pregnant cows at the beginning of the breeding season. Even under ideal conditions with 100% of normal cows and 100% efficiency in detection of estrus, farrowing rates will fail to reach 100%. Only 60-70% of inseminated cows produce a calf born alive and the great majority of failures occur before the second half of pregnancy. This is partly due to the failure of design and partly of embryonic or fetal death. The proportions of embryonic or fetal death are far greater than the failures in the design and the vast majority of these occurred probably by genetic

abnormalities in embryos, but this hypothesis has never been proven. The cause is probably multifactorial, involving interactions between genetics, environment and management.

11. Conclusion

The importance of reproductive efficiency in cattle production systems is directly tied to the success of a program of insemination with calving and breeding seasons predetermined. The records of fertility are complex, but must be done and constantly updated so that all steps of the breeding program of the property are met and at the end of the breeding season, is to obtain good rates with many calves born alive. This chapter dealt with the main steps for the success of a program of artificial insemination, and if they are properly followed, the breeding season will be profitable.

12. References

Baruselli, P.S.; Reis, E.L.; Carvalho, N.A.T. & Carvalho, J.B.P. ECG increase ovulation rate and plasmatic progesterone concentration in Nelore (Bos indicus) heifers treated with progesterone releasing device. In: International Congress on Animal Reproduction, 2004.

Britt, J. H. Impacts of early postpartum metabolism on follicular development and fertility. *Bovine Proceedings*, vol. 24, pp. 39-43, 1992.

Butler, W.R. & Smith, R.D. Interrelationships between energy balance and postpartum reproductive function in dairy cattle. *Journal of Dairy Science*. vol. 72, pp. 767-783, 1989. ISSN 0022-0302.

Caraviello, D.Z.; Weigel, K.A.; Fricke, P.M.; Wiltbank, M.C.; Florent, M.J.; Cook, N.B.; Nordlund, K.V.; Zwald, N.R. & Rawson. C.L. Survey of management practices on reproductive performance of dairy cattle on large U.S. commercial farms. *Journal of Dairy Science*. vol. 89, pp. 4723-4735, 2006. ISSN 0022-0302.

Chebel, R.C., Santos, J.E.P.; Cerri, R.L.A.; Rutigliano, H.M. & Bruno, R.G.S. Reproduction in dairy cows following progesterone insert presynchronization and resynchronization protocols. *Journal of Dairy Science*. vol. 89, pp. 4205-4219, 2006. ISSN 0022-0302.

Dunn, T.G. & Moss, G.E. Effects of nutrient deficiencies and excesses on reproductive efficiency of livestock. *Journal of Animal Science*. vol. 70, pp. 1580-1593, 1992. ISSN 0021-8812.

Embrapa. Planejamento Sanitário de Gado de Corte. Available in http://www.cnpgc.embrapa.br. Access in: 07 de Abril de 2011.

Flipot, P.M.; Roy, G.L. & Dufour, J.J. Effect of peripartum energy concentration on production performance of Holstein cows. *Journal of Dairy Science*, vol. 71, pp. 1840-50, 1988. ISSN 0022-0302.

Galina, C.S.; Orihuela, A. & Bubio, I. Behavioural trends affecting oestrus detection in Zebu cattle. *Animal Reproduction Science*. vol. 42, pp. 465-470, 1996. ISBN 0378-4320.

Geary, T.W.; Ansotegui, R.P.; Roberts, A.J.; Waterman, R.C. Macneil, M.D.; Grings, E.E.; Thompson, B.D. & Lipsey, R.J. Effects of Flunixin Meglumini on pregnancy establishment in beef cattle. Proc. West. Sec. Am. Soc. *Journal of Animal Science*. vol. 56, pp.309-311, 2005. ISBN 0021-8812.

Geary, T.W.; Downing, E.R.; Bruemmer, J.E. & Whitthier, J.C. Ovarian and estrous response of suckled beef cows to the Select Synch estrous synchronization protocol. Prof. *Journal of Animal Science*. vol. 16, pp. 1-5, 2000. ISBN 0021-8812.

Helmer, SD & Britt, JH. Mounting behavior as affected by stage of Estrous cycle in Holstein heifers. *Journal of Dairy Science*. vol. 68, pp. 1290-1296, 1985. ISSN 0022-0302.

Kunkle, W.E.; Sand, R.S. & Era, D.O. Effect of body condition on productivity in beef cattle. In: Fields, M.J. & Sands, R.S. (Ed.). Factors affecting calf crop. Boca Raton: CRC Press, 1994.

Lopez, H.Z.W.; Satter, L.D & Wiltbank, M.C. Effect of dietary phosphorus concentration on estrous behavior of lactating dairy cows. Theriogenology, vol. 61 pp. 437-445, 2004. ISSN 0093-691X.

Lucy, M.C. Reproductive loss in high-producing dairy cattle: Where will it end *Journal of Dairy Science*. vol. 84, pp. 1277-1293, 2001. ISSN 0022-0302.

Mizuta, K. Estudo comparativo dos aspectos comportamentais do estro e dos teores plasmáticos de LH, FSH, progesterona e estradiol que precedem a ovulação em fêmeas bovinas Nelore (Bos taurus indicus), Angus (Bos taurus taurus) e Nelore X Angus (Bos taurus indicus X Bos taurus taurus). 2003. 98 f. Tese (Doutorado em Reprodução Animal) - Faculdade de Medicina Veterinária e Zootecnia, Universidade e São Paulo, São Paulo, 2003.

Moraes, J.C.F.; Jaume, C.M. & Souza, C.J.H. Reproductive management of beef cow. *Journal of Animal Reproduction*, vol. 31, n. 2, pp. 160-166, 2007.

Pinheiro, O.L.; Barros, C.M.; Figueredo, R.A.; Valle, E.R.; Encarnação, R.O. & Padovani, C.R. Estrous behavior and the estrus-to-ovulation interval in Nelore cattle (Bos indicus) with natural estrus or estrus induced with prostaglandin F2 alpha or norgestomet and estradiol valerate. *Theriogenology*, vol. 49, pp. 667-81, 1998. ISSN 0093-691X.

Santos, K.J.G. Estação de monta: Técnica para Melhorar e Eficiência Reprodutiva. Jornal das Cidades. São Luis Montes Belos-GO. 2003.

Short, R.E. & Adams, D.C. Nutritional and hormonal interrelationships in beef cattle reproduction. *Journal of Animal Science*, vol. 68, pp. 29-39, 1988. ISSN 0021-8812.

Short, R.E.; Grings, E.E.; MacNeill, M.D.; Heitschimidt, R.K. & Haferkamp, M.R. Effects of supplement, and sire breed of calf during fall grazing period on cow and calf performance. *Journal of Animal Science*, vol. 74, pp. 1701-1710, 1996. ISSN 0021-8812.

Staples, C.R.; Burke, J.M. & Tatcher, W.W. Influence of supplemental fats on reproductive tissues and performance of lactating cows. *Journal of Dairy Science*. 81: 856-871. 1998. ISSN 0022-0302.

Staples, C.R.; Lucy, F.M.; Michael, M.C. & Thatcher, W.W. Energy balance and size and number of ovarian follicles detected by ultrasonography in early postpartum cows. *Journal of Dairy Science*, vol. 74, pp. 473-482, 1991. ISSN 0022-0302.

Stevenson, J.S. Reproductive management of dairy cows in high milk-producing herds. *Journal of Dairy Science*. vol. 84, pp. 128-143, 2001. ISSN 0022-0302.

Stevenson, J.S.; Kobayashi, Y. & Thompson, K.E. Reproductive performance of dairy cows in various programmed breeding systems including Ovsynch and combination of gonadrotopin-releasing hormone and prostaglandin F2. *Journal of Dairy Science*. vol. 82, pp. 506-515, 1999. ISSN 0022-0302.

Tenhagen, B.A.; Drillich, M.; Surholt, R. & Heuwieser, W. Comparison of timed AI after synchronized ovulation to AI at estrus: Reproductive and economic considerations. *Journal of Dairy Science*. vol. 87, pp. 85-94, 2004. ISSN 0022-0302.

Vailes, L.D., & Britt, J.H. Influence of footing surface on mounting and other sexual behaviors of estrual Holstein cows. *Journal of Animal Science*. vol. 68, pp. 2333-2339, 1990. ISSN 0021-8812.

Walters, A.H. Analysis of early lactation reproductive characteristics in holstein cows. 2000. 83 p. Thesis (M. Sc. in Dairy Science) – Virginia Polytechnic Institute and State University, Blacksburg, Virginia.

Wright, I.A. & Russel, A.J.F. Partition of fat, body composition and body condition score in mature cows. *Animal Production*, Edinburgh, vol. 38, pp. 23-32, 1984.

11

Management Factors Affecting Fertility in Sheep

Pilar Santolaria, Inmaculada Palacin and Jesús Yániz
Instituto Universitario de Ciencias Ambientales y Departamento de Producción Animal y Ciencia de los Alimentos. Escuela Politécnica Superior, Huesca
Universidad de Zaragoza
Spain

1. Introduction

An Arab horse breeder in the early 13th century carried out the first insemination reported, by trapping stallion semen in wool placed in the vagina of a mare and transferring this to the vagina of another mare (Heape, 1898). Later, in 1780, an Italian priest and physiologist named Lazzaro Spallanzani performed artificial insemination with dog semen, and revolutionised the way scientists thought. Since then, scientist and farmers have striven to improve this technology, motivated by the benefits that could be achieved. Sheep is one of the species subsequently linked to this technology and in which many questions still remain to be resolved to improve fertility. However, the potential impact of this technique on the genetic progress of sheep is high and further studies are needed to improve its efficiency.

In Spain, artificial insemination programmes in sheep are linked to the genetic selection schemes of the breeds, but it has not been successfully integrated with reproductive technology on farms as happen in sows or cows. The technical difficulty and weak fertility, ranged between 15 to 60 % for pregnancy rate, limits its application. In Spain, most commercial programmes use refrigerated semen (15 degrees C) by superficial intracervical deposition (cervical), whereas the use of frozen-thawed semen by intrauterine deposition (laparoscopy) is more restricted. Cervical insemination with fresh semen is the main method chosen due to its simplicity and satisfactory results. With the aim of improving its efficiency, this paper focuses on identifying the main management effects affecting AI results when this technology is applied.

2. Female associated factors

Management factors associated with artificial insemination in the ewe can modify fertility. In reproductive planning, intervals between lambings, season, age of ewe, heat stress, nutrition state or breed are some of the factors which have a great effect on fertility results. David et al. (2008), using a joint model combining two main traits, one relative to female and the other relative to the male, reported that the main variation factors of AI success were relative to non-sex-specific effects and to female effect, suggesting that choosing females to inseminate might slightly improve the AI results.

2.1 Season

Seasonal variations are described as a limiting factor in sheep reproduction. In natural conditions, seasonality, which is mediated by photoperiod, modifies hormonal balance and causes seasonal reproductive variations in sheep (Karsch, et al. 1984; Yeates, 1949), giving rise to a decrease in reproductive activity during long days (anoestrous season). Photoperiodic information is translated into neuroendocrine changes through variations in melatonin secretion from the pineal gland (Bittman, et al., 1983). Melatonin, secreted in pineal gland, triggers variations in the secretion of luteinising hormone-releasing hormone (GnRH), luteinising hormone (LH) and follicle stimulating hormone (FSH) (Arendt, et al., 1983, Karsch, et al., 1984). In any case, seasonal changes in reproductive activity are clearly defined in sheep breeds from high latitudes (>40º)(Pelletier, et al., 1987), where the differences in daylight duration between short days and long days are more notable.

As in natural mating, season affects fertility after AI, although hormonal treatment is used to synchronise and induce oestrus. Windsor (1995) reported low cervical AI fertility rates in non-breeding season in Merino ewes, a shallow seasonal breed. According to this, Anel et al. (2005) found a season effect on the AI fertility in Churra ewes, which was more important in cervical than laparoscopic artificial insemination. In cervical AI, semen is deposited in the external portion of the cervix and the sperm transport is affected by cervical mucus quality. Theses authors suggest that photoperiod could alter progestagens and so cervical mucus characteristics, making it scarcer and more viscous. In consequence, sperm transport in the cervix can be interfered with. It is important to note that seasonality affects the ram reproductive parameters in the same way and changes in seminal quality during anoestrous season may decrease the fertility results after AI.

Moreover, subcutaneous melatonin implants are widely used to bring the breeding season forward and improve reproductive performance in non-breeding season (Chemineau, et al., 1991; Haresign, et al., 1990). Melatonin treatments act by mimicking a short-day-like response (O'Callaghan, et al., 1991) and induce oestrus during the non-breeding season. Not only an increase in the percentage of pregnant ewes (fertility) has been described after melatonin implant treatment in anoestrous season, but also the number of lambs born per ewe (litter size) (Abecia, et al., 2007; Arrebola, et al., 2009; Chemineau, et al., 1992). This improvement could be due to a higher rate of embryonic survival, an improvement in luteal function or a reduction in the antiluteolytic mechanisms (Abecia, et al., 2008). In AI, a fertility rate increase has been reported with melatonin implant treatments (Laliotis, et al., 1998; Legaz, et al., 2000) after cervical AI.

2.2 Age

Another important factor affecting fertility after cervical AI is ewe age. In comparison with adult ewes, young and maiden ewes have lower fertility, probably due to impaired sperm transport combined with low mucus production in the cervical canals during oestrus (Selaive-Villarroel & Kennedy, 1983a, b). After that, most studies have described a decrease in AI success with increasing female age. Shackell et al. (1990), predicted 2-3% fertility reduction per year of age for different breeds. Esmailizadeh et al., (2009) reported that as the age of the ewes increased from 2 to 7 years, the proportion of barren ewes significantly decreased from 29 to 5%. In a more recent study in the Spanish Churra dairy breed, Anel et al. (2005), described how, after 1.5 years of age, the lambing rate decreased by 1.74% per year for cervical AI. The highest rates of fertility declining with age were described in the Lacaune breed by Colas et al. (1973), who reported a drop in fertility of 15% per year.

Paulenz et al. (2007), observed that the age of the ewes had a significant effect on the non-return rate, but not on lambing rate, whereas in Fukui et al. (2010), both the pregnancy and lambing rates in the ewes significantly declined as age increased. The detrimental effect of increased fertility age could be explained by the fact that aged ewes have increased risks of reproductive disorders and decreased ovulation rates with quality ovulated oocytes compared with younger ewes.

The question is: what is the optimal age for cervical AI? Alabart et al. (2002) , studied the influence of age on fertility in a total of 3819 Rasa Aragonesa ewes aged 1 to 12 years. In this study, maximum fertility (56.7%) was observed at 3 years, and ewes aged from 2 to 5 years (79.5% of the inseminated ewes) had mean fertility values above 50%. These results partially confirm the observations by Colas et al. (1973), who reported a significant decrease in the fertility of ewes inseminated when over 3.5 years old, and Gabiña and Folch (1987), who observed a strong fall in the fertility of ewes inseminated at 4 or more years of age. Anel et al. (2005) recorded the best fertility rates in ewes aged between 1.5 and 4.5 years; beyond this age, fertility declined remarkably. Fertility also decreased depending on the number of previous parturitions. In other studies, the maximum fertility was obtained at around 2 years of age, with a progressive fall afterwards (Fantova, et al., 1998). It may be concluded that insemination groups should be made up of 2 to 5 year old ewes while younger and older ewes should be used for natural mating.

2.3 Lambing-AI interval

The need for a resting period for the ewe after lambing to allow uterine involution is well known. However, sometimes the increasing reproductive rate imposed by the demanding production system involves short resting periods from lambing to AI, which affects fertility in a negative way. According to Bodin et al. (1999), reducing the lambing-AI interval to below 40-50 days induces a significant decrease in fertility, even after natural mating. Most authors recommend not inseminating ewes any sooner than 50 days post-partum (Anel, et al., 2005).

2.4 Breed

Ewe breed is also a significant source of variation in fertility after AI (Donovan, et al., 2004; Fukui, et al., 2007; Papadopoulos, et al., 2005; Salamon & Maxwell, 1995). Differences in the mean time of ovulation and ovulation rates in different breeds of ewes at differences locations may explain the variation in fertility (Salamon & Maxwell, 1995).

Alternatively, variation may be due to differences in the morphometric characteristics of the cervix (Eppleston, et al., 1994). In this sense, Kaabi et al. (2006), carried out a morphometric study in four ovine breeds (Assaf, Churra, Castellana and Merino) showing important differences in length, width, number of folds and distance between folds, which originates breed variations in the depth of catheter penetration into the cervix during AI. In this study, the breeds yielding lower fertility after AI resulted in higher cervical complexity, and achieved a lesser degree of cervical penetration of the catheter during cervical AI. As explained below, different studies have found a positive correlation between cervical AI depth and fertility (Kaabi, et al., 2006).

2.5 Body weight and body condition score

For an adequate response in a breeding programme, ewes must be suitably nourished and maintained in good body condition. Clearly, ewes with a good nutrient intake respond most rapidly to the onset of the breeding season and continue to respond with an increase in ovulation rate (Keisler & Buckrell, 1997). Flushing is understood as the rapid increase in ovulation rate of ewes receiving a nutrient supplementation before mating. Under harsher nutritional conditions in the semi-arid southern Mediterranean region, where regular food supply is not guaranteed, lambing and twinning rates were shown to be boosted following nutritional flushing (Younis, et al., 1978; Landau & Molle, 1997; Branca, et al., 2000) or when the live weights of the ewes were higher at mating (Gunn & Doney, 1979, Thomson & Bahhady, 1988).

However, Lassoued et al. (2004), showed important interactions between genotype and level of nutrition. In this sense, in highly prolific ewes like D'Man breed, higher levels of nutrition prior to and during mating were associated with improved reproductive performance, but in low prolific breeds such as Queue Fine de l'Ouest, neither ovulation rate nor lambing rate were affected by the dietary treatment. In a recent work by Fukui et al. (2010) body weight did not significantly affect fertility.

Body condition score (BCS) has proved useful as a management tool for subjectively assessing the nutritional status of ewes. In this way, body condition directly affects hypothalamic activity and GnRH secretion, but not pituitary sensitivity to GnRH, and these effects on reproductive performance are also mediated through changes in ovarian hormones or in hypothalamo-pituitary sensitivity to ovarian hormones (Rhind, et al., 1989). The effect of body condition on the ovulation rate of ewes has been extensively reported (Ducker & Boyd, 1977; Morley, et al., 1978; Adalsteinsson, 1979; Gunn & Doney, 1979; Gonzalez, et al., 1997). High body condition score has been associated with an increase of ovulation (Rhind, et al., 1989; Xu, et al., 1989), especially in Mediterranean breeds at the beginning of the breeding season (Forcada, et al., 1992). Most authors recommend a BCS of 2.5 to 3.0 either for natural or artificially breeding (Contreras-Solis, et al., 2009; Husein & Ababneh, 2008). In a study carried out in inseminated Rasa Aragonesa ewes (Bru, et al., 1995), the lowest pregnancy rates (32,7 %) were obtained in sheep with a BCS<2, the average values (48.3%) with BCS between 3 and 2 and the higher values (58.8%) when BCS was >3. The importance of BCS in fertility has been also reported in Spanish Manchega breed (Montoro, 1995).

Fukui et al. (2010), , concluded that body nutritional condition is an important factor, next to ewe age, influencing the fertility of ewes after AI regardless of body weight. Nulliparous ewes less than 3 years old and with a BCS of more than 3.0 are expected to have higher fertility than other types of ewes.

2.6 Farm/Herd

Different ewe farms have different management practices and this may have an impact on fertility after AI. Reproductive planning (intervals between lambings, season, age of first mating, AI technique, etc.) and animal handling (feeding, health, preparation of AI lots, etc.) have a great effect on fertility results (Anel, et al., 2005). The significant effect of the farm has been described in several studies (Anel, et al., 2005, Fantova, et al., 1999, Paulenz, et al., 2002).Thus, in order to improve fertility results, handling conditions on farms must be improved, along with more widespread use of AI techniques.

The geographical area where the farm is located may also have an influence on the success of AI. In a recent study carried out in north-eastern Spain (Palacin et al., 2011), data from 18.528 AI in Rasa Aragonesa ewes belonging to a selection scheme with similar management were recorded in order to analyse the effect of farm geographical location and the theoretical time distance between the farm and insemination centre on the fertility after cervical AI. An average fertility of 54.3% was observed, with significant differences among the 14 regions studied. Fertility rates higher than 60% were found in the northern regions near the Pyrenees Mountains and the lowest results (38.5-48.3%) were obtained in the southern regions. The average time distance of these regions did not differ. The regions nearest to the insemination centre, with similar climatic conditions, showed medium fertility rate (54.0-57.8%). These results showed a huge variability after insemination, taking into account the geographical location of the farm.

2.7 Heat stress

It has been reported than in tropical and sub-tropical areas the local sheep show restricted sexual activity in the summer months (Marai et al., 2004). Marai et al., 2007 reviewed how exposure to high ambient temperature causes impairment of reproductive functions in sheep. The heat effect is aggravated when heat stress is accompanied with high ambient humidity (Marai et al., 2000, 2004, 2006, 2007). Heat stress evokes a series of drastic changes in animal biological functions, which include a decrease in feed intake efficiency and use, disturbances in the metabolism of water, protein, energy and mineral balances, enzymatic reactions, hormonal secretions and blood metabolites. (Shelton, 2000; Marai et al., 2006).

2.8 Synchronization treatment

Oestrous synchronisation and ovulation induction treatments are widely spread in AI in order to control the optimum insemination time. Oestrous behaviour in small ruminants is not clearly shown, so treatments are needed to prevent an asynchrony between ovulation and insemination time, which may be the commonest cause of failure of artificial insemination programmes (Jabbour & Evans, 1991).

Synchronisation treatments are a useful tool not only for AI programmes but also in natural mating, particularly to ensure lambing in anoestrous season. However, many studies report that synchronisation causes reduced fertility after cervical AI (Robinson, et al., 1970; Hawk, 1971) and after natural mating (Quinliva.Td & Robinson, 1969; Hawk & Conley, 1975; Allison & Kelly, 1978). Different hormonal treatments have been used in the control of sheep reproduction, but progestagen analogues (fluorogestone acetate and medroxyprogesterone acetate) are the most commonly used to induce and synchronise oestrus in natural mating or AI of small ruminants (Lunstra & Christenson, 1981; Pearce & Robinson, 1985; Langford, et al., 1982; Baril, et al., 1993, Greyling, et al., 1997). Progestagens produce a mimetic effect of the luteal phase of the oestrous cycle and a sudden progestagen removal followed by administration of an equine chorionic gonadotropin (eCG) dose (FSH- and LH-like stimulation) induces oestrous activity. Currently, intravaginal progestagen-impregnated devices (sponges or CIDR) for 12-14days followed by administration of 250-500IU eCG has been proposed (Abecia, et al., 2011) as a synchronised treatment in sheep, in which insemination can be performed from 47h (intrauterine) to 55 (cervical) hours after device removal.

Although long-term progestagen treatment results in efficient oestrous synchronisation, high variability has been reported in fertility (Vinoles, et al., 2001; Menchaca & Rubianes, 2004;). Progestagen treatment appears to result in an asynchrony between oestrus and ovulation (Scaramuzzi, et al., 1988; Sirois & Fortune, 1990) and reduce sperm transport through the cervix (Killen & Caffery, 1982; Armstrong & Evans, 1984; Pearce & Robinson, 1985). Other studies have reported lower fertility rate caused by the negative effect of long-term progesterone treatment on oocyte development (Vinoles, et al., 2001; Menchaca & Rubianes, 2004) related to subluteal progesterone levels.

According to this, recent research efforts are focused on shortening synchronisation treatments. Shortening treatment (5-6days) with different progestagen devices seems to be enough to achieve efficient oestrous synchronisation in natural mounting both during the anoestrous season (Ungerfeld & Rubianes, 1999) and in breeding season (Vinoles, et al., 1999; Ustuner, et al., 2007) with a similar fertility rate to long-term treatment. Nevertheless, the interval between progestagen device withdrawal and the onset of oestrus was shortened (Ungerfeld & Rubianes, 1999; Vinoles, et al., 2001; Zeleke, et al., 2005; Ustuner, et al., 2007) due to a delay in corpus luteus regression in cyclic ewes (Menchaca & Rubianes, 2004). This asynchrony could decrease the success of artificial insemination programmes, so a treatment that ensures an acceptable luteolysis seems to be necessary to enhance the oestrous synchronisation (Ustuner, et al., 2007).

The luteolytic effect of prostaglandin $F_{2\alpha}$ ($PGF_{2\alpha}$) (McCracke, et al., 1972) and its analogues has been used to control corpus luteus activity. In goats, the use of a short-term progestagen protocol combined with $PGF_{2\alpha}$ administered at progestagen sponge insertion time was successful in artificial insemination with frozen-thawed semen (Corteel, et al., 1988). In sheep, Beck et al (1993) reported acceptable oestrous synchronisation and fertility results in natural mating using $PGF_{2\alpha}$ treatment combined with short-term progestagen. Nowadays, $PGF_{2\alpha}$ treatment use in small ruminant reproduction control has increased because of narrow restrictions on the use of progestagens in animal production both in the United States and the European Union (Martin, et al., 2004; Menchaca & Rubianes, 2004). $PGF_{2\alpha}$ is quickly metabolised with a minimum residue level (Light, et al., 1994). In some South American countries, short progestagen treatment with $PGF_{2\alpha}$ administration is used in goat management (Menchaca & Rubianes, 2004). However, the effectiveness of $PGF_{2\alpha}$ or its analogues depends on the ovary status (Houghton, et al., 1995) and is not very useful during the anoestrous season (Acritopoulou & Haresign, 1980). Moreover, a varied response and low pregnancy rates in AI have been reported with single $PGF_{2\alpha}$ treatment or progestagen combined (Boland, et al., 1978; Hackett, et al., 1981; Olivera-Muzante, et al., 2011), so with the current methods it is not an appropriate synchronisation treatment for AI unless previous oestrous detection is carried out.

Another factor affecting fertility after cervical AI related with hormonal synchronisation is the development of anti-eCG antibodies. Females involved in repeated treatment throughout their reproductive life, particularly those involved in AI genetic programmes or intensive lambing systems, develop anti-eCG antibodies (Baril, et al., 1996; Bodin, et al., 1997; Roy, et al., 1999). These antibodies are associated with low reproductive rates, especially in fixed time AI in sheep (Maurel, et al., 2003) and goats (Baril, et al., 1996), and in multiple ovulated ewes (Forcada, et al., 2011). This is less pronounced when repeated treatment is combined with natural mating. High concentrations of anti-eCG antibodies are reported with a lack or delay in oestrus and pre-ovulatory LH surge (Baril, et al., 1993; Roy, et al., 1999; Maurel, et al., 2003), decreasing the fertility after AI.

Alternatives for reproductive activity control that ensure optimum oestrous synchronisation and successful AI results are needed in sheep, in line with current demands in public and animal welfare.

3. Male associated factors

The ram may greatly influence fertility results after cervical AI. It has been reported that variation in fertility of ram ejaculates exists independently of the sperm quality (Choudhry, et al., 1995; Paulenz, et al., 2002). Variations in the fertility of rams have been reported after cervical inseminations with fresh semen (Anel, et al., 2005; Paulenz, et al., 2002), with frozen semen (Colas, 1979; Windsor, 1997; Soderquist, et al., 1999; Paulenz, et al., 2005, 2007) and after laparoscopic inseminations with frozen semen (Eppleston et al., 1986; Maxwell, 1986; Eppleston, et al., 1991; Eppleston & Maxwell, 1995). In a large scale epidemiological study, Anel et al. (2005) observed that the male factor significantly influenced fertility. Despite the restrictions in the choice of ejaculates, the authors found important differences in fertility among rams, particularly when cervical AI with cooled semen was used. Salamon and Maxwell (1995) proposed that ram differences in fertility could be both genetic and environmental, whereas ejaculate differences are probably due to nutrition, management and previous frequency of ejaculation.

Whereas differences in fertility have been demonstrated among fertile males in different species, the causes of these differences remain unclear (Ostermeier, et al., 2001). Saacke et al. (1988, 1994) have suggested in bulls that factors associated with semen quality which affect fertility can be classified as either compensable or non-compensable. It was suggested that the effects of compensable factors on fertility might be sensitive to the number of sperm inseminated, whereas those of non-compensable factors were not. As the number of sperm inseminated increases, fertility increases until a plateau is reached (den Daas, 1992). At this point, compensable factors no longer have an effect on fertility. Commercial insemination of ovine in Mediterranean Countries provides at least the plateau number of sperm in an insemination dose. It is thus the non-compensable factors that contribute most to the fertility level of a ram. A non-compensable defect in sperm would be one in which a sperm reaches the fertilisation site and initiates the egg activation process, but fails to sustain zygotic, embryonic, or foetal development (Ostermeier, et al., 2001). Evidence of such defects in sperm has been described in bulls with fertility differences (Eid, et al., 1994). Likely candidates for non-compensable factors would be incorrectly assembled chromatin or damaged DNA within the sperm nucleus. It seems logical to assume that the transfer of a complete and intact DNA molecule from sperm to ovum is crucial to obtain fertilisation with certain prospects of success. It is well-known that the presence of defects in the genetic material, such as anomalies in chromatin condensation related with the sperm maturation process, the integrity of the DNA molecule associated with the presence of breaks both of single and double DNA strands, or the presence of chromosomal anomalies, are closely associated with infertility (Aravindan, et al., 1997).

Season

Although seasonality is less marked in male than in female, changes in testicular volume, hormonal profiles, sexual behaviour and semen quality that affect the reproductive performance of rams have been reported (Casao, et al., 2010a). In this sense, the treatment of rams with slow release implants of melatonin during the non-breeding season accounted for increased scrotal diameter and improved the reproductive performance of ewes inseminated during anoestrus with semen from these melatonin-implanted males. A direct beneficial action of melatonin on sperm motility (Casao, et al., 2010c) and on other ram sperm characteristics during the non-breeding season has recently been demonstrated, with decreased apoptotic-like changes and modulating capacitation and fertilisation rates (Casao, et al., 2010b).

Nutrition

Several studies on nutrition in rams have demonstrated that diet may have an effect on testis size and sperm production (Brown, 1994). It also has been described that specific components of the diet, such as Vitamin E, may have a positive effect in increasing semen quality and quantity (Yue, et al., 2010). The effect of diet of the rams on the reproductive success of ewes after AI remains to be determined.

4. Artificial insemination-associated techniques

Inadequate semen preservation and difficulty in passing through the cervix during AI are the major obstacles to the extensive use of cooled or cryopreserved semen in sheep AI programmes (Yaniz, et al., 2010, 2011). Exo-cervical deposition of diluted liquid ram semen, preserved at 15° C for less than 8 h, is currently the AI technique predominantly used in the Mediterranean countries (Lopez-Saez, et al., 2000; Yaniz, et al., 2010, 2011).

4.1 Semen collection

4.1.1 Semen collection frequency

Semen collection frequency may have an impact on sperm quality. Long abstinence periods (Pascual, 1993) and successive ejaculations (Ollero et al., 1994) have been associated with membrane alterations of spermatozoa. A decrease in semen volume and sperm concentration with successive ejaculations has been reported in several studies (Ollero et al., 1996; Kaya et al., 2002). In the study by Ollero et al. (1996), the maximum proportion of viable cells was obtained in the second ejaculate after an abstinence period of 3 days. The authors concluded that the use of the second and/or a mixture of second and third ejaculates would improve the results in artificial insemination. The general recommendation is to establish a routine of semen collection, for example of two-three times per week (two collections per day/per ram) on different and non-consecutive days, independently of the use of the semen obtained. Increased semen collection frequency may have an effect on sperm quality and the composition of the seminal plasma (Kaya et al., 2002), although it remains to be determined whether this has an impact on field fertility. In this sense, the procedure of taking one or two collections per day from each ram during the working week (Monday-Friday), with a 2-day rest period during the weekend, has been described in Ireland (Gordon, 1997).

4.1.2 Hygienic conditions

Semen collection in farm animal species is not a sterile procedure, and some degree of contamination with bacteria cannot be avoided (Clément et al., 1995; Varner et al., 1998; Althouse et al., 2000; Thibier and Guerin, 2000; Althouse and Lu, 2005; Aurich and Spergser, 2007; Bielanski, 2007; Yániz et al., 2010). In rams, semen is usually collected with an open-ended artificial vagina, which may be contaminated with bacteria from the surface of the penis and prepuce, collection area, equipment and people. As a consequence, bacteria might compromise semen quality during storage and contaminate the female's reproductive tract. We have recently described that ram semen is normally colonised by a variety of microorganisms that may reduce semen preservation and fertility (Yániz et al., 2010). In particular, the contamination of ram semen with enterobacterial species reduced sperm quality during storage at 15 °C in a concentration-dependent manner.

Different strategies may be taken to minimise the effects of bacterial contamination on extended semen, as the bacterial concentration remains below a threshold level, so fertility is not affected (Althouse et al., 2000). The first and most viable option is to enhance the hygienic measures during semen collection and processing. Dilution of the ejaculates with sterile diluents will further decrease the concentration of contaminants (Bielanski, 2007), although this aspect has low influence in ovine because of the high sperm concentration employed for AI. Finally, control of bacterial growth is usually performed by the use of semen extenders containing antibiotics with broad-spectrum bactericidal or bacteriostatic activity (Maxwell and Salamon, 1993; Salamon and Maxwell, 2000). Perhaps too much reliance is often placed on this method of bacterial control in ovine semen. In this species, necessarily short storage periods for semen determine that the control of bacterial multiplication may be less important than in other animal species in which successful long-life semen extenders have been developed. Interestingly, in a recent study (Yániz et al., 2010), it was observed that 13% of identified bacteria were simultaneously resistant to penicillin and streptomycin, the most common preservative antibiotic combination used in ovine semen extenders, whereas *E. coli* , the bacteria with the highest impact on sperm quality, was frequently resistant to both antibiotics (31.7 %, 13/41). Antibiotics with higher antimicrobial activities were gentamycin and ceftiofur, and their inclusion in ram semen diluents should be considered.

4.2 Semen evaluation

Semen evaluation is a useful tool in the selection of males and ejaculates for assisted reproduction. Traditional evaluation techniques, based on the subjective assessment of parameters such as sperm motility and morphology, semen volume or concentration, have long been employed in the diagnosis of male subfertility and sterility (Verstegen et al., 2002). An *in vitro* system that could accurately predict field fertility would facilitate stricter selection of AI rams with regard to the semen quality and would provide a valuable tool for increasing conception rate (Donovan et al., 2004). However, finding a laboratory test reliable enough to predict the potential fertility of a given semen sample or a given sire for AI is still considered utopian, as indicated by the modest correlations seen between results obtained in vitro and field fertility (Rodríguez-Martínez, 2003). Male fertility is complex, and depends upon a heterogeneous population of spermatozoa interacting at various levels of the female genital tract, the vestments of the oocyte, and the oocyte itself (Rodríguez-Martínez, 2003). For this reason, laboratory assessment of semen must include the testing of as many relevant sperm attributes for fertilisation and embryo development as possible, not only in individual spermatozoa but also within a large sperm population (Rodríguez-Martínez, 2003). In practice, routine sperm analysis requires fast, objective and accessible methods of assessing different aspects of sperm viability (Yániz et al., 2008). In this sense, the common use of computer-assisted sperm analysis (CASA) methods for sperm motility, of image analysis for the evaluation of membrane integrity (Yániz et al., 2008), of DNA fragmentation with sperm chromatin diffusion techniques (SCD), (Gosalvez et al., 2008; López-Fernández et al., 2008), or fluorimetry, etc., would theoretically improve the predictive capacity of semen analysis, although more studies are needed to determine the utility of these techniques in the practical use of AI.

4.3 Sperm number per AI dose

The difficulty in passing through the cervix during AI due to the type of cervical canal found in this species determines that semen can only be deposited inside the cervix, usually

in the external portion. The retention capacity of the ovine cervix is very low (0,1-0,2 ml) (Gordon , 1997), whereas a large sperm number per dose is required to compensate the huge barrier effect of the cervix (around 400 x 10^6 sperm/dose in Spanish AI).
It is important to determine the minimal sperm dose per insemination in order to maximise the genetic diffusion of males, without decreasing AI success. In the study by Langford and Marcus (1982), fertility after insemination of 400 or 200 x 10^6 spermatozoa was similar to that observed after natural service at progestagen-induced oestrus. However, when less than or equal to 100 x 10^6 spermatozoa were inseminated, fertility fell markedly and the number of lambs per ewe inseminated decreased. These data indicate that insemination of 200 x 10^6 spermatozoa, i.e. less than 10% of the number in a single ram ejaculate, allows normal conception rates in progestagen-treated ewes. It seems that the minimal sperm dose may be between more than 100 and 200 x 10^6 (120 million sperm in Australian works, Gordon, 1997), although a breed-effect should not be discarded, as differences in the cervix anatomy have been described.

4.4 Semen preservation

4.4.1 Diluents

Despite numerous past efforts to improve semen diluents, few new additives have been introduced in the extender composition for ram semen (Yániz et al., 2005). Biological components such as milk or egg yolk in the diluent have not really been effective in the applied use for AI. So, for example, skimmed milk, a complex and variable biological component, is still the main diluent used to preserve sheep semen at 15 °C for AI in numerous countries (López-Sáez et al., 2000; Yániz et al., 2011). The basic components of semi-synthetic diluents for the liquid storage of ram semen (buffers combined with sugars and egg yolk), have changed little since those first used in the early 20th century (Maxwell and Salamon, 1993).
The predominant empirical approach of most of the studies could partially explain the slow advances made in the development of chemically defined extenders for ram semen storage. An individual study on the effect of each extender component on the viability of the sperm cell could greatly contribute to the development of a more rational synthetic diluent. For example, in a recent work (Yániz et al., 2011) we studied the effect of different buffer systems included in the composition of well-defined and synthetic diluents (in vitro), on sperm quality parameters during storage at 15°C. TRIS caused drastic modifications of certain sperm kinematic parameters during storage at 15°C although, along with citrate, it is one of the main buffers included in the composition of semi-synthetic ram semen diluents (López et al.,1999; López-Sáez et al., 2000; Salamon and Maxwell, 2000; Paulenz et al., 2003; Martí et al., 2003; Yániz et al., 2008).
With the available diluents, semen preservation in the non-frozen state is limited to 6-8h without reducing fertility (Maxwell and Salamon (1993); Salamon and Maxwell, 2000). Irrespective of the diluent, dilution rate, storage temperature or conditions, the sperm deteriorated as the storage duration increased. The main changes that occurred during storage included reduction in motility and morphological integrity of sperm. These changes may be attributed to the accumulation of the toxic products of metabolism, mainly of reactive oxygen species (ROS) that cause lipid peroxidation of the sperm plasma membranes. The above events are accompanied by a decline in transport and survival of spermatozoa in the female reproductive tract and reduction in fertility (Salamon and

Maxwell, 2000). When longer period of storage are required, the use of reduced temperature (about 4°C) and egg-yolk-based media is recommended (Gordon, 1997), although in this case the insemination time should also be considered (Fernandez-Abella et al., 2003)

4.4.2 Cold shock

Severe changes in temperature are a common feature of semen storage protocols for assisted reproduction, but are not biological traits to which species have become adapted (López-Fernández et al., 2008). In the ram, as in other mammals, there is a loss of semen quality when cooled semen samples are used for assisted reproduction. Cooled semen undergoes a decrease in sperm quality, which includes reduction in motility, destabilisation of sperm membranes and DNA integrity impairment of sperm function (López-Fernández et al., 2008; Muiño-Blanco et al., 2008). It is well known that ram spermatozoa are more sensitive to cold-shock stress than those of other species (Muiño-Blanco et al., 2008). In fact, the ram exhibits a faster DNA degradation under similar conditions than other species studied (Gosálvez et al., 2007). Temperature excursion episodes in spermatozoa are associated with oxidative stress induced by the generation of reactive oxygen species, which promote DNA fragmentation (López-Fernández et al., 2008). Reactive oxygen species, produced by dead spermatozoa during a sperm temperature reduction, give rise to sperm membrane alterations with the subsequent release into the media of free active enzymes. Then, the accumulation of toxic metabolic products and active free enzymes, such as those contained in the acrosome, is higher in the media as spermatozoa disintegrate. This could facilitate intact sperm degradation in an exponential fashion (López-Fernández et al., 2008). This loss of quality, accompanied by a decline in sperm survival in the female reproductive tract, gives rise to a reduction in fertility and increased embryonic loss (Paulenz et al, 2002). In ovine species, ovulation may take place several hours post-insemination (Cheminau et al., 1992; Romano, 2004) and, consequently, the time that a spermatozoon is able to survive after AI is of critical importance to achieve pregnancy. Consequently, obtained semen samples must be used as quickly as possible with the diluents currently available.

4.4.3 Time from semen recovery to dilution

The role of seminal plasma (SP) in mammalian sperm function remains largely a matter of speculation as both inhibitory and stimulating effects have been found (Muiño-Blanco et al., 2008). It has been reported that exposure of ram spermatozoa to seminal plasma causes a reduction of fertility (Dott et al., 1979), although some components of the seminal plasma, such as certain proteins, seem to have the important function of maintaining the stability of the membrane up to the process of capacitation, and are able to protect and repair the cold-shock damage to sperm (Muiño-Blanco et al., 2008). However, in practice, semen dilution in the ram has to be done as soon as possible after recovery to avoid the inhibitory effects of seminal plasma.

4.5 Insemination technique

4.5.1 Semen deposition site

In mammals, establishing an adequate sperm reservoir in the caudal isthmus and utero-tubaric junction is very important after mounting or AI, as spermatozoa may ascend to the fertilisation site from this reservoir. In ovine species, the cervix is the main anatomical and physiological barrier to the ascent of spermatozoa after mounting or AI. This is particularly relevant after cervical insemination as, in comparison to fresh spermatozoa, a relatively small proportion of the stored cells penetrates the cervical canal and migrates through the uterus of the ewe to the oviducts (Salamon and Maxwell, 2000). Spermatozoa functionally affected during liquid storage may not migrate, or may migrate slowly, and their survival in the female tract is also reduced to about half that of fresh spermatozoa (Salamon and Maxwell, 2000). Attempts to improve the transport of spermatozoa from the posterior cervix to the oviducts of oestrous ewes by prostaglandins added to stored semen have given conflicting results (Maxwell and Salamon, 1993).

In the non-pregnant ewe, the funnel-shaped rings of the cervix, which average around five in number, are not concentrically aligned, and their openings are constricted in most instances to less than 3 mm (King et al, 2004). As explained above, breed is an important determinant of the morphology of the cervix, and that could at least partially explain differences in fertility after cervical AI (Kaabi et al., 2006). Many studies have found a positive correlation between the depth of cervical AI and fertility (Kaabi et al., 2006). In consequence, numerous efforts have been made to develop new methods to deposit the semen as deep as possible into the uterus. Studies based on the use of modified pipettes, or hormones such as oxytocin to dilate the cervical canal, have shown that cervical penetration can be improved. However, fertility results have been very variable (Kaabi, et al., 2006). Special care should be taken to avoid cervical trauma with the catheter during AI, as it has been associated with reductions in pregnancy and lambing rates (Kaabi et al., 2006). Secondary effects of oxytocin may also have an adverse effect on fertility (King, 2004).

4.5.2 Technician

The ability of the inseminator may be another important source of variation of the outcome of sheep AI (Gordon, 1997; Anel et al., 2005). Cervical penetration rates are influenced by operator skill (Eppleston and Maxwell, 1993), and the establishment of training programmes is highly recommended.

4.5.3 Stress around AI

There is some evidence that nutritional or management stress inflicted upon the ewe around AI can markedly reduce fertility by interfering with fertilisation or by increasing early embryo mortality rates (Gordon, 1997). Ewes and rams should be handled with the minimum of disturbance and receive good nutrition around oestrus and the first weeks after AI.

5. Acknowledgements

The authors thank Neil Macowan for assistance with the English translation. This work was supported by the Araid Foundation (grant OTRI 2010-0464), Spanish MICINN (grant IPT-010000-2010-33) and OVIARAGON S.C.L. (grant OTRI OTRI 2010-0465).

6. References

Abecia, J.A., Forcada, F. & Gonzalez-Bulnes, A. (2011). Pharmaceutical Control of Reproduction in Sheep and Goats. *Veterinary Clinics of North America-Food Animal Practice*, Vol.27, No.1, (Mar), pp. 67-+, 0749-0720

Abecia, J.A., Forcada, F., Casao, A. & Palacin, I. (2008). Effect of exogenous melatonin on the ovary, the embryo and the establishment of pregnancy in sheep. *Animal*, Vol.2, No.3, pp. 399-404, 1751-7311

Abecia, J.A., Valares, J.A., Forcada, F., Palacín, I., Martín, S. & Martino, A. (2007). The effect of melatonin on the reproductive performance of three sheep breeds in Spain. *Small Ruminant Research*, Vol.69, No.1-3, (May), pp. 10-16, 0921-4488

Acritopoulou, S. & Haresign, W. (1980). Response of ewes to a single injection of an analog of PGF-2alpha given at different stages of the estrous-cycle. *Journal of Reproduction and Fertility*, Vol.58, No.1, pp. 219-223, 0022-4251

Adalsteinsson, S. (1979). Independent effects of liveweight and body condition on fecundity and productivity of Icelandic ewes. *Animal Production*, Vol.28, No.FEB, pp. 13-23, 0003-3561

Alabart, J.L., Folch, J., Ciudad, M.A., Fantova, E., Sevilla, E. & Quintin, F.J. (2002) Efecto de la edad de la oveja rasa aragonesa sobre la fertilidad en la inseminación artificial (I.A.) dentro del esquema de mejora de la UPRA-OVIARAGÓN S.C.L, Proceedings of: *XXVII Congreso de la Sociedad Española de Ovinotecnia y Caprinotecnia*, Valencia (España)

Allison, A.J. & Kelly, R.W. (1978). Synchronization of estrus and fertility in sheep treated with progestagen-impregnated implants, and prostaglandins with or without intra-vaginal sponges and subcutaneous pregnant mare serum. *New Zealand Journal of Agricultural Research*, Vol.21, No.3, pp. 389-393, 0028-8233

Althouse, G.C., Kuster, C.E., Clark, S.G. & Weisiger, R.M. (2000). Field investigations of bacterial contaminants and their effects on extended porcine semen. *Theriogenology* Vol. 53, pp. 1167-1176, 0093-691X

Althouse, G.C. & Lu, K.G. (2005). Bacteriospermia in extended porcine semen. *Theriogenology* Vol. 63, pp. 573-584, 0093-691X

Anel, L., Alvarez, M., Martinez-Pastor, F., Garcia-Macias, V., Anel, E. & De Paz, P. (2006). Improvement strategies in ovine artificial insemination. Reproduction in Domestic Animals 41 (SUPPL. 2), pp. 30-42, 0936-6768

Anel, L., Kaabi, M., Abroug, B., Alvarez, M., Anel, E., Boixo, J.C., de la Fuente, L.F. & de Paz, P. (2005). Factors influencing the success of vaginal and laparoscopic artificial insemination in churra ewes: a field assay. *Theriogenology*, Vol.63, No.4, (Mar), pp. 1235-1247, 0093-691X

Aravindan, G.R., Bjordahl, J., Jost, L.K. & Evenson, D.P. (1997). Susceptibility of human sperm to in situ DNA denaturation is strongly correlated with DNA strand breaks identified by single-cell electrophoresis. *Experimental Cell Research*, Vol.236, No.1, (Oct), pp. 231-237, 0014-4827

Arendt, J., Symons, A.M., Laud, C.A. & Pryde, S.J. (1983). Melatonin can induce early onset of the breeding-season in ewes. *Journal of Endocrinology*, Vol.97, No.3, pp. 395-400, 0022-0795

Armstrong, D.T. & Evans, G. (1984). Intrauterine insemination enhances fertility of frozen-semen in superovulated ewes. *Journal of Reproduction and Fertility*, Vol.71, No.1, pp. 89-94, 0022-4251

Arrebola, F.A., Abecia, J.A., Forcada, F., García, A., Martín, R.A. & Mesa, O. (2009). Effects of annual rainfall and farm on lamb production after treatment with melatonin implants in Merino sheep: A 4-year study. *New Zealand Veterinary Journal*, Vol.57, No.3, pp. 141-145, 0048-0169

Aurich C. & Spergser J. (2007). Influence of bacteria and gentamicin on cooled-stored stallion spermatozoa. *Theriogenology*, Vol. 67, pp. 912-918, 0093-691X

Baril, G., Leboeuf, B. & Saumande, J. (1993). Synchronization of estrus in goats: The relationship between time of occurrence of estrus and fertility following artificial-insemination. *Theriogenology*, Vol.40, No.3, (Sep), pp. 621-628, 0093-691X

Baril, G., Remy, B., Leboeuf, B., Beckers, J.F. & Saumande, J. (1996). Synchronization of estrus in goats: The relationship between eCG binding in plasma time of occurrence of estrus and fertility following artificial insemination. *Theriogenology*, Vol.45, No.8, (Jun), pp. 1553-1559, 0093-691X

Beck, N.F.G., Davies, B. & Williams, S.P. (1993). Estrous synchronization in ewes. The effect of combining a prostaglandin analog with a 5-day progestagen treatment. . *Animal Production*, Vol.56, (Apr), pp. 207-210, 0003-3561

Bielanski A. (2007). Disinfection procedures for controlling microorganisms in the semen and embryos of humans and farm animals. *Theriogenology*, Vol. 68, pp.1-22, 0093-691X

Bittman, E.L., Dempsey, R.J. & Karsch, F.J. (1983). Pineal melatonin secretion drives the reproductive response to daylength in the ewe. *Endocrinology*, Vol.113, No.6, pp. 2276-2283, 0013-7227

Bodin, L., Drion, P.V., Remy, B., Brice, G., Cognie, Y. & Beckers, J.F. (1997). Anti-PMSG antibody levels in sheep subjected annually to oestrus synchronisation. *Reproduction Nutrition Development*, Vol.37, No.6, (Nov-Dec), pp. 651-660, 0926-5287

Bodin, L., Elsen, J.M., Hanocq, E., Francois, D., Lajous, D., Manfredi, E., Mialon, M.M., Boichard, D., Foulley, J.L., San-Cristobal-Gaudy, M., Teyssier, J., Thimonier, J. & Chemineau, P. (1999). Genetics of reproduction in ruminants. *Productions Animales*, Vol.12, No.2, (May), pp. 87-100, 0990-0632

Boland, M.P., Gordon, I. & Kelleher, D.L. (1978). Effect of treatment by prostaglandin analog (ICI-80,996) or progestagen (SC-9880) on ovulation and fertilization in cycles ewes. *Journal of Agricultural Science*, Vol.91, No.DEC, pp. 727-730, 0021-8596

Branca, A., Molle, G., Sitzia, M., Decandia, M. & Landau, S. (2000). Short-term dietary effects on reproductive wastage after induced ovulation and artificial insemination in primiparous lactating Sarda ewes (vol 58, pg 59, 2000). *Animal Reproduction Science*, Vol.63, No.1-2, (Oct), pp. 123-123, 0378-4320

Brown, B.W. (1994). A review of nutritional influences on reproduction in boars, bulls and rams. *Reproduction Nutrition Development*, Vol.34, No.2, pp. 89-114, 0926-5287

Bru, C., Fantova, E., Sevilla, E., Quintin, F.J. & Alabart, J.L. (1995) Resultados de insemiancion artificial de las ovejas Rasa aragonea de las ganaderías de Carne Aragón, S.C.L. Influencia de la condición corporal, Proceedings of: *XX Jornadas Científicas de la Sociedad Española de Ovinotecnia y Caprinotecnia.*, Madrid (España)

Buckrell, B.C., Buschbeck, C., Gartley, C.J., Kroetsch, T., McCutcheon, W., Martin, J., Penner, W.K. & Walton, J.S. (1994). Further development of a transcervical technique for artificial insemination in sheep using previously frozen semen. *Theriogenology*, Vol.4, No.4, pp. 601-611, 0093-691X

Casao, A., Cebrian, I., Asumpcao, M.E., Perez-Pe, R., Abecia, J.A., Forcada, F., Cebrian-Perez, J.A. & Muino-Blanco, T. (2010a). Seasonal variations of melatonin in ram seminal plasma are correlated to those of testosterone and antioxidant enzymes. *Reproductive Biology and Endocrinology*, Vol.8, (Jun), pp. 1477-7827, 1477-7827.

Casao, A., Mendoza, N., Perez-Pe, R., Grasa, P., Abecia, J.A., Forcada, F., Cebrian-Perez, J.A. & Muino-Blanco, T. (2010b). Melatonin prevents capacitation and apoptotic-like changes of ram spermatozoa and increases fertility rate. *Journal of Pineal Research*, Vol.48, No.1, (Jan), pp. 39-46, 0742-3098

Casao, A., Vega, S., Palacin, I., Perez-Pe, R., Lavina, A., Quintin, F.J., Sevilla, E., Abecia, J.A., Cebrian-Perez, J.A., Forcada, F. & Muino-Blanco, T. (2010c). Effects of Melatonin Implants During Non-Breeding Season on Sperm Motility and Reproductive Parameters in Rasa Aragonesa Rams. *Reproduction in Domestic Animals*, Vol.45, No.3, (Jun), pp. 425-432, 0936-6768

Chemineau, P., Malpaux, B., Delgadillo, J.A., Guerin, Y., Ravault, J.P., Thimonier, J. & Pelletier, J. (1992). Control of sheep and goat reproduction - Use of light and melatonin. *Animal Reproduction Science*, Vol.30, No.1-3, (Nov), pp. 157-184, 0378-4320

Chemineau, P., Vandaele, E., Brice, G. & Jardon, C. (1991). The use of melatonin in improving reproduction performance in sheep. *Recueil De Medecine Veterinaire*, Vol.167, No.3-4, pp. 227-239, 0034-1843

Choudhry, T.M., Berger, T. & Dally, M. (1995). In vitro fertility evaluation of cryopreserved ram semen and its correlation with relative in vivo fertility. *Theriogenology*, Vol.43, No.7, (May), pp. 1195-1200, 0093-691X

Clément, F., Vidament M. & Guérin B. (1995). Microbial contamination of stallion semen. *Biology of Reproduction Monographic*, Vol. 1, pp. 779-786.

Cognié,Y., Bodin, L. & Terqui, M. (1984).The control of the time of ovulation in relation to the use of artificial insemination. In Insémination artificielle et amélioration génétique: Bilan et perspectives critiques ed. JM Elsen and JL Foulley. *Institut National de la Recherche Agronomique*, Paris, France, pp 77-95.

Colas, G. & Brice, G. (1976). Seasonal variations of the fertilizing capacity of the deep frozen ram semen. In: *8th International Congress of Animal Reproduction Artificial Insemination*, Vol.4, pp.977-980.

Colas, G. (1979). Fertility in the ewe after artificial insemination with fresh and frozen semen at the induced oestrous, and influence of the photoperiod on the semen quality of the ram. *Livestock Production Science*, Vol.6, No.2, pp. 153-166, 0301-6226

Colas, G., Thimonie.J, Courot, M. & Ortavant, R. (1973). Fertility and reproductive efficiency during the breeding season of ewes artificially inseminated after treatment with flugestone acetate. *Annales De Zootechnie*, Vol.22, No.4, pp. 441-451, 0003-424X

Contreras-Solis, I., Vasquez, B., Diaz, T., Letelier, C., Lopez-Sebastian, A. & Gonzalez-Bulnes, A. (2009). Efficiency of estrous synchronization in tropical sheep by combining short-interval cloprostenol-based protocols and "male effect". *Theriogenology*, Vol.71, No.6, (Apr), pp. 1018-1025, 0093-691X

Corteel, J.M., Leboeuf, B. & Baril, G. (1988). Artificial breeding of adult goats and kids induced with hormones to ovulate outside the breeding season. *Small Ruminant Research*, Vol.1, No.1, pp. 19-35, 0921-4488

David, I., Robert-Granie, C., Manfredi, E., Lagriffoul, G. & Bodin, L. (2008). Environmental and genetic variation factors of artificial insemination success in French dairy sheep. *Animal*, Vol.2, No.7, (Jul), pp. 979-986, 1751-7311 den Daas, N. (1992). Laboratory assessment of semen characteristics. *Animal Reproduction Science*, Vol.28, No.1-4, pp. 87-94, 0378-4320

Donovan, A., Hanrahan, J.P., Kummen, E., Duffy, P. & Boland, M.P. (2004). Fertility in the ewe following cervical insemination with fresh or frozen-thawed semen at a natural or synchronised oestrus. *Animal Reproduction Science*, Vol.84, No.3-4, (Sep), pp. 359-368, 0378-4320

Dott, H.M., Harrison, R.A.P., & Foster, G.C.A. (1979). The maintenance of motility and the surface properties of epididymal spermatozoa from bull rabbit and ram in homologous seminal and epididymal plasma. *Journal of Reproduction Fertility*, Vol.55, pp. 113-124, 0022-4251

Ducker, M.J. & Boyd, J.S. (1977). The effect of body size and body condition on the ovulation rate of ewes *Animal Production*, Vol.24, No.JUN, pp. 377-385, 0003-3561

Eid, L.N., Lorton, S.P. & Parrish, J.J. (1994). Paternal influence on S-phase in the first cell cycle of the bovine embryo. *Biology of Reproduction*, Vol.51, No.6, (Dec), pp. 1232-1237, 0006-3363

Eppleston, J. & Maxwell, W.C.M. (1993). Recent attempts to improve the fertility of frozen ram semen inseminated into the cervix. *Wool Sheep Breed*, Vol.41, pp 291-302

Eppleston, J. & Maxwell, W.M.C. (1995). Sources of variation in the reproductive performance of ewes inseminated with frozen-thawed ram semen by laparoscopy. *Theriogenology*, Vol.43, No.4, (Mar), pp. 777-788, 0093-691X

Eppleston, J., Evans, G. & Roberts, E.M. (1991). Effect of time of PMSG and GnRH on the time of ovulation, LH secretion and reproductive performance after intrauterine insemination with frozen ram semen. *Animal Reproduction Science*, Vol.26, No.3-4, (Dec), pp. 227-237, 0378-4320

Eppleston, J., Maxwell, W.M.C. , Battye K.M. & Roberts, E.M. (1986). Effect of thawed motility and intrauterine motility of motile sperm on fertility of ewes. *Proceedings of Australian Society of Reproduction Biology*, Vol. 18, pp.19.

Eppleston, J., Salamon, S., Moore, N.W. & Evans, G. (1994). The depth of cervical insemination and site of intrauterine insemination and their relationship to the fertility of frozen-thawed ram semen. *Animal Reproduction Science*, Vol.36, No.3-4, (Sep), pp. 211-225, 0378-4320

Esmailizadeh, A.K., Dayani, O. & Mokhtari, M.S. (2009). Lambing season and fertility of fat-tailed ewes under an extensive production system are associated with liveweight and body condition around mating. *Animal Production Science*, Vol.49, No.12, pp. 1086-1092, 1836-5787

Fantova, E., Bru, R., Sevilla, E., Quintin, F.J., Congost, S., Alabart, J.L. & Folch, J. (1998). Resultados de inseminación artificial en el marco del esquema de selección por prolificidad en las ganaderías de Carne Aragón. ITEA. 94 A (2), 93-100. *ITEA*, Vol.94, No.2, pp. 93-100,

Fantova, E., Ciudad, M.A., Vijil, E., Sevilla, E., Quintin, F.J., Folch, J., Sin, E., Alabart, J.L. & Jurado, J.J. (1999) Evolution of the artificial insemination program in the genetic improvement Schedule of UPRA-Carne oviaragón. Study of flock location and insemination personnal effects, Proceedings of: *XXIV Jornadas Científicas de la Sociedad Española de Ovinotecnia y Caprinotecnia*, Soria (España)

Fernandez-Abella, D., Preve, M.O., & Villegas N. (2003). Insemination time and dilution rate of cooled and chilled ram semen affects fertility. *Theriogenology*, Vol. 60, pp.21-26, 0093-691X.

Forcada, F., Abecia, J.A. & Sierra, I. (1992). Seasonal-changes in estrus activity and ovulation rate in Rasa-Aragonesa ewes maintained at 2 different body condition levels. *Small Ruminant Research*, Vol.8, No.4, (Sep), pp. 313-324, 0921-4488

Forcada, F., Ait Amer-Meziane, M., Abecia, J.A., Maurel, M.C., Cebrián-Pérez, J.A., Muiño-Blanco, T., Asenjo, B., Vázquez, M.I. & Casao, A. (2011). Repeated superovulation using a simplified FSH/eCG treatment for in vivo embryo production in sheep. *Theriogenology*, Vol.75, No.4, pp. 769-776, 0093-691X

Fukui, Y., Kohno, H., Okabe, K., Katsuki, S., Yoshizawa, M., Togari, T. & Watanabe, H. (2010). Factors affecting the fertility of ewes after intrauterine insemination with frozen-thawed semen during the non-breeding season. *Journal of Reproduction and Development*, Vol.56, No.4, (Aug), pp. 460-466, 0916-8818

Fukui, Y., Kohno, H., Togari, T. & Hiwasa, M. (2007). Fertility of ewes inseminated intrauterinally with frozen semen using extender containing bovine serum albumin. *Journal of Reproduction and Development*, Vol.53, No.4, (Aug), pp. 959-962, 0916-8818

Gabiña, D. & Folch, J. (1987) La inseminación artificial ovina. Resultados de su aplicación en un programa de selección en la raza Rasa Aragonesa, Proceedings of: *ITEA*, Zaragoza (España)

Gonzalez, R.E., Labuonora, D. & Russel, A.J.F. (1997). The effects of ewe live weight and body condition score around mating on production from four sheep breeds in extensive grazing systems in Uruguay. *Animal Science*, Vol.64, (Feb), pp. 139-145, 1357-7298.

Gonzalez, R.E., Labuonora, D., & Russel, A.J.F. (1997). The effects of ewe live weight and body condition score around mating on production from four sheep breeds in extensive grazing systems in Uruguay. *Animal Science*, Vol.64, No.1, pp. 139-145, 1357-7298.

Gordon I. (1997). Controlled Reproduction in Sheep and Goats. *Cab International* (U.S.A.).

Gosálvez, J., Fernández, J.L., Gosálbez, A., Arrollo, A., Agarwal, A. & López-Fernández A. (2007). Dynamics of sperm DNA fragmentation in mammalian species as assessed by the SCD methodology. *Fertility and Sterility*, Vol. 88, pp. 365–1365, 1556-5653.

Gosálvez, J., Gosálbez, A., Arroyo, F., Fernández, J.L., & López-Fernández, C. (2008). Assessing sperm DNA fragmentation in the field: an adaptation of sperm chromatin dispersion technology. *Biotechnology and Histochemistry*, Vol.83, No.5, pp 247-52, 1473-7760.

Greyling, J.P.C., Erasmus, J.A., Taylor, G.J. & van der Merwe, S. (1997). Synchronization of estrus in sheep using progestagen and inseminating with chilled semen during the breeding season. *Small Ruminant Research*, Vol.26, No.1-2, (Dec), pp. 137-143, 0921-4488

Gunn, R.G. & Doney, J.M. (1979). Fertility in Cheviot ewes. 1. the effect of body condition at mating on ovulation and early embryo mortality in North and South Country Cheviot ewes. *Animal Production*, Vol.29, No.AUG, pp. 11-16, 0003-3561

Gunn, R.G. (1983). The Influence of Nutrition on the Reproductive Performance of Ewes. In *Sheep production*, ed. Haresign, W., Butterworths, London.

Gunn, R.G., & Doney, J.M. (1979). Fertility in Cheviot ewes. 1. The effect of body condition at mating on ovulation and early embryo mortality in North and South Country Cheviot ewes. *Animal Production*, Vol. 29, pp. 111-121, 0003-3561

Hackett, A.J., Langford, G.A. & Robertson, H.A. (1981). Rertility of ewes after synchronization of estrus with prostaglandin-f2-alpha and artificial-insemination. *Theriogenology*, Vol.15, No.6, pp. 599-603, 0093-691X

Haresign, W., Peters, A.R. & Staples, L.D. (1990). The effect of melatonin implants on breeding activity and litter size in commercial sheep flocks in the Uk. *Animal Production*, Vol.50, (Feb), pp. 111-121, 0003-3561

Hawk, H.W. & Conley, H.H. (1975). Involvement of cervix in sperm transport failures in reproductive-tract of ewe. *Biology of Reproduction*, Vol.13, No.3, pp. 322-328, 0006-3363

Hawk, H.W. (1971). Sperm destruction in sheep vagina. *Journal of Animal Science*, Vol.33, No.1, pp. 255-258, 0021-8812

Heape, W. (1898). On the artificial insemination of mares. *Veterinarian*, Vol.71, pp. 202-212,

Houghton, J.A.S., Liberati, N., Schrick, F.N., Townsend, E.C., Dailey, R.A. & Inskeep, E.K. (1995). day of estrous-cycle affects follicular dynamics after induced luteolysis in ewes. *Journal of Animal Science*, Vol.73, No.7, (Jul), pp. 2094-2101, 0021-8812

Husein, M.Q. & Ababneh, M.M. (2008). A new strategy for superior reproductive performance of ewes bred out-of-season utilizing progestagen supplement prior to withdrawal of intravaginal pessaries. *Theriogenology*, Vol.69, No.3, (Feb), pp. 376-383, 0093-691X

Jabbour, H.N. & Evans, G. (1991). Fertility of superovulated ewes following intrauterine or oviducal insemination with fresh or frozen-thawed semen. *Reproduction Fertility and Development*, Vol.3, No.1, pp. 1-7, 1031-3613

Kaabi, M., Alvarez, M., Anel, E., Chamorro, C.A., Boixo, J.C., de Paz, P. & Anel, L. (2006). Influence of breed and age on morphometry and depth of inseminating catheter penetration in the ewe cervix: A postmortem study. *Theriogenology*, Vol.66, No.8, (Nov), pp. 1876-1883, 0093-691X

Karsch, F.J., Bittman, E.L., Foster, D.L., Goodman, R.L., Legan, S.J. & Robinson, J.E. (1984). Neuroendocrine basis of seasonal reproduction. *Recent Progress in Hormone Research*, Vol.40, pp. 185-232, 0079-9963

Kaya A., Aksoy M. & Tekeli, T. (2002). Influence of ejaculation frequency on sperm characteristics, ionic composition and enzymatic activity of seminal plasma in rams. *Small Ruminant Research*, Vol.44, pp 153-158, 0921-4488.

Keisler, DH. & Buckrell, B.C. (1997). Chapter 88. Breeding strategies. In: *Current therapy in large animal theriogenology*. Edited by Robert s. Youngquist. 1st. edition. ISBN: 0-7216-5396-0.

Killen, I.D. & Caffery, G.J. (1982). Uterine insemination of ewes with the aid of a laparoscope. *Australian Veterinary Journal*, Vol.59, No.3, pp. 95-95, 0005-0423

King, M.E., McKelvey, W.A., Dingwall, W.S., Matthews, K.P., Gebbie, F.E., Mylne, M.J., Stewart, E. & Robinson, J.J. (2004). Lambing rates and litter sizes following intrauterine or cervical insemination of frozen/thawed semen with or without oxytocin administration. *Theriogenology*. Vol.62, pp.1236-44, 0093-691X

Laliotis, V., Vosniakou, A., Zafrakas, A., Lymberopoulos, A. & Alifakiotis, T. (1998). The effect of melatonin on lambing and litter size in milking ewes after advancing the breeding season with progestagen and PMSG followed by artificial insemination. *Small Ruminant Research*, Vol.31, No.1, (Dec), pp. 79-81, 0921-4488.

Landau, S. & Molle, G. (1997). Nutrition effects on fertility in small ruminants with an emphasis on Mediterranean sheep breeding systems. *Proc. FAOrCIHEAM Meeting on the Nutrition of Small Ruminants*, 24–26 October 1996, Rabat, Morocco.

Langford, G.A. & Marcus, G.J. (1982). Influence of sperm number and seminal plasma on fertility of progestagen-treated sheep in confinement. Journal of Reproduction Fertility, Vol.65, pp.325-329, 0022-4251.

Langford, G.A., Ainsworth, L. & Wolynetz, M.S. (1982). Reproductive response of progestogen-treated sheep in confinement to a single and double insemination. *Journal of Animal Science*, Vol.54, No.1, pp. 12-17, 0021-8812

Lassoued, N., Rekik, M., Mahouachi, M. & Ben Hamouda, M. (2004). The effect of nutrition prior to and during mating on ovulation rate, reproductive wastage, and lambing rate in three sheep breeds. *Small Ruminant Research*, Vol.52, No.1-2, (Apr), pp. 117-125, 0921-4488

Legaz, E., Deletang, F. & Martino, A. (2000). Efecto de la utilización de implantes de melatonina sobre los resultados de inseminación artificial en ovejas Manchega x Assaf. *Producción Ovina y Caprina*, Vol.SEOC Teruel, XXV, pp. 555-558,

Light, J.E., Silvia, W.J. & Reid, R.C. (1994). Luteolytic effect of prostaglandin-f2-alpha and 2 metabolites in ewes. *Journal of Animal Science*, Vol.72, No.10, (Oct), pp. 2718-2721, 0021-8812

López, A., Soderquist, L. & Rodriguez-Martinez, H. (1999). Sperm viability in ram semen diluted and stored in three different extenders. *Acta Veterinaria Scandinavica*, Vol.40, pp. 1-9, 0044-605X

López-Fernández, C., Fernández, J.L., Gosálbez, A., Arroyo, F., Vázquez, J.M., Holt, W.V. & Gosálvez, J. (2008). Dynamics of sperm DNA fragmentation in domestic animals III. Ram. *Theriogenology*. Vol.70, pp.898-908, 0093-691X

Lopez-Saez, A., Ortiz, N., Gallego, L. & Garde, J.J. (2000). Liquid storage (5 degrees C) of ram semen in different diluents. *Archives of Andrology*, Vol.44, No.2, (Mar-Apr), pp. 155-164, 0148-5016

Lunstra, D.D. & Christenson, R.K. (1981). Fertilization and embryonic survival in ewes synchronized with exogenous hormones during the anestrous and estrous seasons. *Journal of Animal Science*, Vol.53, No.2, pp. 458-466, 0021-8812

Marai, I.F.M., El-Darawany, A.A., Abou-Fandoud, E.I. & Abdel-Hafez, M.A.M. (2004). Reproductive traits and the physiological background of the seasonal variations in Egyptian suffolk ewes under the conditions of Egypt. Annals of Arid Zone , Vol. 43, No.2, (June), pp. 177-183

Marai, I.F.M., El-Darawany, A.A., Fadiel, A. & Abdel-Hafez, M.A.M. (2007). Physiological traits as affected by heat stress in sheep-A review. Small Ruminant Research Vol. 71, No.1-3, (August), pp 1-12

Marai, I.F.M., Bahgat, L.B., Shalaby, T.H. & Abdel-Hafez, M.A. (2000). Response of Male Lambs to Concentrate Mixtures given with or without Natural Clay under Egypt Conditions. *Annals of Arid Zone*, Vol.39, No.4, pp. 449-460

Marai, I.F.M., El- Darawany, A.A., Abou-Fandoud, E.I. &Abdel-Hafez, M.A.M. (2006). Serun blood components during pre-oestrus, oestru and pregnancy phases in Egyptian

Suffolk as affected by heat stress, under the conditions of Egypt. *Egypt Journal of Sheep and Goats Desertic Animal Science*, Vol.1, No.1, pp. 47-62

Martí, J.I., Martí, E., Cebrián-Pérez, E. & Muiño-Blanco, T. (2003). Survival rate and antioxidant enzyme activity of ram spermatozoa after dilution with different extenders or selection by a dextran swim-up procedure. *Theriogenology* Vol.60, pp. 1025-1037, 0093-691X

Martin, G.B., Milton, J.T.B., Davidson, R.H., Hunzicker, G.E.B., Lindsay, D.R. & Blache, D. (2004). Natural methods for increasing reproductive efficiency in small ruminants. *Animal Reproduction Science*, Vol.82-3, (Jul), pp. 231-246, 0378-4320

Maurel, M.C., Roy, F., Hervé, V., Bertin, J., Vaiman, D., Cribiu, E., Manfredi, E., Bouvier, F., Lantier, I., Boue, P. & Guillou, F. (2003). Réponse immunitaire à la eCG utilisée dans le traitement de l'induction d'ovulation chez la chèvre et la brebisImmune response to equine Chorionic Gonadotropin used for the induction of ovulation in goats and ewes. *Gynécologie Obstétrique & Fertilité*, Vol.31, No.9, pp. 766-769, 1297-9589

Maxwell, W.M.C. & Salamon S. (1993). Liquid storage of ram semen-a review. *Reproduction, Fertility and Development*, Vol. 5, pp. 613-638, 1031-3613.

Maxwell, W.M.C. (1986). Artificial insemination of ewes with frozen-thawed semen at a synchronized oestrus. 2. Effect of dose of spermatozoa and site of intrauterine insemination on fertility. *Animal Reproduction Science*, Vol.10, No.4, (Apr), pp. 309-316, 0378-4320

McCracke.Ja, Samuelss.B, Goding, J.R., Glew, M.E., Green, K., Carlson, J.C. & Baird, D.T. (1972). Prostaglandin-f2-alpha identified as a luteolytic hormone in sheep. *Nature-New Biology*, Vol.238, No.83, pp. 129-135, 0090-0028.

Menchaca, A. & Rubianes, E. (2004). New treatments associated with timed artificial insemination in small ruminants. *Reproduction Fertility and Development*, Vol.16, No.4, pp. 403-413, 1031-3613

Montoro, V. (1995). La inmemiancón artificial con semen refrigerado en el esquema de seleccion de la raza ovina manchega. *Tesis Doctoral*, pp. 148,

Morley, F.H.W., White, D.H., Kenney, P.A. & Davis, I.F. (1978). Predicting ovulation rate from liveweight in ewes *Agricultural Systems*, Vol.3, No.1, pp. 27-45, 0308-521X

Muiño-Blanco, T., Pérez-Pé, R. & Cebrián-Pérez, J.A. (2008). Seminal plasma proteins and sperm resistance to stress. *Reproduction in Domestic Animals*, Vol.4, pp.18-31, 1439-0531.

O'Callaghan, D., Karsch, F.J., Boland, M.P. & Roche, J.F. (1991). Role of short days in timing the onset and duration of reproductive activity in ewes under artificial photoperiods. *Biology of Reproduction*, Vol.44, No.1, (January 1, 1991), pp. 23-28, 0006-3363.-3363

Olivera-Muzante, J., Fierro, S., López, V. & Gil, J. (2011). Comparison of prostaglandin- and progesterone-based protocols for timed artificial insemination in sheep. *Theriogenology*, Vol.In Press, Corrected Proof, pp. 0093-691X

Ollero, M., Muiño-Blanco, T., López-Pérez, M.J. & Cebrián-Pérez, J.A. (1996).Viability of ram spermatozoa in relation to the abstinence period and successive ejaculations. *International Journal of Andrology*, Vol.19, pp. 287-92, 1365-2605

Ollero, M., Pascual, M.L., Muiño-Blanco, T., Cebrián-Pérez, J.A. & López-Pérez, M.J. (1994). Revealing surface changes associated with maturation of ram spermatozoa by centrifugal counter-current distribution in an aqueous two-phase system. *Journal of Chromatography*, Vol. 668, pp.173-178, 0021-9673.

Ostermeier, G.C., Sargeant, G.A., Yandell, B.S., Evenson, D.P. & Parrish, J.J. (2001). Relationship of bull fertility to sperm nuclear shape. *Journal of Andrology*, Vol.22, No.4, (Jul-Aug), pp. 595-603, 0196-3635

Palacin, I., Abecia, J.A., Forcada, F., Casao, A., Cebrian, J.A., Muino, T., Palacios, C. & Pontes, J.M. (2008). Effects of exogenous melatonin treatment on out-of-season ram fertility. *Italian Journal of Animal Science*, Vol.7, No.2, pp. 199-206, 1594-4077

Palacín, I., Santolaria, P., Fantova, E., Blasco, M.E., Quintín-Casorrán, F.J., Sevilla-Mur, E., & Yániz, J.L. (2011). Efecto de la localización geográfica sobre los resulados de fertiilidad en el programa de inseminación artificial de la unión de productores de rasa aragonesa (UPRA). *ITEA*, en prensa

Papadopoulos, S., Hanrahan, J.P., Donovan, A., Duffy, P., Boland, M.P. & Lonergan, P. (2005). In vitro fertilization as a predictor of fertility from cervical insemination of sheep. *Theriogenology*, Vol.63, No.1, (Jan), pp. 150-159, 0093-691X

Pascual, M.L., Muino-Blanco, T., Cebrian-Perez, J.A., & Lopez-Perez, M.J. (1993). Sperm cell heterogeneity revealed by centrifugal counter-current distribution in an aqueous two-phase system. Journal of Chromatography - Biomedical Applications Vol. 617, No.1, pp. 51-57, 1570-0232.

Paulenz, H., Söderquist, L., Adnøy, T., Fossen, O.H., & Berg, K.A. (2003). Effect of milk- and TRIS-based extenders on the fertility of sheep inseminated vaginally once or twice with liquid semen. *Theriogenology*, Vol.60, pp. 759-766, 0093-691X

Paulenz, H., Adnoy, T. & Soderquist, L. (2007). Comparison of fertility results after vaginal insemination using different thawing procedures and packages for frozen ram semen. *Acta Veterinaria Scandinavica*, Vol.49, (Sep), pp. 0044-605X

Paulenz, H., Adnoy, T., Fossen, O.H., Soderquist, L. & Berg, K.A. (2002). Effect of deposition site and sperm number on the fertility of sheep inseminated with liquid semen. *Veterinary Record*, Vol.150, No.10, (Mar), pp. 299-+, 0042-4900

Paulenz, H., Soderquist, L., Adnoy, T., Soltun, K., Saether, P.A., Fjellsoy, K.R. & Berg, K.A. (2005). Effect of cervical and vaginal insemination with liquid semen stored at room temperature on fertility of goats. *Animal Reproduction Science*, Vol.86, No.1-2, (Mar), pp. 109-117, 0378-4320

Pearce, D.T. & Robinson, T.J. (1985). Plasma progesterone concentrations, ovarian and endocrinological responses and sperm transport in ewes with synchronized estrus. *Journal of Reproduction and Fertility*, Vol.75, No.1, pp. 49-62, 0022-4251

Pelletier, J., Chemineau, P., Thimonier, J. & Vollandnail, P. (1987). Environment and changes in reproductive activity in sheep and goat. *Ed. P.Pevet. Karger Basel. Proc. 8th ESPC Conf. Strasbourg*, Vol.3, pp. 121-135,

Quinliva.Td & Robinson, T.J. (1969). Numbers of spermatozoa in genital tract after artificial insemination of progestagen-treated ewes. *Journal of Reproduction and Fertility*, Vol.19, No.1, pp. 73-&, 0022-4251

Rhind, S.M., McMillen, S., McKelvey, W.A.C., Rodriguezherrejon, F.F. & McNeilly, A.S. (1989). Effect of the body condition of ewes on the secretion of LH and FSH and the pituitary response to gonadotrophin-releasing hormone. *Journal of Endocrinology*, Vol.120, No.3, (Mar), pp. 497-502, 0022-0795

Robinson, T.J., Moore, N.W., Lindsay, D.R., Fletcher, I.C. & Salamon, S. (1970). Fertility following synchronization of oestrus in sheep with intravaginal sponges .1. effects of vaginal douche, supplementary steroids, time of insemination, and numbers and dilution of spermatozoa. *Australian Journal of Agricultural Research*, Vol.21, No.5, pp. 767-&, 0004-9409

Rodríguez-Martínez, H. (2003). Laboratory Semen Assessment and Prediction of Fertility: still Utopia?. *Reproduction in Domestic Animals* Vol.38, pp. 312–318, 0936-6768.

Romano, J.E. (2004). Synchronization of estrus using CIDR. FGA or MAP intravaginal pessaries during the breeding season in Nubian goats. *Small Ruminant Research*, Vol.55, pp.15–19, 0921-4488

Roy, F., Combes, B., Vaiman, D., Cuibiu, E.P., Pobel, T., Deletang, F., Combarnous, Y., Guillou, F. & Maurel, M.C. (1999). Humoral immune response to equine chorionic gonadotropin in ewes: Association with major histocompatibility complex and interference with subsequent fertility. *Biology of Reproduction*, Vol.61, No.1, (Jul), pp. 209-218, 0006-3363

Saacke, R.G., Bame, J., Karabinus, D.S., Mulins, J. & Whitman, S. (1988). Transport of abnormal sperm in the artificially inseminated cow based upon accessory sperm in the zona pellucida, Proceedings of: *Proceedings of the 11th International Congress on Animal Reproduction and Artificial Insemination. Dublin, Ireland,* Dublin, Ireland

Saacke, R.G., Nadir, S., Dalton, J., Bame, J., DeJarnette, J.M., Defelos, S. & Nebel, R.L. (1994). Accessory sperm evaluation and bull fertility—an update. , Proceedings of: *Proceedings of the 15th NAAB Technical Conference on Animal Reproduction and Artificial Insemination,* Milwaukee, Wisc

Salamon, S., & Maxwell, W.M.C. (2000). Storage of ram semen. *Animal Reproduction Science*, Vol.62, pp. 77-111, 0378-4320

Salamon, S. & Maxwell, W.M.C. (1995). Frozen storage of ram semen I. Processing, freezing, thawing and fertility after cervical insemination. *Animal Reproduction Science*, Vol.37, No.3-4, (Feb), pp. 185-249, 0378-4320

Scaramuzzi, R.J., Downing, J.A., Campbell, B.K. & Cognie, Y. (1988). Control of fertility and fecundity of sheep by means of hormonal manipulation. *Australian Journal of Biological Sciences*, Vol.41, No.1, pp. 37-45, 0004-9417

Selaive-Villarroel, A.B. & Kennedy, J.P. (1983a). Fertility studies in young and mature merino ewes. 1. Cervical mucus production. *Theriogenology*, Vol.20, No.5, pp. 537-541, 0093-691X

Selaive-Villarroel, A.B. & Kennedy, J.P. (1983b). Fertility studies in young and mature merino ewes. 2. Sperm transport. *Theriogenology*, Vol.20, No.5, pp. 543-547, 0093-691X

Shackell GH, Kyle B, Littlejohn RP. Factors influencing the success of a large scale artificial insemination programme in sheep. Proc. New Zeal Soc Anim Prod 1990:50:427-430

Shelton, M. (2000). Reproductive performance of sheep exposed to hot environments. Malik R.C., Razzaque M.A., and Al-Nasser A.Y. (Eds), Published by the Kuwait Institute for Scientific Research. *Sheep Production in Hot and Arid Zones*, pp. 155-162.

Sirois, J. & Fortune, J.E. (1990). Lengthening the bovine estrous-cycle with low-levels of exogenous progesterone - a model for studying ovarian follicular dominance. *Endocrinology*, Vol.127, No.2, (Aug), pp. 916-925, 0013-7227

Soderquist, L., Lundeheim, N. & Nilsson, B. (1999). Assessment of fertility after using different procedures to thaw ram spermatozoa frozen in mini straws. *Reproduction in Domestic Animals*, Vol.34, No.2, (May), pp. 61-66, 0936-6768

Thibier, M. & Guerin, B. (2000). Hygienic aspects of storage and use of semen for artificial insemination. *Animal Reproduction Science*, Vol.62, pp. 233-251, 0378-4320

Thiéry, J.C. , Chemineau, P., Hernandez, X., Migaud, M. & Malpaux, B. (2002). Neuroendocrine interactions and seasonality. Domestic Animal Endocrinology, Vol.23, No.1-2, pp 87-100

Thomson, E.F. & Bahhady, F.A. (1988). A note on the effect of live weight at mating on fertility of Awassi ewes in semi-arid northwest Syria. *Animal Production*, Vol.47, (Dec), pp. 505-508, 0003-3561

Ungerfeld, R. & Rubianes, E. (1999). Effectiveness of short-term progestogen primings for the induction of fertile oestrus with eCG in ewes during late seasonal anoestrus. *Animal Science*, Vol.68, (Apr), pp. 349-353, 1357-7298

Ustuner, B., Gunay, U., Nur, Z. & Ustuner, H. (2007). Effects of long and short-term progestagen treatments combined with PMSG on oestrus synchronization and fertility in awassi ewes during the breeding season. *Acta Veterinaria Brno*, Vol.76, No.3, (Sep), pp. 391-397, 0001-7213

Vázquez, M.I., Abecia, J.A., Forcada, F. & Casao, A. (2010). Effects of exogenous melatonin on in vivo embryo viability and oocyte competence of undernourished ewes after weaning during the seasonal anestrus. *Theriogenology*, Vol. 74, pp. 618-26, 0093-691X

Verstegen, J., Iguar-Ouada, M. & Onclin, K. (2002). Computer assisted semen analyzers in andrology research and veterinary practice. *Theriogenology*. Vol.57, pp. 49-79, 0093-691X

Vinoles, C., Forsberg, M., Banchero, G. & Rubianes, E. (2001). Effect of long-term and short-term progestagen treatment on follicular development and pregnancy rate in cyclic ewes. *Theriogenology*, Vol.55, No.4, (Mar), pp. 993-1004, 0093-691X

Vinoles, C., Meikle, A., Forsberg, M. & Rubianes, E. (1999). The effect of subluteal levels of exogenous progesterone on follicular dynamics and endocrine patterns during the early luteal phase of the ewe. *Theriogenology*, Vol.51, No.7, (May), pp. 1351-1361, 0093-691X

Windsor, D.P. (1995). Factors influencing the success of transcervical insemination in merino ewes. *Theriogenology*, Vol.43, No.6, (Apr), pp. 1009-1018, 0093-691X

Windsor, D.P. (1997). Variation between ejaculates in the fertility of frozen ram semen used for cervical insemination of Merino ewes. *Animal Reproduction Science*, Vol.47, No.1-2, (May), pp. 21-29, 0378-4320

Xu, Z., McDonald, M.F. & McCutcheon, S.N. (1989). The effects of nutritionally-induced liveweight differences on follicular development, ovulation rate, oestrus activity and plasma follicle-stimulating hormone levels in the ewe. *Animal Reproduction Science*, Vol.19, pp 67-78, 0378-4320

Yániz, J., Marti, J.I., Silvestre, M.A., Folch, J., Santolaria, P., Alabart, J.L. & Lopez-Gatius, F. (2005). Effects of solid storage of sheep spermatozoa at 15 degrees C on their survival and penetrating capacity. *Theriogenology*, Vol 64, pp. 1844-1851, 0093-691X

Yániz, J.L., Santolaria, P., Marco-Aguado, M.A. & López-Gatius, F. (2008). Use of image analysis to assess the plasma membrane integrity of ram spermatozoa in different diluents. *Theriogenology* Vol.15, No.70(2), pp.192-8, 0093-691X

Yaniz, J.L., Marco-Aguado, M.A., Mateos, J.A. & Santolaria, P. (2010). Bacterial contamination of ram semen, antibiotic sensitivities, and effects on sperm quality during storage at 15 degrees C. *Animal Reproduction Science*, Vol.122, No.1-2, (Oct), pp. 142-149, 0378-4320

Yaniz, J.L., Mateos, J.A. & Santolaria, P. (2011). Zwitterionic buffers preserve ram semen quality more efficiently than TRIS during storage at 15 degrees C. *Small Ruminant Research*, Vol.95, No.1, (Jan), pp. 54-60, 0921-4488

Yeates, N.T.M. (1949). The breeding season of the sheep with particular reference to its modification by artificial means using light. *Journal of Agricultural Science*, Vol.39, No.1, pp. 1-&, 0021-8596

Younis, A.A., Alkamali, A.A. & Eltawil, E.A. (1978). Effect of flushing on fertility of Awassi and Hamdani ewes. *World Review of Animal Production*, Vol.14, No.2, pp. 41-48, 0043-8979

Yue, D., Yan, L., Luo, H., Xu, X. & Jin, X. (2010). Effect of Vitamin E supplementation on semen quality and the testicular cell membranal and mitochondrial antioxidant abilities in Aohan fine-wool sheep. *Animal Reproduction Science*, Vol.118, No.2-4, pp. 217-222, 0378-4320

Zeleke, M., Greyling, J.P.C., Schwalbach, L.M.J., Muller, T. & Erasmus, J.A. (2005). Effect of progestagen and PMSG on oestrous synchronization and fertility in Dorper ewes during the transition period. *Small Ruminant Research*, Vol.56, No.1-3, (Jan), pp. 47-53, 0921-4488

12

Effect of Cryopreservation on Sperm Quality and Fertility

Alemayehu Lemma
Addis Ababa University, School of Veterinary Medicine, Debre Zeit, Ethiopia

1. Introduction

Geographical barriers to breeding animals have long been reduced because of possibilities of semen transportation. In modern cattle breeding, where artificial insemination (AI) is the most widely applied tool facilitating extensive utilization of frozen semen from genetically superior sires, cryopreservation has been an invaluable technique. In order to extend the time span of the viability of spermatozoa, their metabolic rate has to be slowed down thereby reducing the rate at which substrates are used and toxins are produced. As a general rule cooling of spermatozoa is the simplest method that can successfully depress spermatozoal metabolic rate and therefore, prolong sperm survival. The use of carbon dioxide and other metabolic inhibitors like proteinase inhibitors are also known to produce a similar but less successful effect (Colenbrander *et al,* 2003; Cremades *et al,* 2005; Curry *et al,* 2000).

Semen stored after cooling to 5-8°C will survive for 24-48 h without a significant decline in motility and even up to 96 h without a significant drop in fertilization rates. Though chilling semen provides an efficient and successful means of short-term storage, it has yet some adverse effects on the spermatozoa manifested as a depression in viability rate, structural integrity, depressed motility and conception rates (Batellier *et al,* 2001; Medeiros *et al,* 2002; Watson, 2000). Preferably, the spermatozoa of many species can now be stored indefinitely at -196°C in liquid nitrogen for future use, while still retaining acceptable fertilization rates postthaw. The techniques for successful cryopreservation of spermatozoa have also slowly progressed over the past several decades (Hammerstedt *et al,* 1990) and are now fairly standardized. However, cryopreservation is also known to be detrimental to sperm function and fertility even with the most up to date techniques. Generally, sperm viability is decreased by 50%, whereas fertilizing capacity is affected by a factor of sevenfold after cryopreservation (Lessard *et al,* 2000).

The effects of cryopreservation on sperm function and fertility have been widely studied, particularly in bovine. Various sperm organelles have been known to be affected due to the detrimental effects of cryopreservation. Induction of premature acrosomal reaction, altered mitochondrial function, reduction of motility and failure of chromatin decondensation, all of which influence the viability and fertility of the sperm cells have been reported by different authors (Chaveiro *et al.* 2006; Cooter *et al,* 2005; Watson, 2000; Wongtawan *et al,* 2006). Cooling is a major stressor, as a result of which membrane bound phospholipids reorient themselves into a different configuration that disrupt membrane function and permeability

(Amman and Graham, 1993; Lessard *et al,* 2000). The stress response shown by spermatozoa as a reaction to a drop in temperature is referred as cold shock. Generally, cold shock damage manifests itself as a decline in cell metabolism, altered membrane permeability, loss of intracellular components, irreversible loss of spermatozoan motility and an increase in the number of dead spermatozoa. The damage to the cellular membranes is of most significance because it has a carry-over effect on other cellular structures and functions.
The severity of the cold shock depends upon the final temperature and the rate of temperature drop. The cellular damage resulting from cooling or freezing affecting both the structure and function of the cells can be categorized as direct or indirect (Amann and Pickett, 1987; Watson, 1990). Direct damage is more definable and is the type usually associated with cold shock evident shortly after the drop in temperature and is affected by the rate of cooling. Indirect or latent damage is more difficult to quantify and may not be initially apparent; it tends not to be dependent upon the rate of cooling. Addition of cryoprotectant agent (CPA) such as glycerol, or of other components such as egg yolk, milk, bovine serum albumin, polyvinyl alcohol and liposomes in extenders have been used in an attempt to providing some protection to spermatozoa and minimizing the adverse effects of cryopreservation (Katila, 1997). Direct cellular damage is irreversible and is usually apparent at later stage during postthaw analysis particularly in samples that are to rapidly frozen (Bildeau *et al,* 2000; Pommer *et al,* 2002; Samper, 2001). Hence, the ability to predict postthaw sperm quality and fertility from a routine sperm function assay would be greatly beneficial to the success of cryopreservation.

2. Cryopreservation of semen

In order to realize many of the potential advantages of AI, long-term storage of semen is necessary. This is only possible by freezing, a system which halts the metabolic processes of the spermatozoa, allowing indefinite storage without a significant loss of fertility. The discovery of the cryoprotectant properties of glycerol has made cryopreservation possible. Among the many benefits resulting from the process of cryopreservation are the genetic improvement of important farm species and control of diseases affecting them both of which have a highly significant impact on the sustainability of the agri-food industry (Bailey *et al,* 2000). Cryopreservation has been widely used in the modern cattle industry and AI has been the most widely applied tool in facilitating the extensive utilization of frozen semen. Today, cryopreservation has enabled producers to have the ability to access superior genetics for a fraction of the price of buying a bull. Increased breeding efficiency and exploitation of sires through AI programs has become widespread in both the dairy and equine industry. However, the development of a reliable method to cryopreserve sperm is extremely important for preservation of superior genes from valuable animals. The maximum time allowed from semen collection to insemination varies considerably, ranging from immediate insemination requirements to an indefinite in vitro semen storage period. As a result of the growing popularity of these artificial breeding programs, the need to maintain fertility of sperm after varying periods of storage has become increasingly important. In addition to this cryopreservation has enabled the storage of animal genetics to keep allele variation and keep hope for endangered species. Genome resource banking to preserve the biodiversity of rare and endangered species or valuable transgenic lines would also benefit from sperm cryopreservation. Moreover, reproductive research with non-domestic animals particularly those involving cryopreservation of sperm, oocytes, and embryos can also provide insight and direction into establishing more effective genetic and conservation management programs.

The success of cryopreservation depends upon many other factors, including interactions between cryoprotectant, type of extender, cooling rate, thawing rate and packaging, as well as the individual animal variation (Andrabi, 2007; Clulow *et al*, 2008; Cooter *et al*, 2005). Some loss in spermatozoan viability is inevitable due to the processing procedures prior to freezing as well as during the actual freezing process. Research reports of the success of cryopreserved semen vary significantly often affected by the method of experimentation and recording, which is unstandardized in many reproductive researches. Information about pregnancy rate to a single insemination, timing of insemination, the number of spermatozoa inseminated, volume of inseminate used or type of extender used are still incomplete for some farm animals. Moreover, motility of spermatozoa has proven to be an even poorer indicator of fertility in frozen–thawed samples (Samper *et al*, 1991). Regardless of all these considerations, for cryopreservation to be considered a success the process should enable a spematozoon to retain its fertilizing capacity at postthaw. To achieve this it must retain its ability to produce energy via metabolism; to maintain normal plasma membrane configuration and integrity; retain its motility; and enzymes, such as acrosin, within the acrosome to allow penetration of the ova. Disruption of any of these functions or abilities will significantly affect the spermatozoon's ability to achieve fertilization. The greatest risk to the maintenance of these attributes is presented by the formation of ice crystals and the resultant movement of water up osmotic gradients during the process of cryopreservation.

During the process of freezing, several biophysical changes are evident within the semen sample. As the temperature drops to below freezing the sample undergoes supercooling. As the temperature drops further beyond supercooling, extracellular ice crystals begin to form from the water within the surrounding medium. This ice formation increases the concentration of solutes, such as sugars, salts and proteins. In response to this newly developed osmotic pressure gradient and the fact that water within the spermatozoon is slower to form ice crystals than the water in the surrounding medium, water passes out of the spermatozoa, particularly from the spermatozoon head, across the semi-permeable plasma membrane. Consequently, the spermatozoon becomes increasingly dehydrated (Andrabi, 2007; Watson, 2000; Woelders, 1997). The rate of efflux of water from the spermatozoa also depends upon the speed of temperature drop: the slower the drop, the greater would be the time needed for the efflux of water, and hence a much greater dehydration. This does reduce the chance of ice crystal formation within the spermatozoon, which could cause considerable physical damage (Amann and Pickett, 1987; Hammerstedt *et al*, 1990), but an even greater damage occur due to increased intracellular dehydration and solute concentration. On the other hand, if the cooling rate is rapid, water has little time to move out of the spermatozoon and hence large intracellular ice crystals form, causing physical damage to cell membranes and other intracellular components. However, the problems of dehydration and solute concentration are less evident with rapid cooling. A successful cryopreservation should, therefore, aim at arriving at an optimum cooling rate that will provide a compromise between all these factors.

There are two main temperature ranges of concern regarding damage to spermatozoa during freezing: the period of supercooling (0°C to -5°C) and the formation of ice crystals (-6°C to -15°C) (Woelders, 1997). Excessive supercooling results in a rapid ice formation, with the possibility of physical damage. In samples other than semen, this problem can be overcome by a technique termed seeding, which is designed to induce ice formation more gradually over a greater temperature range. However, there is little or no evidence that seeding a semen sample during the freezing process has any advantageous effects. The second area of concern is known to have a significant effect on spermatozoan function post thaw. In an attempt to overcome some of these problems, the use of CPA has been investigated. Cryoprotectants may be divided into either penetrating or non-penetrating depending on their action. Penetrating cryoprotectants are able to penetrate the plasma membrane of the spermatozoa and, therefore, act intracellularly as well as extracellularly. The second type of CPA is non-penetrating and can only act extracellularly.

Glycerol remains to be one of the most favored CPA, especially with bovine semen. It is a penetrating cryoprotectant, acting as a solvent and readily taken up by spermatozoa, entering the cell within one minute of addition to the surrounding medium (Pickett and Amann, 1993). Its presence, both intra- and extracellularly, acts to lower the freezing point of the medium to a temperature much lower than that of water. This in turn reduces the proportion of the medium which is frozen at any one time, reducing the effect of low temperature on solute concentrations and hence on osmotic pressure differences (Amann and Pickett, 1987; Medeiros *et al*, 2002; Watson and Duncan, 1988). It also provides channels of unfrozen medium, between ice crystals, in which spermatozoa may exist while at low temperatures. A further effect of glycerol may be a salt buffering action. Other penetrating CPAs include dimethyl sulphoxide (DMSO) and propylene glycol. Non-penetrating CPAs include sugars like lactose, mannose, raffinose, trehalose and proteins, such as egg yolk lipoprotein. These CPAs are believed to act by increasing the osmotic pressure of the extracellular fluid and hence drawing water out of the spermatozoa, thereby decreasing the risk of formation of ice crystals and hence physical damage. However, they do not alleviate, and may even exacerbate the problem of dehydration and increases in solute concentration (Steinmann, 1996).

Other alternatives have been used as CPA, including Orvus ES paste, a mix of anionic detergents, and the synthetic detergent OEP, an amino-sodium lauryl sulphate. OEP apparently alters the composition of egg yolk, improving its cryprotectant properties. Its inclusion was initially tried in extenders for use with boar semen with some success. It was used in an extender containing 5% egg yolk, 2.5% glycerol at 0.4% proportion of OEP, along with lactose, fructose, glucose, ethylenediamine tetraacetic acid (EDTA), sodium citrate and sodium bicarbonate (Christanelli *et al*, 1984).

Both penetrating and non-penetrating CPAs themselves were later on known to cause some form of damage to the spermatozoa (Fiser *et al*, 1991). This was believed to be either due to physical damage as a result of the changes in osmotic pressure gradients or to biochemical disruption of subcellular components. The addition of cryoprotectant such as glycerol has a more adverse effect on motility than on mortality or fertility (Blach *et al*, 1989). A study was carried out in stallion semen sample (n=41) to compare two freezing techniques (cooling at +4°C for 2.5 hrs, suspending the straws on a rack in a Styrofoam box 3cm above liquid nitrogen for 7 minutes followed by plunging the straws in to the liquid nitrogen; and programmable freezer; IceCube 14S, Vers. 1.30, SY-LAB Gerate GmbH, Austria) using an extender containing egg yolk and glycerol (Gent extender, Minitube Int., Germany). The mean (±SD) total motility for samples frozen in liquid nitrogen was 32.8 ±13% (range=5-55%) while the mean (±SD) live percent was 43.3 ±13% (range=14-63%). Total motility and live sperm percent were also highly correlated (Fig.-1) in the samples frozen by liquid nitrogen. Though greater numbers of sperms were live, not all were found to be motile in both methods of freezing. Conversely, other studies indicate that the use of motility as an indication of viability is not a very accurate assessment in post-thaw samples. This is believed to be because of a greater detrimental effect of cryopreservation agent on the mitochondria than on the acrosome region of the spermatozoan head. The detrimental effect of glycerol on such function is apparently more evident in stallions than in other species such as bull.

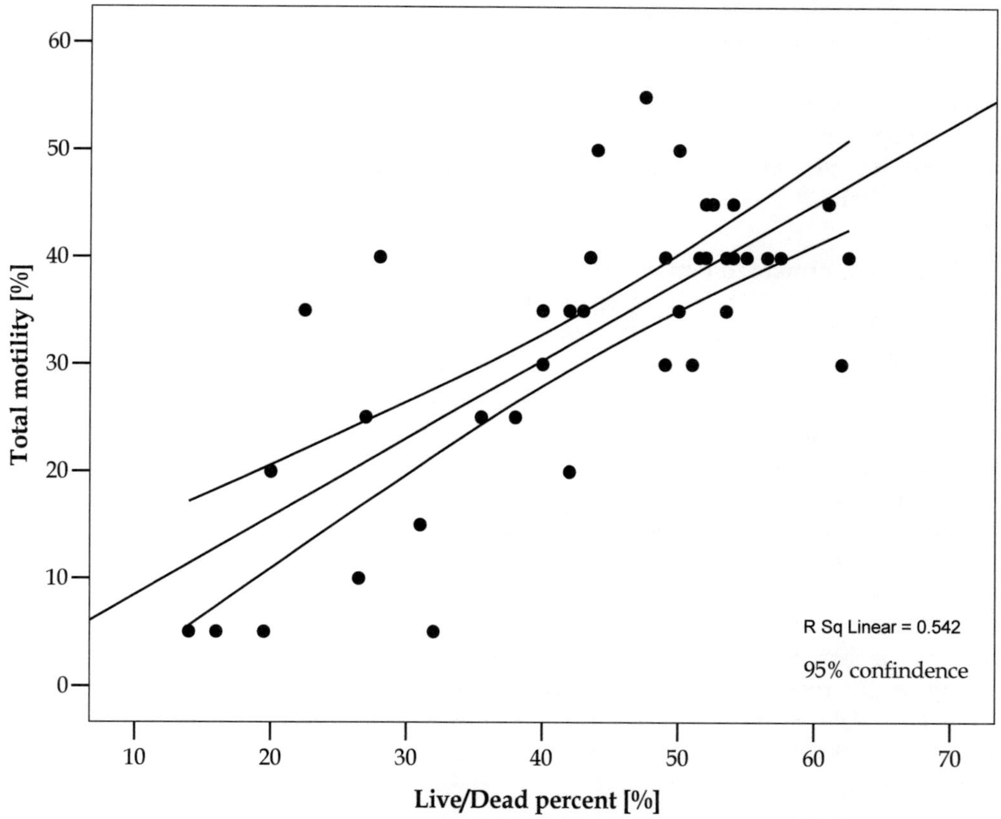

Fig. 1. Correlation between total motility and live/dead percent of stallion semen preserved in Gent extender containing egg yolk and glycerol preserved using liquid nitrogen

A further detrimental effect of the use of glycerol is the rapid efflux of glycerol from the spermatozoa into the glycerol-free secretions of the female's tract at insemination. This rapid exit across the plasma membrane is also believed to cause damage to the spermatozoa and, hence, loss of sperm function (Pickett and Amann, 1993). This accounts in part for the apparent poor positive correlation between motility and fertilization rates in post thaw equine spermatozoa. Computer-automated sperm head morphometry has been used to determine the effects of cryopreservation on bovine sperm head. The protocol for the use of cryoprotectants is ultimately a compromise between the advantages and detrimental effects of their incorporation. Consequently, the exact protocol may vary with individual breeding males in order to obtain optimal results. However, such individual tailoring is not practical in a commercial situation and hence further compromise is normally required.

3. Effect of cryopreservation on spermatozoa

Spermatozoa continuously change and develop from their origins as somatic cells until their destination as highly specialized cells capable of fertilization. They have basically three functional regions comprising a head that contain the condensed nuclear material, a mid piece serving as a powerhouse and a tail which is the propulsive region. Subsequent maturation occur within the epididymis, followed by further development induced first by contact with seminal plasma and then by the secretions of the female tract (Varner and Johnson, 2007). The final stages of spermatozoon development are induced by the immediate environment of the oocyte and its zona. In the process, most of the organelles are lost together with the cytoplasm, and the spermatozoal chromatin is remodeled. This specialization, though, is achieved at a cost, reducing the spermatozoon's ability to repair itself leading to a greater susceptibility to environmental change. Hence, even under ideal conditions, it is inevitable that some damage will occur to spermatozoa during the freezing process (Andrabi, 2007).

3.1 Effect on spermatozoal metabolism

The structural changes produced in the postthaw sperm cells membrane are primarily linked to altered abilities for energy sourcing. This would later on influence both cellular metabolism and other sperm functions such as motility (Cerolini *et al,* 2001; Dziekonska *et al,* 2009; Gillan *et al,* 2004). A spermatozoon is one of the smallest cells in the body specifically designed for propagation of genetic material achieved through fertilization. Like many other cells in the body, it requires a constant supply of energy for maintenance of cellular order and functions needed for survival and accomplishment of its task. This energy requirement increases significantly with the onset of activated motility, and becomes even more pronounced when hyperactivated motility is initiated (Granish and Suarez, 2002; Varner and Johnson, 2007). Plenty of exogenously derived nutrients are required by the spermatozoa to gain the strength needed for the long journey from the epididymis to the ovum in the female reproductive tract. These nutrients are metabolized intracellularly, resulting in the release of useable energy available for cellular processes primarily in the form of ATP. Like many metabolically active body cells, spermatozoa possess the metabolic machinery required for glycolysis, the citric acid cycle, and oxidative physphorylation. ATP for spermatozoa is mainly derived either by glycolysis in the cytoplasm or through oxidative phosphorylation in the mitochondria (Dziekonska *et al,* 2009; Januskauskas, and Zillinskas, 2002). The relative contributions of the two processes to ATP generation are as yet unclear. A gradual reduction in the metabolic activity of spermatozoa during storage at cold shock temperature could limit the production of detrimental by-products, which might compromise sperm function but metabolic activity altered in this way does also influence essential sperm functions such as motility. Among the different alterations of activity of the intracellular enzymes, glucose-6-phosphate-dehydrogenase is the first enzyme which leaves the cell when the cellular membrane is damaged during cold shock. Generally, the intracellular concentration of ATP is decreased or lost and the AMP/ADP-rate is increased by the cryopreservation.

Spermatozoal motility, considered to be one of the most frequently used characteristics for evaluating the fertility potential of ejaculated spermatozoa, is known to be dependent on mitochondrial function. The ATP generated by oxidative phosphorylation in the inner mitochondrial membrane is transferred to the microtubules to drive motility. Hence reduced sperm motility induced by cryopreservation is believed to be mainly associated with mitochondrial damage (Januskauskas, and Zillinskas, 2002; Ruiz-Pesini *et al,* 2001). In human spermatozoa, mitochondrial enzymatic activities were shown to be correlated with spermatozoal motility (Ruiz-Pesini *et al,* 2001). Male infertility can result from a significant decrease in the number of motile forms and/or from movement quality disorders. Some studies reported a significant correlation between computer assessed spermatozoal motility and field fertility (Januskauskas *et al,* 2003) however, in a more recent study (Garcia-Macias *et al,* 2007), spermatozoal total and progressive motilities and velocity parameters were known to have no correlation with fertility though the authors noticed that velocity parameters were highest in the high-fertility group in their study. The decrease in correlation between motility and fertility has been suggested to be due to a difference in the change of permeability of the acrosome and mitochondrial membranes to calcium ions. The acrosome membrane suffers most from cold shock which accounts for most of the fertility failure (Deneke N., Lemma A., and Yilma T., 2010, Unpublished information). Vesiculation of the acrosomal and plasma membranes occurs during sperm cell death which is termed as false acrosomal reaction. A true acrosome reaction, which precedes fertilization, occurs only in live, intact spermatozoa. Thus, it is important not only to analyze semen for sperm viability but also to determine the alteration of acrosomal integrity simultaneously. HOST and acrosomal integrity tests were employed to evaluate sperm membrane integrity in Holstein Friesian AI bulls belonging to the National Artificial Insemination Centre (Ethiopia). The proportion of sperm cells that reacted to HOST (n=36) was 60.6±9.2% and the proportion of sperm with altered acrosome in the same sample was 50.6%. HOST reaction was highly correlated ($r = 0.82$, $p<0.001$) to higher percent live sperm in frozen sample indicating that live sperms whose membrane is relatively intact will react to the HOST solution. When the two tests are performed simultaneously, acrosomal alteration seem to be directly correlated with membrane integrity as evidenced in the correlation study (Fig.-2). Similar correlation result between the incidence of swollen tails after incubation for 20-30 min, and of altered acrosomes and total spermatozoan motility has also been previously reported for horses (Cueva *et al,* 1997).

Storage of spermatozoa outside the body cavity can impact availability of oxygen and metabolic processes. Cryopreservation of spermatozoa is associated with both oxidative stress and physical stress (Chatterjee *et al,* 2001; Mazur *et al,* 2000). If raw or extended semen is left undisturbed in a laboratory setting, use of dissolved O_2 by aerobic respiration leads to depletion of O_2 and the need to resort to glycolysis for meeting energy demands. Spermatozoa such as that of a stallion are highly susceptible to extreme oxidative stress in view of their absolute reliance on the aerobic metabolism to meet their ATP requirements. Moreover, their inability to synthesize antioxidants, their exuberant content of polyunsaturated fatty acid, their unique capacity to generate superoxide anions (O_2^-) and hydrogen peroxide (H_2O_2) through mitochondrial respiration, and their restricted endogenous antioxidant defense mechanism which is lost with the cytoplasm during the final stages of spermatogenesis all contribute to the extreme oxidative stress also observed during cryopreservation (Aitken and Baker, 2004; Parks and Lynch, 1992;). Compared to the raw fresh semen, cryoprserved spermatozoa experience a shorter lifespan and a lower fertility (Andrabi, 2007; Samper, 2001). This was partially attributed to the great difference between fresh and frozen sperm in the generation rate of O_2^- and H_2O_2 or in the intracellular concentration of free calcium ions (Ca^{2+}) (Ball and Vo, 1999; Pommer et al 2002; Samper, 2001). Protection against the effects of reactive oxygene species like O_2^- and H_2O_2 in

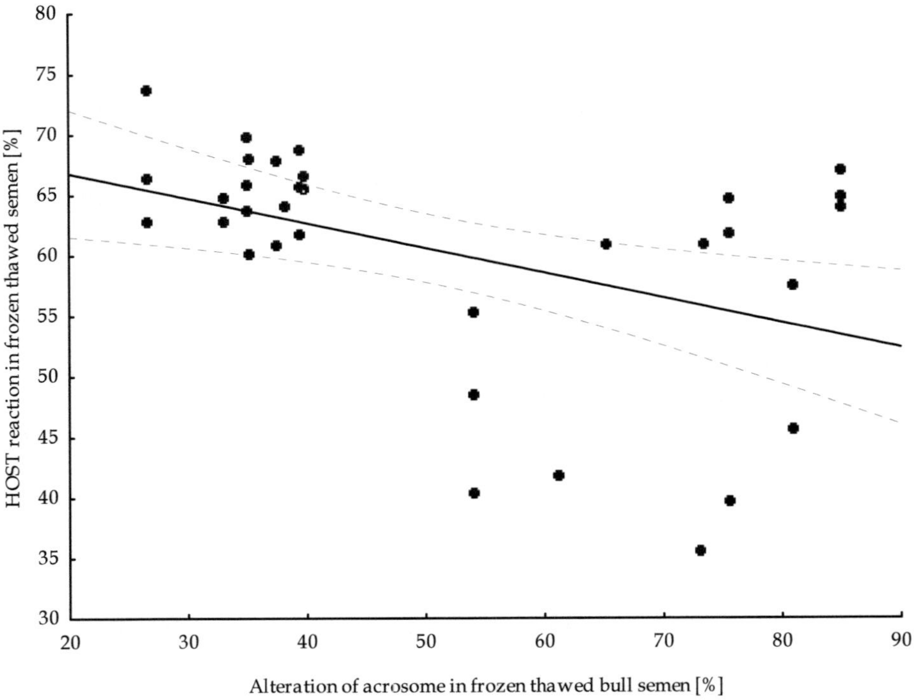

Fig. 2. Correlation between HOST reaction and alteration of acrosomal integrity in frozen-thawed bull semen (n = 36; r= -0.45; p<0.001)

spermatozoa is afforded by a variety of scavenging molecules. Pyruvate, for instance, is a potent scavenger of H_2O_2 and its supplementation to a chilled stored stallion semen or to a frozen thawed bull semen resulted in a significant augmentation of sperm motility and ATP levels. Oxidation of thiols in sperm proteins by O_2^- and H_2O_2 was found to be associated with inhibition of sperm motility and fertilizing ability (Mamoto *et al*, 1996). Cryopreservation of bull sperm in egg yolk based extenders significantly reduced the intracellular level of thiols and post-thaw treatment of frozen semen with thiols containing antioxidants prevented H_2O_2 -mediated loss of sperm motility (Bilodaeu *et al*, 2001).

3.2 Effect on spermatozoal ultra-structure

Mammalian sperm are very sensitive to lower temperature past body temp down to the freezing point of water mainly due to the sensitivity of the plasma membrane which is the primary site of injury in cryopreserved spermatozoa. The freezing induces membrane alteration, which when thawed, causes changes in protein activity and subsequently altered permeability to water and solutes. This results in a substantial loss of viable spermatozoa (Bailey *et al*, 2003). The characteristics of membranes that affect their sensitivity include cholesterol/phospholipid ratio, content of non-bilayer-preferring lipids, degree of hydrocarbon chain saturation and protein/phospholipid ratio (Medeiros *et al*, 2002). Each species of animal contains a different membrane composition. This causes different effects from cooling and subsequently different cryosensitivity of sperm across various species.

Membranes are naturally fluid, a prerequisite for their efficient function. The two main factors known to affect fluidity are the relative concentrations of phospholipids and cholesterol in which higher concentration of phospholipids results in a more fluid membrane, and the temperature of the membrane. As membranes are cooled, lipids undergo transition from their normal fluid state to a liquid crystalline state, in which the fatty acyl chains become disordered (Medeiros *et al*, 2002; Parks and Lynch, 1992; Watson, 2000). During freezing this liquid crystalline state is transformed to a gel state where the fatty acyl chains become re-ordered in a parallel fashion producing a rigid structure. The phase transition temperature for these changes varies with different lipids and depends upon their structures. In general, the longer the fatty acyl chains, the higher is the phase transition temperature. As each lipid class within a membrane reaches its phase transition temperature it conforms to the gel configuration and tends to aggregate together with other similarly conformed lipids within the membrane (Parks and Graham, 1992). The remainder of the lipids within the membrane may still be fluid, so areas of gel membrane can be identified within a mainly fluid structure. In addition, the junction areas between the gel and the other lipid and protein fractions become areas of weakness, subject to fusion and rupture as well as being permeable to ions (Hammerstedt *et al*, 1990).

The peak phase transition temperature for phospholipids within the membrane of boar's, bull's and stallion's spermatozoa are 24.0°C, 25.4°C and 20.70°C, respectively. Similarly, the peak transition temperature for glycolipids in stallion spermatozoon membranes is 33.4°C, compared with 36.2°C and 42.8°C for boars and bulls, respectively (Parks and Lynch, 1992). These differences in peak transition temperatures account for the variable tolerance to cold shock exhibited by spermatozoa from these species of domestic animals. The membrane configuration has a roughly even distribution of phospholipids in both the outer and inner layers for reasons of stability. The major phospholipids within the spermatozoon plasma membrane namely phosphatildylcholine, sphingomyelin and phosphatidylethanolamine have differing positions within the membrane bilayer. Phosphatidylcholine and sphingomyelin are associated with the outer layer of the bilayer, whereas phosphatidylethanolamine has an affinity for the inner, cytosolic layer. These affinities are not normally evident except when the membrane is under stress. Hence, cold shock causes changes to the distribution of the phospholipids across the bilayer which results in altered membrane function (Amann and Pickett, 1987; Hammerstedt *et al*, 1990). Generally, changes in plasma membrane integrity and motility are both indicators of sperm viability and metabolic intactness. In this regard boar spermatozoa are known to suffer extensive membrane and tail damage during freezing and thawing, and those spermatozoa that survive suffer from a shortened lifespan, requiring AI to be carried out with large numbers of spermatozoa closely timed to the moment of ovulation (Wongtawan *et al*, 2006).

Another major component of the spermatozoon membrane is protein. The protein-lipid interactions are critical for the efficient functioning of the membrane. It is important to ensure even distribution and molding of proteins into the bilayer, thus eliminating pores and membrane faults. These interactions may also be required for the efficient functioning of these proteins as enzymes, receptors or channels for the movement of ions like calcium ions. These configurations of the membrane and interactions between its components function ideally at a normal body temperature. Hence, freezing beyond the transition phase temperature results in a change to the gel state and a gradual aggregation of specific lipids within the membrane. Consequently, these protein-lipid interactions are disrupted and therefore, the proteins no longer act efficiently as enzymes, receptors or ionic channels (Medeiros *et al*, 2002). The membrane as a whole loses some of its structural and functional integrity. Disruption of the membrane configuration also interferes with the function of the glycocalyx components, peripheral proteins known to confer stability to the spermatozoa in their passage through the female system. This will influence peripheral protein attachment, causing them to aggregate in the areas of membrane still in the fluid state once gel formation has begun (Andrabi, 2007; Housley and Stanley, 1982). Many of these changes to membrane configuration involving lipids are known to be irreversible and subsequent warming of the spermatozoa does not restore the original membrane configuration.

Another sperm alteration linked to freezing is related to the transfer of proteins through the cell, which is modulated by the distribution of lipids along the membrane, altering the response to induction of capacitation and the acrosome reaction of frozen/thawed spermatozoa during fertilization (Guthrie and Welch, 2005). Dislocation of proteins in the plasma membrane, such as those belonging to the glucose transporter (GLUT) family have also been reported as major problem related to cryopreservation. These GLUT proteins are mainly responsible for the transport of hexose across mammalian sperm membranes (Kokk *et al*, 2005). GLUT proteins have been detected in the spermatozoa membrane of dog (Rigau *et al*, 2002), human (Kokk *et al*, 2005) and boar (Medrano *et al.*, 2006), highlighting their important role in the regulation of sperm glucose and fructose metabolism.

Ultrastructural studies have shown the presence of detrimental effects of cryopreservation on various sperm organelles such as altered spermatozoal mitochondria (Nishizono *et al*, 2004). Microscopic examination of stallion spermatozoa indicates that the function of the mitochondrial cristae is also affected by cold shock. This damage to mitochondrial structure and hence its function within the spermatozoa is likely to account for the decrease in motility observed after freezing (Ruiz-Pesini *et al*, 2001). Moreover, swelling of the acrosomal area was observed to be a consequence of cold shock, which indicates a loss of integrity as membranes are normally unable to stretch. Freezing is also known to change motion characteristics of spermatozoa due to the irreversible changes to the mid-piece and coiling of the tail (Watson, 1990). Particularly in donkeys, spermatozoa show an increased incidence of backward motion because of an over-bending of the tail area (Ayalew E. and Lemma A., 2010; Tsega A. and Lemma A., 2009; Unpublished observation).

Cryopreservation has also been shown to induce the acrosome reaction in spermatozoa. DNA integrity of sperm is essential for accurate transmission of paternal genetic information. Normal condensation and stabilization of sperm chromatin in the nucleus followed by decondensation after sperm penetration and injection into the cytoplasm of the oocyte are pre-requisites for fertilization. However, sperm chromatin structure and DNA are known to be altered or damaged during cryopreservation (Donnelly *et al*, 2001; Fraser and Strzezek 2004; Hammadeh *et al*, 2001; Peris *et al*, 2004). It is reported that the cryopreservation process of freezing and thawing can increase abnormal chromatin condensation in human (Donnelly *et al*, 2001; Hammadeh *et al*, 2001; Royere *et al*, 1991), boar (Fraser and Strzezek, 2004), and ram (Peris *et al*, 2004) sperm. Normal chromatin packaging is also known to significantly decrease after the freeze-thawing procedure in human sperm. The chromatin structure of a mature spermatozoon is normally highly condensed, making about 5-10% in volume of that of a somatic cell. This packing is a result of a marked alteration in the composition of nucleoproteins that occurs during epididymal transit. The spermatid genome encodes for protamines, a unique type of spermatozoal protein, which predominate as nucleoproteins during spermatozoal maturation in the epididymis. The cysteine residues of this protein establish intramolecular and intermolecular disulfide linkages that result in compaction and stabilization of the associated DNA. This design is believed to provide protection to the chromosomes during their transport within the female reproductive tract (Varner and Johnson, 2007). It has been postulated that a reduction of sperm surface area due to alteration of sperm chromatin may ultimately be manifested in abnormal morphology of the sperm head. A decrease in the percentage of normal sperm heads in the ejaculate has been correlated with lowered fertility in bulls and over-condensation of chromatin appears to be associated with reduced fertility in men (Royere *et al*, 1991). Moreover, cryopreservation appears to reduce the ability of sperm chromatin to decondense. The adverse effects of cryopreservation on sperm chromatin and head morphology may be responsible for lowered fertility of spermatozoa observed after cryopreservation.

3.3 Cpacitaion-like effect of cryopreservation

Once spermatozoa reach the site of fertilization, there appear to be highly coordinated cellular and molecular events that should happen before the actual fertilization. The sperm cells first attach temporarily to oviductal epithelial cells, a process that requires specific cell to cell attachment, possibly mediated through spermatozoal surface carbohydrate-binding proteins, termed lectins (Varner and Johnson, 2007). They then undergo capacitation and hyperactivation, bind to the oocyte zona pellucida, undergo the acrosome reaction, penetrate the zona, and finally fuse with and penetrate the oolemma. Intracellular calcium levels increase in sperm during capacitation, hyperactivation and the zona pellucida-induced acrosome reaction. Increased concentrations of calcium ions are believed to trigger an intracellular signalling way associated with capacitation. Capacitaion and cryopreservation induce several similar changes to the sperm including calcium influx in to the cells (Bailey *et al*, 2000). However, during cryopreservation sperm cells fail to properly moderate normal internal calcium levels. Restructured membranes and distorted lipid-protein associations are believed to favour further calcium ion influx during cryopreservation. Disruption of the normal capacitation and/or the acrosome reaction due to abnormal concentrations of calcium ion would severely compromise the fertilizing potential of spermatozoa post-thaw. On the other hand, cryopreserved sperm cells exhibit a capacitaion-like behaviour and appear to be in a partially capacitated state due to the cryopreservation-induced membrane changes that makes the cells to be more active to their environment after thawing. As demonstrated by different authors, capacitaion normally creates a state of destabilization with which the sperm cell acquires the fertilizing capacity while remaining susceptible to membrane degeneration and spontaneous acrosomal reaction when fertilization fails (Bailey *et al*, 2000). Cryopreservation creates a subpopulation of killed and partially or fully capaciatated sperm thereby reducing the heterogeneity of the sperm population. This will produce a sperm subpopulation with a shortened lifespan in vivo and whose fertilization potential has been severely compromised reducing the fertility of the semen sample as a whole.

Capacitaion like effect or 'Cryo-capacitation' is one of the major factors associated with reduced longevity and poor survivability of cryopreserved spermatozoa in female reproductive tract (Bailey *et al*, 2000; Watson, 2000), resulting in reduced fertility of frozen-thawed semen. At present, it is generally accepted that poor survival of spermatozoa in the female reproductive tract is among the most important consequences of sperm cryoinjury caused by cryopreservation. This concept of premature capacitation and reduced longevity of sperm cells in the female reproductive tract has led to the routine use of oviductal insemination by laparscopy rather than vaginal or even transcervical insemination in different animals (Bailey *et al*, 2000). The capacitation-like changes have been demonstrated by greater proportion of chlortetracycline fluorescent pattern "B" due to freezing thawing in bull (Cormier *et al*, 1997), boar (Maxwell, and Johnson, 1997), equine spermatozoa (Thomas, *et al*, 2006), and in buffalo bull semen (Kadirvel *et al*, 2009). Impaired sperm membrane function due to cryopreservation inevitably diminishes the successful union of the oocyte and spermatozoa during in vivo fertilization. The structural reorganization of the sperm head plasma membranes after cryopreservation appears to disrupt the ability of the sperm to interact normally with cells of the female genital tract (Lessard *et al*, 2000; Medeiros *et al*, 2002; Watson, 2000). Poorly motile spermatozoa are also less likely to arrive at the site of fertilization in vivo or to penetrate the zona. Moreover, the proportion of motile sperm population itself is adversely affected by cryopreservation (Cerolini *et al*, 2001; Gillan *et al*, 2004). Reduced sperm binding is likely a result of membrane injury, possibly by structural damage to the sperm receptors or by incomplete receptor aggregation.

4. Evaluation of post-thaw semen quality

The semen quality and its relationship with fertility have great importance in animal production. Hence, in vitro tests are frequently applied to determine the quality of semen for its approval and use in both AI and other biotechnology procedures. Conventional laboratory tests for assessment of semen quality include light microscopic study of spermatozoal morphology, and estimation of spermatozoal motility which in turn encompass percentages of motile and progressively motile sperm; velocity of spermatozoal movement; and longevity following in vitro storage. Other features of semen quality include concentration, volume, detection of the presence of urine, blood, or potentially pathogenic bacteria and functional integrity tests. The choice of adequate parameters by reproducible, fast and sensitive methods is of increasing concern. This is because the predictive value of the standard seminal parameters is limited or insufficient for the identification of subfertile individuals (Clement, 2001; Love *et al*, 2000).

The nucleus, acrosome, the flagellum, mitochondria, and the plasma membrane are the most important regions of the spermatozoa that need to be assessed during postthaw semen evaluation. A series of laboratory tests devised to evaluate these various compartments will aid in the improved localization of spermatozoal dysfunction thereby improving the predictive values of laboratory-based semen evaluation to a relatively more accurate level. More specific techniques such as testing the mitochondrial function, flagellar substructure, and plasma membrane integrity are already available (Graham and Moce, 2005; Gravance *et al*, 2001; Thomas *et al*, 1998). A variety of laboratory procedures used today in the assessment of the integrity of the plasma membrane are important components of the postthaw semen evaluation. Among them is the evaluation of the ability of spermatozoa to exclude extracellular dyes, such as eosin, which are non permeable when the membrane is intact. Another approach is the hypo-osmotic swelling test (HOST) in which the spermatozoa are exposed to a hypotonic media (50 to 100-mOsm range) to test their osmoregulatory function (Davies-Morel, 1999; Neild *et al*, 1999). Dyes that can traverse the membrane and those that are membrane-impermeable can be combined in a solution before spermatozoal exposure to provide a more accurate reflection of membrane integrity. For instance, fluorescent plasma-membrane dyes can be combined with mitochondrial dyes or acrosomal dyes to provide more thorough coverage of the functional regions in the assay (Garner *et al*, 1994; Kavak *et al*, 2003; Love *et al*, 2003). More recently, a computer assisted semen analysis (CASA) is in use and gives extensive information about the kinetic property of the ejaculate based on measurements of the individual sperm cells. Using CASA, motility and movement characteristics of spermatozoa have been correlated to in vivo fertility. Still, CASA-assessed motility is done on a rather limited number of spermatozoa and is predisposed to a certain degree of human bias.

An understanding of how molecular and ultra-structural basis of spermatozoal function, spermatozoa-oviductal interactions, and gamete engagement are influenced by cryopreservation will undoubtedly lead to many practical applications in semen evaluation. From this may arise possibilities for detailed laboratory tests to assess spermatozoal function, to introduce improved methods of semen preservation, options for applications of assisted reproductive technologies and even treatment options for subfertile animals. The chromatin structure assay (SCSA) tests, for instance, is a flow cytometric procedure that uses the metachromatic fluorochrome to test the denaturability of spermatozoal chromatin that is not normally monitored by conventional methods in various species (Evenson *et al,* 1995; Love 2005; Makhlouf and Niederberger, 2006). Chromatin susceptibility to denaturation is correlated with the level of actual DNA strand breaks and might be indicative of genetically defective spermatozoa (Evenson *et al,* 1995). Several types of defective sperm organelles and DNA can be detected in large number of sperm by immunochemical assays and flow cytometry. Microarray profiling of sperm mRNA has been shown to indicate gene expression associated with both fertile and infertile males (Evenson *et al,* 2002; Thomas *et al,* 1998). More importantly, spermatozoa affected by such damage might show no apparently detectable alteration in motility or membrane integrity, but may induce embryonic failure after fertilization (Fatehi *et al,* 2006). Further DNA damages are not evident until the time of fertilization making the chromatin defect clinically significant as it represents a potential non repairable defect. This becomes quite important clinically, because affected spermatozoa in an ejaculate may not be impaired from fertilization, and hence performing repeated insemination may not increase pregnancy rate.

The search for the identification of biochemical markers of spermatozoal function is still ongoing. Such finding will improve the efficiency of laboratory-based detection of infertility induced by the process of freezing/thawing by targeting specific cellular components. However, incorporation of detailed tests such as SCSA for semen evaluation should not replace or reduce the value of the conventional methods of spermatozoal motility or morphology tests. More recently, much attention has been given to the test of capacitation process, as an immediate precursor to fertilization. However, on the path to fertilization there are many preliminary steps prior to capacitation leading to the need for sperm evaluation involving tests of spermatozoal response to particular environmental conditions related to the overall fertilization process (Petrunkina *et al,* 2007).

5. Fertility of cryopreserved spermatozoa

The process of cryopreservation represents an artificial interruption of the progress of the spermatozoon towards post-ejaculation maturation and fertilization. Even with the best preservation techniques to date, cryopreservation process still causes harmful damage to the spermatozoa. As it has been discussed earlier in this chapter, cryopreservation affects fertility by virtue of its effect on sperm membranes, cytoskeleton, motile apparatus and nucleus, and cell metabolism. Moreover, freezing and subsequent thawing procedures render the remaining surviving spermatozoa physiologically different from spermatozoa before cryopreservation. Sprmatozoa become very sensitive to any form of stress in their environment in vivo as well as in vitro. As a result, fertility from frozen thawed semen is poorer than that obtained from fresh semen. For this reason, proper evaluation of the post-thaw quality of spermatozoa is of utmost interest for AI industry to obtain information on the fertilizing capacity of the cryopreserved semen.

Many tests of sperm motility, morphology, acrosomal status, defective sperm organelles and DNA, and metabolism have been correlated with fertility (Evenson *et al*, 2002; Larsson and Rodriquez-Martinez, 2000; Muller, 2000; Saacke *et al*, 2000; Thomas *et al*, 1998). All of these spermatozoal attributes have been shown to be either directly or indirectly affected by cryopreservation or the thawing process. The correlation between fertility and percentage of motile sperm in a semen sample has already been demonstrated. In one study, after insemination of 55 cows with frozen semen a 30.9% (17 cows) pregnancy rate with an average number of services per conception of 2.7 was found. Conception rate to first service was only 7.2%. The mean (±SD) alteration of acrosome and positive reaction to HOST for successful (pregnant) and failed insemination (non pregnant) were 47.6 ± 9.9% and 64.7 ± 3.0%, and 62.7 ± 7.3% and 42.1 ± 3.9%, respectively with a highly significant ($p<0.001$) difference in both tests between the successful and failed inseminations. Semen that did not impregnate contained the highest proportion of sperm with altered acrosome that did not react well to HOST. This shows the significance of the use of combination of semen evaluation methods to avoid the use of poor quality semen and hence reduce the male factor from fertility assessments (Deneke N., Lemma A., and Yilma T., 2010, Unpublished information). Significant variation in the success rates for frozen semen has been reported with an apparently much wider variation in the performance of equine semen post freezing and thawing than is with bovine semen. For instance, one-cycle pregnancy rates of 32-51% have been reported in mares (Muller, 1987; Pickett and Amann, 1993).

In general, pregnancy rates for frozen semen at best reach values approaching those of natural service but may also result in complete failure, despite the protocol for freezing apparently being unchanged (Pickett and Amann, 1993). It is very difficult, therefore, to predict likely conception rates with any certainty and it is also very difficult to compare, with accuracy, the pregnancy rates obtained in different research work using frozen semen. In most of the research carried out there are many variables, the details of which are often not specified. The results reported for pregnancy rates depend, among other things, upon: the individual animal and the quality of semen produced; the minimum standard set for semen quality prior to acceptance for freezing; the number of spermatozoa per straw and straws per insemination; the freezing protocol; the thawing protocol; post-thaw semen quality control; the numbers and reproductive ability of the females used for insemination; the timing of the insemination; the number of inseminations per cycle; and the number of cycles and inseminations per pregnancy. Hence, no absolute figure has been arrived at for pregnancy rates using frozen semen (Pickett and Amann 1993). Fertility of an ejaculate from a male is also highly dependent on the fertility of the females. Conversely, a more recent review indicates that male fertility should not be evaluated independently of female fertility (Amann, 2005). The same author reported that a stallion with 95% fertility can have an observed fertility as high as 90% if bred to mares with 95% fertility, and as low as 24% if bred to mares with 25% fertility. Subsequently lower fertility is seen if the stallion's fertility is lower. Because of this female factor in fertility using a single male on a group of females to ascertain fertility is not sufficient to extrapolate the results to a population.

6. Extenders used in freezing semen

The addition of a cryoprotectant in to the semen sample is needed in order to protect spermatozoa from cold shock. A large variety of extenders combining various components (sugars, electrolytes, buffers, egg yolk, milk and milk products), have been proposed and used for extending sperm. Milk and milk-based extenders are known to be practical and efficient in protecting spermatozoa of various species (Batellier *et al*, 2001; Varner *et al*, 1989). Based on the composition and dynamics of the spermatic membranes, some substances such as lipids, fatty acids and proteins have been incorporated to the semen with the goal of decreasing sperm damages related to cryopreservation. Glycerol and egg yolk extenders are amongst the first to be used for freezing semen (Curry, 2000; Garner *et al*, 1999; Holt, 2000; Medeiros *et al.*, 2002), and today many extenders use glycerol as the major cryoprotectant. Glycerol is used at a relatively high concentration which can be detrimental to spermatozoan viability at higher temperatures hence it is added after the semen has been cooled (Fahy, 1986). The deleterious effects are due to osmotic stress, changes in membrane organization, fluidity and permeability, as well changes in the lipid composition. Thus, a compromise has to be reached with regards to the concentration of glycerol and the length of time that the glycerol is in contact with the spermatozoa prior to freezing, in order to maximize the beneficial effects of glycerol as a cryoprotectant but minimize its toxic effects. In one study, the inclusion rate of 4% glycerol in an extender containing 20% egg yolk was found to be superior to 2% or 6% glycerol as regards to progressive motility (Cochran *et al*, 1984). In addition, the efficiency of glycerol may be affected by the diluents to which it is added, as well as the method of storage.

The cryoprotectant nature of many other substances, including sugars and liposomes has also been demonstrated. In equines, it is a common practice today that the preparation of semen for cryopreservation involves the use of two extenders: a primary extender for initial dilution, which is aspirated off after centrifugation, prior to the addition of a secondary extender for freezing. Numerous extenders have been used as primary or secondary extenders. Examples of extenders for freezing include egg yolk and those based on skimmed milk with egg yolk (Pickett and Amann, 1993). Good success has been reported with the use of trehalose as a cryoprotectant within a skimmed milk-egg yolk extender. It is suggested that trehalose has a stabilizing effect on the spermatozoon plasma membrane (Steinmann, 1996).

Unlike the bull and the ram in which fructose is the major energy source, most extenders use glucose as the major source of energy for metabolic activity and movement of spermatozoa in equines (Katila, et al, 2001). In this regard, three extenders were evaluated for their efficiency of sustaining the viability of jack sperm as measured by motility characteristics (Ayalew E. and Lemma A., 2010; Unpublished observation). The first extender was a heated skimmed milk (95°C for 10 minutes and cooled to 37°C before use). The second extender was prepared from glucose (4gm), glycerol (4%), and crystalline penicillin (150,000 IU) diluted in heated skimmed milk to make up 100ml extender (represented as SMGLU). The third extender contained 4% glycerol in skimmed milk (represented as SMGLY). SM was used for storage in Equitainer (Agtech Inc, Manhattan, USA) while SMGLU and SMGLY were used for liquid nitrogen storage after a 2.5hr optimization at +4°C, suspension over liquid nitrogen vapour for 7 minutes and plunging the straws immediately into the liquid nitrogen. SMGLU preserved sperm showed superior results ($p<0.05$) for both total and forward progressive motility than either SM alone or SMGLY (Table 1).

Semen parameter	SM [Equitainer] n=15	SMGLY [Liquid nitrogen] n=32	SMGLU [Liquid nitrogen] n=13
Live sperm after 24hr [%]	36.2±24.3	10.2±11.7	34.3±7.5
Total Motility after 24hr [%]	24 ±17.4	8.8 ±9.6	30±10.6
Progressive motility at 24hr [%]	19.3 ±14.5	7.2±7	24.6±10.5

Table 1. Mean (±SD) of semen parameters for three different extenders used to dilute jack semen

In another study, insemination of 34 animals (17 mares and 17 jennys) with jack semen extended in heated skimmed milk and stored in Equitainer (Agtech Inc, Manhattan, USA) for 24 hrs resulted in 38.2% pregnancy rate (Tsega A. and Lemma A., 2009; Unpublished observation). Addition of trehalose to bull semen extenders is known to provide a modest improvement in fertility when used in combination with glycerol, which remains the cryoprotective agent of choice. Egg yolk phospholipids can also lessen chilling injury on bull sperm by binding to low density lipoproteins of the membrane and by increasing the permeability of the membrane, although they do not alter intrinsic membrane composition and/or physical properties (Holt, 2000). The addition of concanavalin-A to the freezing diluent, a substance that has the ability to coat and thus protect spermatozoa membrane, has been suggested to provide additional protection for acrosome membranes and help to preserve motility post freezing and during thawing (Koskinen *et al*, 1989). The inclusion of liposomes, which have proved successful in bulls, has been tried with some success in equine semen (Heitland *et al*, 1995).

7. Freezing and thawing rates

Storage of semen at ambient temperature does not in itself significantly reduce the spermatozoan metabolic rate, thus limiting the potential length of storage and demanding cryopreservation at -196°C in liquid nitrogen for long term storage. The cooling/freezing rate in the critical temperature range is of considerable importance during cryopreservation process because this determines whether the spermatozoa will remain in equilibrium with their extracellular environment or become progressively supercooled with the increasing possibility of intracellular ice formation (Kumar *et al*, 2003). During slow cooling, the dehydration of the spermatozoa can proceed to the point of osmotic equilibrium between intracellular and extracellular space with maximal, often detrimental, cellular dehydration. However, raising the cooling rate too much will not prevent the formation of intracellular ice because of the slow dehydration. Therefore, the survivability of the spermatozoa depends upon the optimum cooling rate. Optimal cooling rate will reduce the excessive concentration of intracellular solutes and intracellular dehydration thereby reducing excessive shrinkage of the sperm cells. However, even at optimum cooling rates, spermatozoa remain vulnerable to the unfavorable conditions for a shorter period of time (Woelders, 1997).

The type of extender used and the speed of temperature drop are known to have an effect on susceptibility of spermatozoa to cold shock and the success rate of freezing semen. Moreover, the freezing rate depends on the method of processing and of storage. The cooling of straws can be conveniently done by either initial suspension in racks over a tank of liquid nitrogen or a computer-controlled programmable freezer followed by plunging into liquid nitrogen for long-term storage (Clulow *et al*, 2008). The extent of damage to a spermatozoon as a result of cold shock depends not only on the drop in temperature but also the speed with which this drop is attained. The rate of temperature drop was found to be most critical over the specific temperature range of 0-5°C when motility was evaluated later. In general, the faster the rate of cooling, the more severe is the damage (Kayser, 1990). There is further evidence which suggests that the rate of temperature drop also determines the subsequent active life of the spermatozoa (Andrabi, 2007).

Frozen spermatozoa are further injured during the thawing process, which has been regarded as being due to re-crystallization of ultra-microscopic ice crystals to form comparatively large ice crystals (Watson, 2000; Woelders, 1997). The warming damage occurs when the spermatozoa pass through the critical temperature zone of -5°C to -15°C (Kumar *et al*, 2003). Water bath temperatures between 4°C and 75°C can be used to successfully thaw semen however, the temperature chosen for the water bath depends on the desired rate of thawing. During fast thawing (optimum; at 37°C for at least 45 sec) the time for re-crystallization to occur is limited and this increases the survivability of spermatozoa. However, when the duration of thawing is insufficient for the out-flow of excess cryoprotectant from the cell it suffers osmotic stress and the spermatozoa swells and lyses as the medium becomes abruptly diluted by the melting of extracellular ice (Pegg, 2002). The thawing rate can be influenced by factors such as the temperature and nature of the environment (air or water bath) and the thermal conductivity of the packaging as related to the diameter of the lumen of the packing. Some semen thawing protocols involve the addition of warmed extender to aid the process of thawing which will also increase the volume of the inseminate and aid preservation of spermatozoan viability. Thawing extenders may be used for semen stored in pellets, vials or straws, and are added as part of the thawing process.

8. Packaging for frozen semen

To maximally utilize the genetics of desired sires on a commercial basis, attempts are made to package a minimal number of spermatozoa per insemination unit without sacrificing fertility (Foote and Parks, 1993; Shannon and Vishwanath, 1995). Ultimately, the number of motile spermatozoa per insemination is determined by the postthaw motility evaluations and non return to estrus rates from a large number of inseminations. The ability to predict postthaw sperm quality and fertility from a routine sperm function assay is beneficial when one considers the extended period of progeny testing.

Several methods are available for the packaging of spermatozoa for freezing in different species. They include glass ampoules or vials, polypropylene, polyvinyl or plastic round or flat straws (usually 0.5-1.0 ml in volume), flat aluminium packets (10-15 ml); pellets (0.1-0.2 ml), and macrotubes (Heitland *et al*, 1996; Kneissl, 1993; Park *et al*, 1995). Both ampoules and straws are traditionally frozen by suspension over liquid nitrogen, followed by plunging into liquid nitrogen at -196°C. Subsequent work investigating the effect of the rate of freezing led to the current application of the use of computer-controlled programmable freezers at different packaging sizes (Clulow *et al*, 2008). Although pellets have the advantage of allowing a rapid drop in temperature to be achieved, they are not suited for easy identification after freezing. In addition, the re-use of the carbon dioxide block or metal plate carries the potential risk of cross contamination with spermatozoa from the previous freezing batch. On the other hand, the use of vials or straws readily allows the accurate identification of samples and considerably reduces the risk of cross-contamination during cryopreservation.

As different methods of storage have been used, the question of whether the means of storage has any effect on the success rate of cryopreservation has been raised. In this regard, different authors have compared spermatozoa stored in different packages (Heitland *et al*, 1996; Kneissl 1993; Park *et al*, 1995). Their results showed an effect on spermatozoa quality manifested through reduced motility and conception rate. The reports further stressed the roles of different extenders used, the interaction between extender, and means of packaging. However, the reasons for these discrepancies was not fully explained, and it was also not clear in all work how the dimensions of the straws change with volume, in addition to which different extenders and concentration of spermatozoa were used. On the other hand, a more recent work in stallion demonstrated that stallion spermatozoa can be frozen at a concentration as low as 40×106 mL^{-1} in 0.25mL straws without a negative effect on sperm motility, morphology or acrosome integrity (Clulow *et al*, 2008).

9. Recent advances in cryopreservation

The application of frozen-thawed semen technology is currently increasing worldwide. Several studies have focused on identifying damages during freezing and thawing, tests to screen sperm quality post-thaw, evaluation of alternative cryoprotectants and other additives, and freezing procedures to improve sperm viability and fertility (Clulow *et al*, 2008; Goolsby *et al*, 2004; Medeiros *et al*, 2002; Squires *et al*, 2004;). Most of the progress in improving survival of frozen-thawed spermatozoa centers on minimizing the oxidative damage and decreasing the osmotic stress on spermatozoa. Equine sperm are particularly known to be susceptible to oxidative stress, relative to other species, because of their high content of unsaturated fatty acids. In addition to membrane effects, lipid peroxidation can also damage DNA. The addition of antioxidants to extenders has been used as a method to decrease lipid peroxidation and oxidative stress associated with cryopreservation (Bilodaeu *et al*, 2001; Pe˜na *et al*, 2003; Roca *et al*, 2004). Different amides, compounds with lower molecular weight than glycerol and penetrate the sperm plasma membrane more readily, have been evaluated as alternative cryoprotectants to glycerol in different animals (Bianchi *et al*, 2008; Medeiros *et al*, 2002; Squires *et al*, 2004;). These compounds include methyl formamide (MF), dimethyl formamide (DMF) or ethylene glycol (EG) and dimethyl acetamide. They were known to provide greater post-thaw motility when used at different concentrations. Particularly, MF and DMF or EG have been used as alternative cryoprotectants for individual males whose sperm has lesser post-thaw motility when frozen in glycerol (Bianchi *et al*, 2008; Squires *et al*, 2004). The use of low-density lipoproteins (LDLs), most often isolated from egg-yolk from different species, as additive has proven beneficial for sperm function post-thaw, particularly for DNA-integrity(Rodriguez-Martinez and Wallgren, 2011). Attempts to minimize osmotic stress during cryopreservation have included step-wise dilution of cryoprotectants, by incorporating cholesterol-loaded cyclodextrins (CLC) in freezing diluents (Wessel and Ball, 2004). As an alternative to adding CLC to extenders provision of polyunsaturated fatty acids in the feed as a means of altering the sperm-lipid membrane profile has been tried with some success in boars and stallions (Brinsko *et al*, 2005; Purdy and Graham, 2004).

Different kinds of freezing procedures have also been reported in the last several years in an attempt to controlling the rates of cooling. Recent results indicate that the cryopreservation

of bull, stallion and boar semen could be improved by using a programmable freezer (Bianchi *et al*, 2008; Clulow *et al*, 2008; Woelders and Chaveiro, 2004). An interaction between glycerol concentration and cooling rate has been described for boar semen. Current cryopreservation methods based on optimal combinations of glycerol and cooling rate has allowed consistent sperm survival in the frozen semen, with acceptable variation among individuals. Another method, termed multi-thermal gradient (MTG), that aims to overcome the problems of conventional freezing protocol has also been reported (Arav *et al*, 2002). This freezing technology is based on directional freezing in which the spermatozoa are moved through a linear temperature gradient so that, theoretically, the cooling rate and ice front propagation are precisely controlled. Thus, the spermatozoa are preserved gently between horizontal columns of ice thereby avoiding the damaging effects of the random ice crystal formation observed in conventional freezing. The technique is also known to allow the incorporation of controlled seeding into the freezing process and prevent the dehydration of sperm commonly seen in conventional freezing while halving the level of glycerol required (Arav *et al*, 2002). A slightly different technique, termed unique freezing technology (UFT) which was originally designed to freeze foodstuffs, has been recently tested for semen cryopreservation (Goolsby *et al*, 2004). The UFT involves placing extended samples in a bath that contains an organic fluid with a heat capacity similar to water with a freezing rate of -6.1°C /min. Similar results of post-thaw motilities with sperm frozen in traditional liquid nitrogen procedures have been reported for four UFT treatments (Goolsby *et al*, 2004).
Another front of investigation in the last decade has been the development of methods of examining sperm ultrastructural characteristics and alterations. Amongst these are sperm kinematics assessed by computer-assisted motility analysis, osmotic resistance tests, plasma membrane integrity evaluation with fluorescent membrane-impermeable dyes, evaluation of acrosomal status with fluorescein isothiocyanate-conjugated lectins, investigation of DNA integrity using the SCSA, or assessment of membrane architectural status (Gillan *et al*, 2004; 2005). Most methods require the application of fluorescence microscopy and/or flow cytometric techniques. Because of their highly quantitative, repeatable, and sensitive nature, the techniques are already getting their place in many modern semen laboratories.

10. Conclusion

Cryopreservation continues to be one the most frequently employed technique for use in modern animal production. Commercial AI will inevitably use this technique to preserve and transport semen over a wider area around the world. However, even with the most up to date procedure cryopreservation still causes detrimental effect on sperm compartments and their function. To ensure that semen used for AI are of a relatively uniform, and of high quality, artificial breeding organizations should discard ejaculates based on seminal quality tests immediately after ejaculation and after freezing and thawing. There are evidences resulting from different investigation that different sperm compartments are interrelated, the defect in one will invariably affect the other compartment. The success of sperm cell in its ability to fertilize is also affected at different level during its course from its origin until it reaches the ovum. Cryopreservation would be an additional artificial interruption in this journey. Therefore, the knowledge of the biochemical basis of the detrimental effects of cryopreservation and the means to detect these changes easily, cheaply and accurately during semen evaluation would be of great significance. The use of combination of tests, rather than the employment of a single test, would give superior and more complete information about the status of the spermatozoa. There are already successes in improving the methods of detection of high quality sperm with good fertility using combination of tests addressing different functions and compartments of the sperm. Tests addressing integrity of sperm chromatine structure are able to identify sperm defects not normally detected during conventional semen analysis. They are highly useful in that their application can avoid carryover problems reflected in the embryo after fertilization has taken place. While most of the investigations were carried out in bovine and equine, the lack of complete information for other species has led to extrapolation of knowledge which in some instances has not given acceptable results. For this reason, the evaluation of different extender combinations, freezing techniques, and developing new methods of semen evaluation should be undertaken for various species of animals worldwide.

11. Reference

Aitken, RJ and MA Baker, 2004. Oxygene stress and male reproductive biology. Reprod. Fertil. Dev.; 16:581 - 588

Amann RP, 2005. Weaknesses in reports of 'fertility' for horses and other species. Theriogenol.; 63:698-715

Amann RP and JK Graham, 1993. Spermatozoal function. In: DiRienzi D, ed. Equine reproduction. Philadelphia: Lea and Febiger; 715-745

Amann RP and BW Pickett, 1987. Principals of cryopreservation and a review of cryopreservation of stallion spermatozoa. J. Equine Vet. Sci. 7:145-173.

Andrabi SMH, 2007. Fundamental principles of cryopreservation of *Bos taurus* and *Bos indicus* bull spermatozoa. Mini review. Int. J. Agri. and Biol.; 9:367-369

Arav, A., S. Yavin, Y. Zeron, D. Natan, I. Dekel and H. Gacitu, 2002. New trends in gamete's cryopreservation. Mol. Cell. Endocrinol.; 187:77-81

Ayalew E and A Lemma, 2010. Evaluation of cryopreservation methods and extender types for storage of donkey semen. As part of DVM thesis, Faculty of Veterinary Medicine, Addis Ababa University

Bailey JL, JF Bilodeau and N Cormier, 2000. Semen cryopreservation in domestic animals: A damaging and capacitating phenomenon. J. Androl.; 21:1-7

Bailey JL, A Morrie and N Cormier, 2003. Semen cryopreservation: success and persistent in farm species. Canadian J. Anim. Sci.; 83:393-401

Ball BA, and A Vo, 1999. Reactive oxygene species generation by equine spermatozoa. Biol. Reprod.; 60:136-137

Batellier F, M Vidament, J Fauquant, G Duchamp, G Arnaud, JM Yvon, and M Magistrini, 2001. Advances in cooled semen technology. Anim. Reprod. Sci.; 68:181-190.

Bianchi I, K Calderam, and K Calderam, 2008. Evaluation of amides and centrifugation temperature in boar semen cryopreservation. Theriogenol.; 69:632-638.

Bilodeau, JF, S. Blanchette, C. Gangnon, and MA Sirard, 2001. Thiols prevent H_2O_2-mediated loss of sperm motility in cryopreserved bull semen. Theriogenol.; 56:275-286.

Blach, EL, RP Amann, RA Bowen, and D Frantz, 1989. Changes in quality of stallion spermatozoa during cryopreservation: plasma membrane integrity and motion characteristics. Theriogenol.; 31:283–298.

Brinsko SP, DD Varner, CC Love, TL Blanchard, BC Day and ME Wilson, 2005. Effect of feeding a DHA-enriched nutriceutical on the quality of fresh, cooled and frozen stallion semen. Theriogenol.; 63:1519-1527

Cerolini S, A Maldjian, F Pizzi and TM Gliozzi, 2001. Changes in sperm quality and lipid composition during cryopreservation of boar semen. Reproduction; 121: 395-401.

Chatterjee S, E De Lamirande, and C Gagnon, 2001. Cryopreservation alters membrane sulphydryl status of bull spermatozoa: Protection by oxidized glutathione. Mol. Reprod Dev.; 60:498-506.

Chaverio A, L Machado, A Frijters, B Engel, and H Woelders, 2006. Improvement of parameters of freezing protocol for bull sperm using two osmotic supports. Theriogenol.; 65:1875-1890.

Christanelli MJ, EL Squires, RP Amann, and BW Pickett, 1984. Fertility of stallion semen processed, frozen and thawed by a new procedure. Theriogenol.; 22:39-45.

Clement F., Y. Ladonnet, and M. Magistrini, 2001. Sperm morphology and fertility. Anim. Reprod. Sci.; 68:362-363.

Clulow JR., L.J. Mansfield, LHA. Morris, G. Evans, and WMC. Maxwell, 2008. A comparison between freezing methods for the cryopreservation of stallion spermatozoa, Anim. Reprod. Sci. 108:298-308

Cochran JD, RP Amann, DP Froman, and BW Pickett, 1984. Effects of centrifugation, glycerol level, cooling to 5^{0}C, freezing rate and thawing rate on the post thaw motility of equine spermatozoa. Theriogenol.; 22:25-38

Colenbrander B, BM Gadella, and TA Stout, 2003. The predictive value of semen analysis in the evaluation of stallion fertility. Reprod. Dom. Anim.; 38:305-311.

Cooter PZ, HA Goolsby, and SD Prien, 2005. Preliminary evaluation of a unique freezing technology for bovine spermatozoa cryopreservation. Reprod. Dom. Animal; 40:98-99

Cormier N, MA Sirard and JL Bailey, 1997. Premature capacitation of bovine spermatozoa is initiated by cryopreservation. J. Androl.; 18:461-467.

Cremades T, J Roca, H Rodriguez-Martinez, T Abaigar, MJ Vazquez and EA Martine 2005. Kinematic Changes during the cryopreservation of boar spermatozoa. J. Andrology; 26:610-618

Cueva, FI de la C, Rigau T, Bonet S, Briz M and Rodriguez-Gill JE, 1997. Subjecting horse spermatozoa to hypoosmotic incubation: effects of ouabain. In: Davies-Morel MCG, 1999. Equine artificial insemination. CAB International, Wallingford, UK; Pp 229-230

Curry MR, 2000. Cryopreservation of semen from domestic livestock. Rev. Reprod., 5: 46–52

Davies-Morel MCG, 1999. Equine artificial insemination. CAB International, Wallingford, UK; Pp 416

Deneke N, A Lemma, and T Yilma, 2010. Study on the efficiency of conventional semen evaluation procedure employed at Kaliti National artificial insemination center and fertility of frozen-thawed bull semen. As part of MSc thesis, Faculty of Veterinary Medicine, Addis Ababa University

Donnelly ET, N McClure, and SE Lewis, 2001. Cryopreservation of human semen and prepared sperm: effects on motility parameters and DNA integrity. Fertil. and Steril. 76:892-900.

Dziekońska A, L Fraser, and J Strzeżek, 2009. Effect of different storage temperatures on the metabolic activity of spermatozoa following liquid storage of boar semen. J. Anim. and Feed Sci.; 18:638-649

Evenson DP, BL Sailer, and LK Jost 1995. Relationship between stallion sperm deoxyribonucleic acid (DNA) susceptibility to denaturation in situ and presence of DNA strand breaks: implications for fertility and embryo viability. Biol. Reprod. Mono. 6:655-659.

Evenson DP, KL Larson, and LK Jost, 2002. Sperm chromatin structure assay: its clinical use for detecting sperm DNA fragmentation in male fertility and comparison with other techniques. J. Androl. 23:25-43.

Fahy GM, 1986. The relevance of cryoprotectant 'toxicity' to cryobiology. Cryobiology 23:1-13.

Fatehi AN, MM. Bevers, and E Schoevers, 2006. DNA damage in bovine sperm does not block fertilization and early embryonic development but induces apoptosis after the first cleavages. J. Androl; 27:176-188.

Fiser PS, C Hansen, KL Underhill, and JNB Shrestha, 1991. The effect of induced ice nucleation (seeding) on the post thaw motility and acrosomal integrity of boar spermatozoa. Anim. Reprod. Sci.; 24:293-304.

Foote RH and JE Parks, 1993. Factors affecting preservation and fertility of bull semen: a brief review. Reprod. Fertil. Dev.; 5:665-73

Fraser L and J Strzezek, 2004. The use of comet assay to assess DNA integrity of boar spermatozoa following liquid preservation at 5 and 16 ^{0}C. Folia Histochemica et Cytobiologica; 42:49-55.

Garcia-Macias V, de Paz P, Martinez-Pastor F, Alvarez M, Gomes-Alves S, Bernardo J, Anel E and Anel L, 2007. DNA fragmentation assessment by flow cytometry and Sperm-Bos-Halomax (bright-field microscopy and fluorescence microscopy) in bull sperm. Int. J. Androl.; 30:88-98

Garner DL, LA Johnson, ST Yue, BL Roth, and RP Haugland, 1994. Dual DNA Staining Assessment of Bovine Sperm Viability Using SYBR-14 and Propidium Iodide. J Androl.; 15:620-629.

Garner DL, CA Thomas, and CG Gravance, 1999. The effect of glycerol on the viability, mitochondrial function and acrosomal integrity of bovine spermatozoa. Reprod. Dom. Anim., 34:399-404

Gillan L, WMC Maxwell, and G Evans, 2004. Preservation and evaluation of semen for artificial insemination. Reprod. Fertil. Dev.; 16:447-454.

Gillan L, G Evans and WM Maxwell, 2005. Flow cytometric evaluation of sperm parameters in relation to fertility potential. Theriogenol.; 63: 445-457

Goolsby HA, JR Elanton, and SD Prien, 2004. Preliminary comparisons of a unique freezing technology to traditional cryopreservation methodology of equine spermatozoa. J. Equine Vet. Sci.; 314-318

Graham JK, and E Moce, 2005. Fertility evaluation of frozen/thawed semen. Theriogenol.; 64:492-504

Granish Ho HC, and Suarez SS KA, 2002. Hyperactivated motility of bull sperm is triggered at the axoneme by Ca^{2+} and not cAMP. Dev. Biol.; 250:208-217.

Gravance CG, DL Garner, MG Miller, and T Berger, 2001. Fluorescent probes and flow cytometry to assess rat sperm integrity and mitochondrial function. Reprod. Toxicol.; 15: 5-10

Guthrie HD and Welch GR, 2005. Effects of hypothermic liquid storage and cryopreservation on basal and induced plasma membrane phospholipid disorder and acrosome exocytosis in boar spermatozoa. Reprod. Fertil. and Dev.; 17:467-477

Hammadeh ME, S Greiner, P Rosenbaum, and W Schmidt, 2001. Comparison between human sperm preservation medium and TEST-yolk buffer on protecting chromatin and morphology integrity of human spermatozoa in fertile and subfertile men after freeze-thawing procedure. J Androl.; 22:1012-1018

Hammerstedt RH, JK Graham, and JP Nolan, 1990. Cryopreservation of mammalian sperm: what we ask them to survive. J. Androl.; 11:73–88.

Heitland AV, DJ Jasko, JK Graham, EL Squires, RP Amann, and BW Pickett, 1995. Motility and fertility of stallion spermatozoa cooled and frozen in a modified skim milk extender containing egg yolk and liposome. Biol. Reprod. Mono.; 1:753-759.

Heitland AV, Jasko DJ, Squires EL, Graham JK, Pickett BW and Hamilton C, 1996. Factors affecting motion characteristics of frozen–thawed stallion spermatozoa. Equine Veterinary Journal; 28: 47-53.

Holt WV, 2000. Fundamental aspects of sperm cryobiology: the importance of species and individual differences. Theriogenol.; 53:47-58

Housley MD and KK Stanley, 1982. Dynamics of Biological Membranes. John Wiley and Sons, New York, pp. 51-81

Januskauskas A, and H Zillinskas, 2002. Bull semen evaluation post-thaw and relation of semen characteristics to bull's fertility. Veterinarija ir zootechnika; 17:1392-2130

Januskauskas A, A Johannisson, and H Rodriguez-Martinez, 2003. Subtle membrane changes in cryopreserved bull semen in relation with sperm viability, chromatin structure, and field fertility. Theriogenol.; 60:743-758

Kadirvel, G, S Kumar, A Kumaresan and P Kathiravan, 2009. Capacitation status of fresh and frozen-thawed buffalo spermatozoa in relation to cholesterol level, membrane fluidity and intracellular calcium Anim. Reprod. Sci., 116: 244-253

Katila T, GB Combes, DD Varner and TL Blanchard, 1997. Comparison of three containers used for the transport of cooled stallion semen. Theriogenol.; 48:1085-1092.

Kavak A, A Johannisson, N Lundeheim, H Rodriguez-Martinez, M Aidnik, S Einarsson, 2003. Evaluation of cryopreserved stallion semen from Tori and Estonian breeds using CASA and flow cytometry. Anim. Reprod. Sci; 76:205-216.

Kayser JPR, 1990. Effects of linear cooling rates on motion characteristics of stallion spermatozoa. MSc Thesis, Colorado State University.

Kneissl S, 1993. Tiefgefrierkonservierung von Pferdesperma: Einfluss der Samenentnahmetechnik, Zentrifugation, Konfektionierungsform und Einfriermethode auf die Motilität und Membranintegrität der Samenzellen. (Cryopreservation of stallion semen: The influence of semen collection techniques, centrifugation, packaging forms, and methods of freezing on the motility and plasma membrane integrity of spermatozoa). Thesis, Tierärztliche Hochschule Hannover.

Kokk K, E Verajankorva, M Laato, XK Wu, H Tapfer and P Pollanen, 2005. Expression of insulin receptor substrates 1-3, glucose transporters Glut-1-4, signal regulatory protein 1 alpha, phosphatidylinositol 3-kinase and protein kinase B at the protein level in the human testis. Anatomical Sci. Int.; 80: 91-96

Koskinen E, M Junnila, T Katila and H Soini, 1989. A preliminary study on the use of betaine as a cryoprotective agent in deep freezing of stallion semen. J. Vet. Med.-A, 36: 110-114.

Kumar S, JD Millar and PF Watson, 2003. The effect of cooling rate on the survival of cryopreserved bull, ram and boar spermatozoa: a comparison of two controlled-rate cooling machines. Cryobiology; 46:246-53

Larsson, B and H Rodriquez-Martinez, 2000. Can we use in vitro fertilization tests to predict semen fertility? Anim. Reprod. Sci.; 60: 327-336.

Lessard C, S Parent, P Leclerc, JL Bailey, and R Sullivan, 2000. Cryopreservation Alters the Levels of the Bull Sperm Surface Protein P25b. J Androl., 21:700-707

Love CC, 2005. The sperm chromatin structure assay: a review of clinical applications. Anim. Reprod. Sci; 89:39-45.

Love CC, JA Thompson, SP Brinsko, SL Rigby, TL Blanchard, VK Lowry, and DD Varner, 2003 Relationship between stallion sperm motility and viability as detected by two fluorescence staining techniques using flow cytometry. Theriogenol.; 60:1127-1138.

Love CC, DD Varner, JA Thompson, 2000. Intra- and interstallion variation in sperm morphology and their relationship with fertility. J. Reprod. Fertil. Suppl; 56:93-100.

Makhlouf AA, and C Niederberger, 2006. DNA integrity tests in clinical practice: it is not a simple matter of black and white (or red and green). J. Androl.; 27:316-323.

Mammoto A, N Masumoto, M Tahara, Y Ikebuchi, M Ochmichi, K Tasaka, and A Miyake, 1996. Reactive oxygen species block sperm-egg fusion via oxidation of sperm sulhydryl protein in mice. Biol. Reprod. 55:1063-68

Maxwell, WM and LA Johnson, 1997. Chlortetracycline analysis of boar spermatozoa after incubation; flow cytometric sorting, cooling, or cryopreservation. Mol. Reprod. Dev.; 46: 408-418

Mazur P, N Katkova, and JK Critser, 2000. The enhancement of the ability of mouse sperm to survive freezing and thawing by the use of high concentrations glycerol and the presence of an Escherichia coli membrane preparation (Oxyrase) to lower the oxygen concentration. Cryobiology; 40:187-209

Medeiros CMO, F Forell, ATD Oliveria, and JL Rodrigues, 2002. Current status of sperm cryopreservation: why isn't it better? Theriogenol.; 57: 327-44

Medrano A, Garcia-Gil N, Ramió L, Rivera MM, Fernández-Novell JM, Ramírez A, Peña A, Briz MD, Pinart E, Concha II, Bonet S, Rigau T and Rodríguez-Gil JE, 2006. Hexose-specificity of hexokinase and ADP-dependence of pyruvate kinase play important roles in the control of monosaccharide utilization in freshly diluted boar spermatozoa. Mol. Reprod. and Dev.; 73:1179-1194

Muller Z, 1987. Practicalities of insemination of mares with deep frozen semen. J. Reprod. Fertil., Suppl.; 35:121-125.

Muller CH, 2000. Rationale, interpretation, validation, and uses of sperm function tests. J. Androl.; 21:10-30.

Neild D, G Chaves, M Flores, N Mora, M Beconi, A Aguero, 1999. Hypoosmotic test in equine spermatozoa. Theriogenol.; 51:721-727

Nishizono H, M Shioda, T Takeo, T Irie and N Nakagata, 2004. Decrease of fertilizing ability of mouse spermatozoa after freezing and thawing is related to cellular injury. Biol. Reprod.; 71: 973-978

Park NK, WY Oh, SS Lee, CA Oh, SW Kang, SB Ko, MS Kang and HS Kim, 1995. Studies on semen freezing in Cheju native stallions. J. Agri. Sci., 37: 459-463.

Parks JE, and JK Graham, 1992. Effects of cryopreservation procedures on sperm membranes. Theriogenol.; 38:210-223.

Parks JE and DV Lynch, 1992. Lipid composition and thermotropic phase behavior of boar, bull, stallion and rooster sperm membrane. Cryobiology; 29:255-266.

Pegg DE, 2002. The history and principles of cryopreservation. Semi. Reprod. Med.; 20: 5-13.

Pe˜na FJ, A Johannisson, M Wallgren, and H Rodriguez-Martinez, 2003. Antioxidant supplementation in vitro improves boar sperm motility and mitochondrial membrane potential after cryopreservation of different fractions of the ejaculate. Animal Reprod. Sci.; 78:85–98

Peris SI, A Morrier, M Dufour and JL Bailey, 2004. Cryopreservation of ram semen facilitates sperm DNA damage: relationship between sperm andrological parameters and the sperm chromatin structure assay. J. Androl.; 25: 224-233.

Petrunkina AM, D Waberski, AR Gu¨nzel-Apel, and E To¨pfer-Petersen, 2007. Focus on determinants of male fertility: Determinants of sperm quality and fertility in domestic animals. Reproduction; 134:3-17

Pickett BW and RP Amann, 1987. Extension and storage of stallion spermatozoa. A review. Equine Veterinary Science; 7:289-302.

Pickett BW and RP Amann, 1993. Cryopreservation of semen. In: McKinnon, AO and Voss, EL (eds) Equine Reproduction. Lea and Febiger, Philadelphia, pp. 768–789.

Pommer AC, JJ Linfor and SA Mayers, 2002. Capacitation and acrosomal exocytosis are enhanced by incubation of stallion of spermatozoa in commercial semen extender. Theriogenol.; 57:1493-1501

Purdy, PH and JK Graham, 2004. Effect of cholesterol-loaded cyclodextrin on the cryosurvival of bull sperm. Cryobiology; 48:36-45

Rigau T, M Rivera, MJ Palomo, JM Fernandez-Novell, T Mogas, J Ballester, A Pen˜a, PJ Otaegui, JJ Guinovart and JE Rodriguez-Gil, 2002. Differential effects of glucose and fructose on hexose metabolism in dog spermatozoa. Reproduction; 123: 579-591.

Roca J, MA Gil, M Hernandez, I Parrilla, JM Vazquez, EA Martinez, 2004. Survival and fertility of boar spermatozoa after freeze-thawing in extender supplemented with butylated hydroxytoluene. J Androl; 25:397-405

Rodriguez-Martinez H and M Wallgren, 2011. Advances in Boar Semen Cryopreservation Review article; Vet. Med. Int.; 2011:1-5

Royere D, S Hamamah, JC Nicolle and J Lansac, 1991. Chromatin alterations induced by freeze-thawing influence the fertilizing ability of human sperm. Int. J. Androl.; 14:328-332

Ruiz-Pesini E, E Alvarez, J Enriquez, and M Lopez-Perez, 2001. Association between seminal plasma carnitine and sperm mitochondrial enzymatic activities. Int. J. And.; 24:335-340.

Saacke RG, JC Dalton, S Nadir, RL Nebel, JH Bame, 2000. Relationship of seminal traits and insemination time to fertilization rate and embryo quality. Anim. Reprod. Sci.; 60: 663-677.

Samper JC, JC Hellander and BG Crabo, 1991. Relationship between the fertility of fresh and frozen stallion semen and semen quality. J. Reprod. Fertil. Suppl.; 44:107-114.

Samper JC, 2001. Management and fertility of mares bred with frozen semen. Anim. Reprod. Sci; 68:219-228

Shannon P, and R Vishwanath, 1995. The effect of optimal and suboptimal concentrations of sperm on the fertility of fresh and frozen bovine semen and a theoretical model to explain the fertility differences. Anim. Reprod. Sci.; 39:1-10.

Squires, EL, SL Keith, and JK Graham, 2004. Evaluation of alternative cryoprotectants for preserving stallion spermatozoa. Theriogenol.; 62:1056-1065

Steinmann H, 1996. Use of trehalose as a cryoprotectant in the freezing of stallion semen. A laboratory study. Thesis, Tierärztliche Hochschule Hannover, Germany.

Thomas CA, DL Garner, JM DeJarnette, and CE Marshall, 1998. Effect of cryopreservation on bovine sperm organelle function and viability as determined by flow cytometry. Biol Reprod 58:786-793.

Thomas, AD, SA Meyers and BA Ball, 2006. Capacitation-like changes in equine spermatozoa following cryopreservation. Theriogenol., 65: 1531-1550

Tsega A and A Lemma, 2009. Study on breeding soundness and fertility of senar jackass *(Equus asinus)* in North Gondar. As part of MSc thesis, Faculty of Vet. Medicine, Addis Ababa University.

Varner DD, TL Blanchard, PJ Meyers, SA Meyers, 1989. Fertilizing capacity of equine spermatozoa stored for 24 h at 5 or 20°C. Theriogenol.; 32: 515-525

Varner DD and L Johnson, 2007. From a Sperm's Eye View: Revisiting our perception of this intriguing cell. AAEP Proceedings; 53:104-177

Watson PF and AG Duncan, 1988. Effect of salt concentration and unfrozen water fraction on the viability of slowly frozen ram spermatozoa. Cryobiology; 25:131-142.

Watson PF, 1990. AI and the preservation of semen. In: Lamming, GE (ed.) Marshall's Physiology of Reproduction, Volume 2, Male Reproduction. Churchill, Livingstone, London, pp. 747-869

Watson PF, 2000. The causes of reduce fertility with cryopreserved semen. Anim. Reprod. Sci.; 60:481-92,

Wessel, MT and BA Ball, 2004. Step-wise dilution for removal of glycerol from fresh and cryopreserved equine spermatozoa. Anim. Reprod. Sci.; 84:147-156

Woelders H, 1997. Fundamentals and recent development in cryopreservation of bull and boar semen. Vet. Quart.; 19:135-138

Woelders H and A Chaveiro, 2004. Theoretical prediction of 'optimal' freezing programmes. Cryobiology; 49:258-271

Wongtawan T, F Saravia, M Wallgren, I Caballero and H Rodriguez-Martinez, 2006. Fertility after deep intra-uterine artificial insemination of concentrated low-volume boar semen doses. Theriogenol.; 65:773-787.

13

Effect of Fatty Acids on Reproductive Performance of Ruminants

Herrera-Camacho, José[1], Soberano-Martínez, Alejandra[1], Orozco Durán, Karlos Edmundo[2], Aguilar-Pérez, Carlos[2] and Ku-Vera, Juan Carlos[2]
[1]Instituto de Investigaciones Agropecuarias y Forestales
Universidad Michoacana de San Nicolás de Hidalgo
[2]Campus de Ciencias Biológicas y Agropecuarias
Universidad Autónoma de Yucatán
México

1. Introduction

Different types of fats have been utilized in an attempt to improve reproductive function in ruminant animals. Fatty acids derived from plants and oil seeds have exerted a major impact on reproductive performance, some of the most common sources include sunflower, linseed, cottonseed, rapeseed and soyabean. Animal fat (tallow) and calcium salts of saturated fatty acids may escape in a significant percentage rumen hydrogenation to be incorporated into adipose tissue and milk. Fish by-products contain a high proportion of polyunsaturated fatty acids (PUFAs) and pass without being altered in the rumen exerting no effects on rumen fermentation. Each dietary source of fat varies regarding composition of specific fatty acids (Table 1).

Early studies of the effect of fat in the ration on reproductive performance were carried out by Burr & Burr (1930), who observed that fat deficiency in the ration of growing rats induced alterations in ovulation rate and on the onset of oestrus, while lipid supplementation reestablished reproductive performance of the females, coining the concept of essential fatty acids. In later studies, research was aimed at evaluating the effect of fat supplementation in different animal species both ruminant and non-ruminant, on reproductive aspects such as the establishment of puberty (Smith et al., 1989), semen production (Castellano et al., 2010), maternal recognition of pregnancy (Abayasekara & Wathes, 1999, Filley et al., 2000, Lopes et al., 2009) by means of the suppression of luteolytic signals (Mattos et al., 2000), restart of ovarian activity after parturition (de Fries et al., 1998), follicle development, quality of oocytes (Staples & Thatcher, 2005; Bilby et al., 2006c), and of the embryo (Cerri et al., 2009), modification in the mechanism of synthesis and secretion of hormones involved in reproductive processes (Staples et al., 1998) and on production aspects such as quality of milk (Rego et al., 2004; Bernal et al., 2010) or meat (Wood et al., 2003). Due to the fact that some fatty acids (FA) are essential for mammals and to the role of fatty acids on reproductive processes, it is possible that cattle reproduction will be influenced more by the type of lipids consumed than for the total lipid intake. This is particularly important since ruminants hydrogenate PUFAs in the rumen, limiting the amount of PUFAs that are absorbed from the small intestine (Thatcher & Staples, 2007,

Santos et al., 2008, Doreau et al., 2011). However, it is possible that some specific PUFAs may pass intact the reticulo-rumen and be absorbed from the small intestine, allowing in this way the improvement of reproductive efficiency directly on the target tissue of the reproductive system of the female (autocrine or paracrine) or by an indirect effect mediated by the endocrine system (Staples & Thatcher, 2005).

Fat source	**Fatty acid**						
	C14:0	C16:0	C16:1	C18:0	C18:1	C18:2	C18:3
	Myristic	Palmitic	Palmit-oleic	Stearic	Oleic	Linoleic	Linolenic
Tallow	3	25	3	18	43	3.8	<1
Yellow grease	2	21	4	11	44	14	<1
Energy Booster 100[1]	3	40	1	41	10	2	<1
Megalac: EnerG-II[1]	1	50	<1	4	36	8	<1
Megalac- R[1]	1	36	<1	4	26	29	3
Canola oil	<1	4	<1	2	63	19	9
Cottonseed oil	1	23	<1	3	18	54	1
Flaxseed oil	<1	5	1	3	20	16	55
Extruded Linseed	<1	7.6		5.2	20	14.5	51.3
Rapeseed oil	<1	5	<1	2	54	22	11
Safflower oil	<1	7	<1	2	12	78	<1
Soyabean oil	<1	11	<1	4	23	54	8
Sunflower oil	<1	7	<1	5	19	68	1
Menhaden fish oil[2]	7	16	8	3	12	1	2

Table 1. Fatty acid composition of selected dietary fat sources. [1]Commercial preparations considered partially inert in the rumen; [2]Also contain 14% C20:5 and 9% C22:6 (Thatcher & Staples, 2007).

Several studies have shown that PUFAs of the ω-3 family such as eicosapentaenoic acid (C20:5, ω-3) and docosahexaenoic acid (C22:6, ω-3) suffer insignificant biohydrogenation in the rumen (Thatcher & Staples, 2007). These fatty acids are usually found in feedstuffs derived from fish (and other marine products), such as the oil and the meal which are considered non essential since they can be synthesized from linoleic acid (ω-3), and apparently play an important role in animal performance (Thatcher & Staples, 2007). Furthermore, lipid supplements partially resistant to biohydrogenation in the rumen have been developed such as calcium salts of long chain fatty acids (Ca-LCFA) with the aim of increasing the amount of unsaturated FA which can be absorbed by limiting biohydrogenation (Mattos et al., 2000). PUFAs act as mediators in a series of processes in several reproductive tissues, including fluidity of cell membrane, intracellular signaling and susceptibility to oxidative damage (Wathes et al., 2007). Changes in chain length, degree of unsaturation and position of the double bonds in the acil chain of fatty acids may have a major impact on reproductive function and play a role in livestock reproduction (Mattos et al., 2000). Potential mechanisms may include increment of energy density of the ration (Ferguson et al., 1990), even when for some workers (Williams & Amstalden, 2010), the effect of fat supplementation on reproduction is independent of the energy density of ration or of changes in live weight of animals. Considering all the above described, the aim of this review is to examine some of the reproductive processes in the bovine and ovine females which could be regulated or modified by the inclusion of lipids in the ration.

2. Effect of lipid supplementation on pregnancy rate

Incorporation of lipids in rations for dairy cattle usually increases energy density of ration and improves lactation and reproductive performance (Funston, 2004). However, when they are supplied in early lactation, frequently there is a reduction in feed intake due to a reduction in dry matter digestibility and to an increase in energy of greater availability, so when lipids are supplied in the early postpartum period, there is little alteration in the energy status of the animal even when a higher energy density ration is consumed (Santos et al., 2008).

Then, if dietary fat does not alter the energy status of dairy cows, reproductive response results more from the supply of some fatty acids, than from the effect of the energy supply *per se* (Staples et al., 1998, Williams & Amstaldem, 2010).

There are several studies that report a better reproductive performance in cows fed supplementary lipids. In this respect, Staples et al. (1998), showed that lipid consumption exerted a positive effect on reproductive aspects in dairy cows (Table 2). In beef cattle, the same trend has been observed. It is in this context that, de Fries et al. (1998) reported that Brahman cows consuming 5.2% lipids in the ration showed a trend towards an increase in pregnancy rate than those cows which consumed only 3.7% lipids in the ration. Ferguson et al. (1990) observed a 2.2 times increase in the possibility of pregnancy in lactating cows consuming 0.5 kg lipids per day. In another study, it was demonstrated that grazing cows supplemented with fat, pregnancy rate at first service was 16% higher than in cows which did not receive fat in the ration (Bader et al., 2000).

Bellows et al., (2001) observed that supplementation with safflower seed, soyabeans, or sunflower seed (4.7, 3.8 and 5.1% fat in the ration, respectively) for the last 65 days before calving increased subsequent pregnancy rates (94%, 90% and 91%, respectively) of first-calf beef heifers compared with the control (79 %) that received only 2.4 % fat in the ration. In another study Bellows et al., (2001), using good quality forage and a higher amount of fat in the ration (6.5%) during 68 days before calving, was unable to improve pregnancy rates relative to a control ration (2.2% fat), this result indicates that when adequate nutrients are available, the effect of supplemental fat may be masked.

Grazing Holstein cows which were supplemented for 103 days, as from day 10 post-partum, with two sources of bypass fat Megalac plus 3% (MP; 0.4 kg/day, containing Ca salts of palm fatty acids and Ca salts of methionine hydroxy analogue) and Megapro Gold (MPG; 1.5 kg/day, containing Ca salt of palm fatty acids, extracted rapeseed meal and whey permeate), MPG increased ($P<0.05$) conception rate to first service compared to control group (CG). Conception rate to first service was similar ($P=0.14$) on MP compared to CG. For pregnancy to second service, CG had a higher ($P<0.05$) conception rate than MP. There were no significant differences between treatments in overall pregnancy rate, services per conception, number of cows served in the first three weeks of the breeding season or the 6-

weeks in-calf rate. Comparing the combined fat treatments to CG resulted in a higher ($P<0.05$) conception rate to first service for the fat treatments but no significant difference in overall pregnancy rate (McNamara et al., 2003).

Reference	Fat source	Percent inclusion	Pregnancy rate
Fergunson et al., 1990	Ca-Palm oil	2.0 %	59[1]
Sklan et al.,1991	Ca-Palm oil	2.6 %	82
Scott et al., 1995	Ca-Palm oil	1 lb d^{-1}	98
Garcia-Bojalil et al., 1998	Ca-Palm oil	2.2 %	86
Son et al., 1996	Tallow	3 %	62
Espinoza et al., 2010	Tallow	9.5%	Herd A 70; Herd B 55%
Frajblat and Butler, 2003	Energy Booster	1.7 %	86
Petit et al., 2001	Flaxseed	17%	87
Ambrose et al., 2006[a]	Flaxseed	9%	48[1]
Ambrose et al., 2006b	Flaxseed	9%	26[1]
Fuentes et al., 2007	Extruded Linseed	1.7 kgd^{-1}	39
McNamara et al., 2003	MegaPro Gold	3.3 lb d^{-1}	54
Juchem et al., 2004	Soy + Trans C18:1	1.5%	34[1]
Cullens, 2005	Megalac-R	2%	58[1]
Aguilar-Pérez et al., 2009	ByFat ®	1.8%	33
Espinoza et al., 2010	Megalac®	9.6%	Herd A 80; Herd B 58%
Castañeda-Gutierrez et al., 2005	Ca-CLA	0.3 lb d^{-1}	81
Bernal-Santos et al., 2003	Ca-CLA	0.3 lb d^{-1}	42
Bruckental et al., 1989	Fish meal	7.3%	72
Armstrong et al., 1990	Fish meal	1.8 lb d^{-1}	64
Carroll et al., 1994	Fish meal	3.5 %	89
Burke et al., 1997	Fish meal	2.8	41

Table 2. Reproductive performance of beef cows supplemented with fat in the ration. [1]First insemination (Adapted from Thatcher & Staples, 2007).

In another study, Aguilar-Pérez et al., (2009) observed that pregnancy rate of F_1 (Holstein x Zebu) cows grazing under tropical conditions in Mexico, was not affected by supplementation with bypass fat (33.3%), relative to a control group (41.7%) at 90 days postpartum. In conclusion, fat supplementation increased conception rate to first service but did not significantly affect the proportion of cows pregnant at the end of the breeding season, these results suggest that the higher quality of the forage supplied in the different seasons that the trial lasted, may have been a factor that masked the effect of fat supplementation. Juchem et al. (2010) evaluated the effect of supplementation before and after parturition with Ca-LCFA of palm oil or with a mixture of linoleic and *trans*-octadecenoic acids and observed that cows fed PUFAs showed a higher pregnancy rate than those supplemented with palm oil at 27 and 41 days (37.9 *vs* 28.6% and 35.5 *vs* 25.8%, respectively) after artificial insemination. Recently, Lopes et al. (2009) fed Nellore cows with 0.1 kg $cow^{-1}day^{-1}$ of PUFAs and observed that pregnancy rate was improved. In this respect, Mattos et al. (2000) suggested that the positive effect of fat on fertility may not be due to improvement in energy balance of the cows but rather to the specific effect of some dietary fatty acids on the physiology of the hypothalamus-hypophysis-ovary axis and even the uterus.

In a review of previous studies in which conjugated linoleic acids (CLA) were supplemented to dairy cows during early lactation, de Veth et al. (2009) demonstrated that the probability of pregnancy increases in 26% when CLA are increased in the ration and that the optimum CLA amount is 10.0 g d^{-1}, after which the beneficial effects are reduced. It is possible that the positive effect of lipid supplementation may be due to specific fatty acids (Staples & Thatcher, 2005), and the absorption of unsaturated FA in ruminants is limited due microbial biohydrogenation in the rumen (Lopes et al., 2009). Some studies have evaluated the possibility that unsaturated FA intake, particularly those of the *n*-6 (linoleic acid) and *n*-3 (α-linolenic, eicosapentaenoic, docosahexaenoic acids) families, may have some influence on reproduction in cows, even when reports in the literature are not always consistent (Santos et al., 2008). In this respect, when cows were fed 0.75 kg of linseed rich in α-linolenic acid (*n*-3), or sunflower rich in linoleic acid (*n*-6), pregnancy rate tended to increase in cows of the first treatment (Ambrose et al., 2006a).

In other studies, no response was observed with linseed (Fuentes et al., 2008). Similarly, feeding *n*-3 fatty acids from fish oil in the form of Ca-LCFA did not improve pregnancy rate postpartum at first service in beef cows when compared to supplementation with beef tallow (Juchem, 2007) or with Ca-LCFA from palm oil (Silvestre, quoted by Santos et al., 2008), even when pregnancy rate at second service postpartum was higher in cows fed *n*-3 fatty acids (Silvestre, quoted by Santos et al., 2008). In grazing F_1 (*Bos taurus* x *Bos indicus*) cows, Aranda-Ávila et al. (2010) observed a 15.4% increase in pregnancy rate when cows were supplemented with corn oil, relative to a control group (54.5 *vs* 41.7 % respectively) after 35 day supplementation; however, differences were not statistically significant. It is possible that the poor response observed in those studies may be due to an increase in milk production along with a loss of body weight, which occurs in greater or lesser degree in cows during the early postpartum period (Sklan et al., 1994).

3. Effect of lipid supplementation on the hypothalamus-hypophysis-ovary axis

The major objective of cow-calf enterprises is to produce one calf per cow annually. Thus, management strategies that enhance reproductive performance of milk and beef cows are beneficial to the productivity of cow-calf operations. Previous studies reported that utilization of dietary fat as a nutraceutical, particularly PUFAs, positively influenced reproductive function in both milk and beef cows (Williams & Stanko, 2000). Furthermore, these positive effects were independent of the additional energy contribution from the PUFAs sources (Funston, 2004). Different mechanisms have been proposed by means of which fat supplementation may affect functioning of the hypothalamus-hypophysis-ovary axis. Early work in this respect suggested that fat supplementation may affect secretion of reproductive and metabolic hormones and further research demonstrated that fat addition to the ration modified ovarian activity in heifers and adult cows postpartum.

The mechanism (or mechanisms) by which dietary fat improves reproductive performance has not been elucidated. Several hypotheses have been proposed: 1) an amelioration of a negative energetic balance, thus leading to an earlier return to oestrus postpartum and, therefore, improved fertility; 2) an increase in steroidogenesis favorable to improved fertility; 3) manipulation of insulin so as to stimulate ovarian follicle development; and 4) a stimulation or inhibition of the production and release of $PGF_{2\alpha}$, which influences the persistence of the corpus luteum (Staples et al., 1998)

3.1 Hormonal secretion and lipid metabolites

Some studies showed that dietary fat supplementation in dairy heifers increased circulating concentrations of progesterone (Talavera et al., 1985), and enhanced lifespan of induced corpus luteum during early postpartum in beef cows (Williams, 1989; Ryan et al., 1995). Other studies suggest that when lipids are included in the ration of cows to increase energy density, caloric balance is improved which directly influences hypophysis-gonadal activity postpartum (Harrison et al., 1995), increasing, in principle, the amplitude and frequency of secretion of luteinizing hormone (LH) in animals (Sklan et al., 1994). In this respect, de Luna et al. (1982), reported an increase in the secretion of luteinizing hormone in ovariectomized cows treated with GnRH and supplemented with beef tallow. In sheep, secretion of luteinizing hormone in response to the injection of GnRH at day 10 of the oestrus cycle was greater in Pelibuey sheep supplemented with Ca-LCFA from palm oil during 30 days than in the control group (Espinoza et al., 1997).

Other studies, using isocaloric and isonitrogenous diets in cows of poor body condition indicated that the increase in dietary fat consumption augmented the number of follicles of medium-size by 1.5- to 5-fold within 3 to 7 weeks and these changes occurred coincident with changes in serum insulin, growth hormone and intraovarian insulin-like growth factor (IGF-1) (Wehrman et al., 1991; Ryan et al., 1992; Thomas et al., 1997). Table 3 summarizes the effects of dietary fat supplementation on follicular physiology and growth as observed in different studies.

Reference	Effect
Wehrman et al., 1991; Ryan et al., 1992; Hightshoe et al., 1991; Lucy et al., 1991; Thomas & Williams, 1996; Thomas et al., 1997; Lammoglia et al., 1996; Stanko et al., 1997; de Fries et al., 1998	Increased number of medium-sized follicles (polyunsaturated fat > saturated and highly polyunsaturated fat effects)
Lucy et al., 1989, 1991	Milk cows supplemented with Ca-LCFA palm oil, the basal level of LH was increase
Wehrman et al., 1991; Ryan et al., 1992	Increased granullosa cell progesterone production *in vitro*, increased follicular fluid progesterone
Lopes et al., 2009, Salas-Razo et al., 2011	Cows supplemented with rumen inert polyunsaturated fat had greater mean serum progesterone concentrations compared with control
Ryan et al., 1992; Thomas & Williams, 1996	No effect on superovulation rate
de Fries et al., 1998; Bilby et al., 2006a; Garnsworthy et al., 2008	Increased number of large follicles; increased size of largest follicle

Table 3. Summary of the effect of dietary fat supplementation in cattle on ovarian follicular growth and steroid production. (Modified from Williams & Amstalden, 2010)

On the other hand, it has been shown that hiperlipidic rations supplied both to dairy as well as to beef cows, induced and increase in the levels of blood cholesterol, as it was observed by Hightshoe et al. (1991) in cows supplemented postpartum with Ca-LCFA from palm oil. Similar results, were reported in Angus and Hereford cows which consumed a supplement which contained 125 g of Ca-LCFA from palm oil (Espinoza et al., 1995), in Chinampas (*Bos taurus*) cows consuming Ca-LCFA from palm oil or beef tallow (Espinoza-Villavicencio et al., 2010); this is particularly important since cholesterol is the main precursor for progesterone synthesis in the corpus luteum as well as of other steroid hormones at the follicular level (Childs et al., 2008c). Thus, when supplementation with protected fats from rumen biohydrogenation is augmented, it is possible to increase concentration of plasma progesterone in cows (Lopes et al., 2009), which is associated positively with pregnancy rate (Santos et al., 2008). When endometrial secretions are modified (Gray et al., 2001) changes are induced in endometrial architecture which are fundamental for the appropriate development of the embryo (Wang et al., 2007). Nonetheless, in other studies, no response has been observed of fat supplementation on progesterone synthesis. In this respect, Robinson et al. (2002), using cows fed a ration rich in linoleic acid showed a reduction of up to 50% in the serum levels of progesterone between days 4 and 8 of the oestrus cycle, while those cows consuming a ration rich in linolenic acid showed a lower concentration of this hormone, but in days 4 and 15 of the oestrus cycle (Robinson et al., 2002). Recent work (Huante, 2010), demonstrated that secretion of progesterone in Brahman cows with low body condition at calving and during the postpartum (2.0 points, in the scale 1-5) was unaffected by supplementation with oilseeds with 60% of unsaturated fatty acids, relative to the control group (0.065±0.013 *vs* 0.054±0.013 ng/ml, respectively). These results suggest that due to the low body condition, the cow uses feed energy for its maintenance and not for reproductive processes. Those results suggest that the above mentioned fatty acid, exert different effects in the synthesis of ovarian steroids (Hinckley et al., 1996). Childs et al. (2008b) fed beef heifers a ration enriched with fish oil (*n*-3) and even when no increase in serum progesterone was achieved at day 7 of the oestrus cycle, they postulated that there was evidence of a greater synthesis of progesterone during the whole oestrus cycle due to the increase in the serum concentration of cholesterol and to the greater size of the corpus luteum.

While in sheep, concentration of progesterone in the follicular fluid was greater than in sheep which consumed the ration enriched with *n-3* fatty acids, than those which were fed with a greater amount of *n*-6 fatty acids (Wonnacott et al., 2010). Some *in vitro* studies have demonstrated that progesterone metabolism can be inhibited by high concentrations (300 μM) of α-linolenic acid in the culture media (Piccinato et al., 2010). This is perhaps related to the fact that certain PUFAs may also increase serum concentration of insulin and this in turn, reduce hepatic expression of some enzymes of the cythocrome P_{450} complex which catabolize progesterone (Lemley et al., 2008). Oestradiol, another hormone derived from cholesterol has stimulatory effects on the uterine secretion of $PGF_{2\alpha}$ (Knickerbocker et al. 1986) and can increase sensibility of the corpus luteum to prostaglandins by intensifying its regression (Howard et al., 1990). Previous studies demonstrate that intra-abomasal infusion of yellow fat induced a reduction in blood levels of oestradiol between days 15 and 20 of the oestrus cycle, compared to cows which were infused with glucose intra-abomasally. The relationship between dietary fatty acids and synthesis of steroid hormones may be direct through a direct effect on steroidogenesis (acute regulatory protein of steroids; STAR, cythocrome P450 protein, family 11; subfamily A polypeptide enzyme 1; CYP11A1) etc. or indirectly through prostaglandins. STAR plays a fundamental role in the synthesis of steroid hormones (Stocco et al., 2005). In previous work, it has been observed that in beef heifers there was a reduction in the concentration of arachidonic acid in the endometrial tissue when they were fed *n*-3 PUFAs (Childs et al., 2008a; Childs et al., 2008b). On the other hand, there is evidence that supplementation with linoleic acid (*n*-6) increased uterine secretion of $PGF_{2\alpha}$ (Cullens, 2005), which could derive in a greater availability of arachidonic acid in the endometrium. Under such conditions it could be speculated that a possible way to act of the *n*-3 and *n*-6 fatty acids in steroidogenesis is by reducing or increasing the availability of arachidonic acid, respectively and as a consequence, the expression of RNAm for STAR synthesis.

3.2 Lipids on ovarian activity

These results suggest that another of the mechanisms by means dietary lipids may improve reproductive performance of cattle is influencing follicular development and ovulation. In this, respect, Lucy et al. (1991), replaced corn with Ca-LCFA from palm oil in the ration of dairy cows at calving, and increased the number of medium size follicles (6-9 mm) and of follicles greater than 15 mm within 25 days postpartum. Furthermore, the diameter of the greatest follicle was superior in cows fed Ca-LCFA from palm oil (18.2 *vs* 12.4 mm). When this study was repeated with isocaloric diet, observed effects were similar (Lucy et al. 1993).
The greatest increase in medium follicle populations occurred in response to plant oil consumption, which is likely a direct result of the effects of high levels of linoleic acid in the rumen. Maximum follicular growth responses to plant oil supplementation have occurred when plant oils were fed at 4 to 6% of dietary dry matter, with lesser increases observed at lower levels of added fat. Animal tallow, calcium salts of saturated fatty acids or fish oil have been shown to have less clear effects on follicular growth than plant-derived oils. Moreover, postpartum beef cows which calved in a very poor body condition (BCS of 3; 1-9 scale) were unable to develop medium or large follicles at a rate equal to those with a body condition score of 4 or greater after 3 weeks of fat consumption (Ryan et al., 1994).
The number of medium size follicles (5 to 10 mm) was higher in beef cows which consumed feed with a greater content of PUFAs (Thomas et al., 1997) and in dairy cows which consumed a diet enriched with 5% *n*-3 fatty acids derived from fish oil (Heravi-Moussavi et al., 2007). Similar results were observed in cows fed with diets enriched with *n*-3 or *n*-6 fatty acids (Robinson et al., 2002). Staples & Thatcher (2005) summarized the effect of increasing lipids in the ration on the size of the dominant follicle: on average, the size of the dominant follicle was 3.2 mm greater than in females fed with some source of fat, which represents a 23% increase. Other studies (Bilby et al., 2006d; Garnsworthy et al., 2008) showed that the size of the dominant follicle is increased in cows fed diets rich in PUFAs. In sheep, the use of Ca-LCFA from palm oil (El-Shahat & Abo-El maaty, 2010) or from corn oil (Herrera et al., 2008) in the feed improved the number and size of the preovulatory follicles, as well as rate of ovulation and the superovulatory response in Pelibuey sheep (Herrera et al., 2008). These evidences demonstrate that consumption of lipids accelerate follicular growth (de Fries et al., 1998), which may influence the restart of ovulation postpartum, as it was shown by Marín-Aguilar et al. (2007) who observed that Holstein cows supplemented with plant oil (60% PUFAs) reduced by 7 days the restart of ovarian activity relative to a control group. de Veth et al. (2009) observed that time at first ovulation in dairy cows was reduced by 8 days when they were supplemented with 8 g/d of *trans*-10, *cis*-12 CLA.

4. Lipids and its effect on endometrial secretion of prostaglandins

Studies in a variety of species have shown that dietary PUFAs can modulate prostaglandin synthesis and metabolism. Eicosanoids, comprising prostaglandins, thromboxanes, leukotrienes and lipoxins, are all synthesized from C20 fatty acids (Mattos et al., 2000). The most biologically active two series prostaglandins are derived from arachidonic acid, but the less active three series prostaglandins can be produced from eicosapentaenoic acid by the action of the same enzymes (Robinson et al., 2002).

Prostaglandins play an important role in reestablishing oestrus cycles both immediately after parturition and thereafter until conception. Prostaglandin $F_{2\alpha}$ ($PGF_{2\alpha}$) is responsible for uterine involution after parturition. The uterus releases $PGF_{2\alpha}$ during each oestrus to regress each new corpus luteum if the cow is not pregnant and initiate a new oestrus cycle. During the period of corpus luteum regression, concentrations of $PGF_{2\alpha}$ and progesterone are inversely related. If the cow does conceive, release of $PGF_{2\alpha}$ from the uterus is prevented in order to preserve the corpus luteum and maintain pregnancy (Funston & Filley, 2002).

Linoleic acid is a substrate for the synthesis of $PGF_{2\alpha}$. Linoleic acid can be desaturated and elongated to arachidonic acid (C20:4, *n*-6), which is a precursor for $PGF_{2\alpha}$. Regulatory enzymes for this conversion include delta 6 desaturase and cyclooxygenase. Linoleic acid can inhibit prostaglandin synthesis by competitive inhibition with these key enzymes. Arachidonic, and two fatty acids found in fishmeal, eicosapentaenoic (C20:5) and docosahexanoic (C22:6), have been shown to inhibit cyclooxygenase activity as well. It is important to note that linolenic acid (C18:3) was also present in the endometrial prostaglandin synthesis inhibitor isolated by Thatcher et al. (1994), and that linolenic acid has been shown to be a strong inhibitor of prostaglandin synthesis (Mattos et al., 2000). The amount and probably type of particular fatty acids reaching the target tissues likely influence if prostaglandin synthesis is going to be stimulated or inhibited (Thatcher & Staples, 2000).

Figure 1 shows the schematic metabolic pathway of dietary n-6 and n-3 PUFAs and potential mechanisms for regulation of $PGF_{2\alpha}$ secretion. Absorbed PUFAs are desaturated and elongated in organs such as the mammary gland, adipose tissue, testis, brain, placenta and the liver (of non-ruminants). Dietary PUFAs and their desaturation and elongation products are incorporated into phospholipids of the plasma membrane. The amount of each fatty acid incorporated depends on the amount of precursor present in the diet. External stimuli such as the binding of oxytocin (OT) to the oxytocin receptor (OTr) stimulates the activity of phospholipase A2 (PLA2) and phospholipase C (PLC), which cleave phospholipids from the plasma membrane and ultimately increase availability of diacylglycerol (DAG) and fatty acids for processing by prostaglandin H synthetase (PGHS). Eicosapentaenoic acid (EPA; C20:5, n-3) is processed by PGHS to generate prostaglandins of the 3 series. Arachidonic acid (AA; C20:4 *n*-6) can be processed by PGHS, epoxygenase and lipoxygenase to generate prostaglandins of the 2 series, epoxyeicosatrienoic acids (EETs), leukotrienes and hydroxyeicosatetraenoic acids (di-HETEs), respectively (Mattos et al., 2000).

In vitro studies have demonstrated that some *n*-3 (eicosapentaenoic and docosahexaenoic) fatty acids reduce biosynthesis of prostaglandins of the series 2 in cells and tissues (Mattos et al., 2003). Similarly, some isomers from conjugated linoleic acid inhibited synthesis of $PGF_{2\alpha}$ and the effect was independent of the concentration of linolenic acid and the ratio *n*-6:*n*-3 (Harris et al., 2001). The above results are interesting due to the fact that most

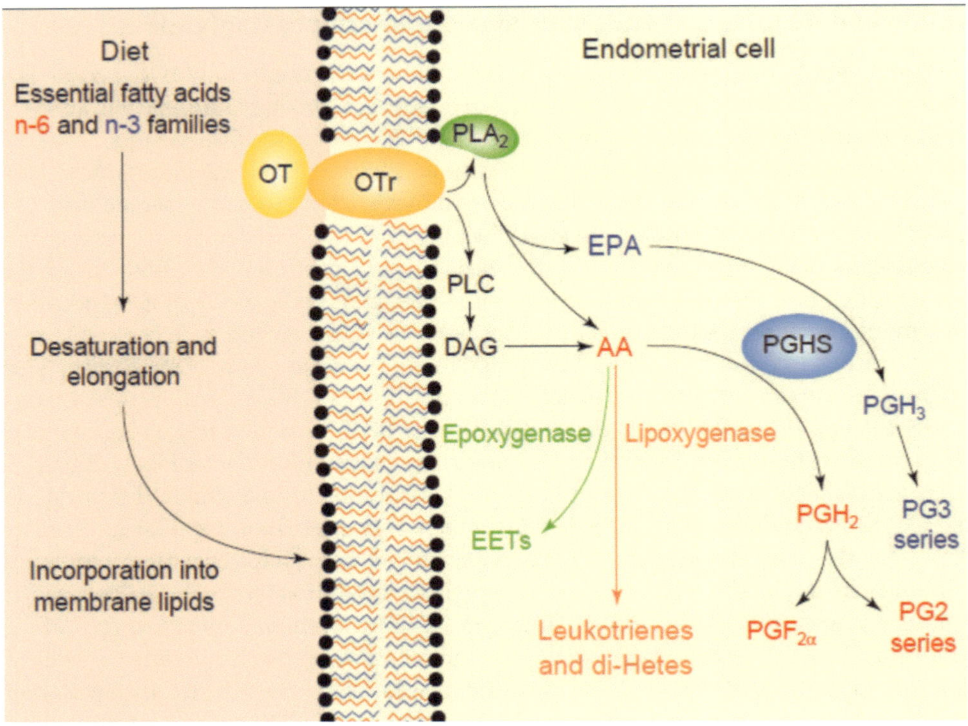

Fig. 1. Schematic representation of the metabolism of dietary *n*-6 and *n*-3 polyunsaturated fatty acids and potential mechanisms for regulation of $PGF_{2\alpha}$ secretion (Mattos et al., 2000).

embryonic losses in cattle occur during days 8-16 after artificial insemination (Sreenan et al., 2001), which leads to believe that some embryos may not reach the appropriate size at that moment to inhibit synthesis of $PGF_{2\alpha}$ for luteolysis to occur (Thatcher et al., 1994), showing the inability to inhibit luteolytic action by $PGF_{2\alpha}$ during the critical period of maternal recognition of pregnancy (Childs et al., 2008a). In this context, inhibition of the synthesis of $PGF_{2\alpha}$ could increase the rates of embryo survival and pregnancy (Binelli et al., 2001). PUFAs (*n*-3) such as eicosapentaenoic acid may inhibit uterine synthesis of $PGF_{2\alpha}$ by competing with arachidonic acid by means of COX, or in the case of docosahexaenoic acid, by competence with arachidonic acid by phospholipase A2 enzymes (Mattos et al., 2000).

Fish meal has relatively high concentrations of eicosapentaenoic and docosahexaenoic acids, in such a way that their incorporation in the ration of cattle may reduce the synthesis of $PGF_{2\alpha}$ and delay regression of the corpus luteum, improving embryo survival and herd fertility (Staples et al., 1998)

Previous studies showed that the infusion of a fat source rich in linoleic acid (17%) into the abomasum of lactating dairy cows resulted in a significant reduction in the release of PGFM, as measured in peripheral plasma, in response to an injection of oxytocin on day 15 of a synchronized oestrous cycle (Oldick et al., 1997). These results indicate that high concentrations of PUFAs in the diet can decrease endometrial secretion of prostaglandins.

In this respect, in cows, fed with *n*-3 fatty acids derived from fish meal, a reduction was observed in endometrial secretion of arachidonic acid, increasing in this same tissue the levels of eicosapentaenoic acid and total *n*-3 fatty acids (Burns et al., 2003; Bilby et al., 2006b). Similar effects were observed in dairy cows which consumed increasing amounts of fish meal or Ca-LCFA from fish oil (Bilby et al. 2006a). Due to the addition of *n*-3 and *n*-6 in the phospholipid component of endometrium, it is possible that changes in the content of fatty acids in the endometrial tissue may modulate secretion of $PGF_{2\alpha}$ in cows (Santos et al., 2008). In further studies, Burns et al. (2003) reported an increase in eicosapentaenoic acid at day 18 postpartum, as well as a reduction in arachidonic acid in the caruncules of beef cows fed fish meal. In another study, supplementing the diet with fish oil during the periparturient period reduced uterine secretion of $PGF_{2\alpha}$ in lactating dairy cows. In this sense, beef heifers fed *n*-3 PUFAs reduced production of arachidonic acid in endometrial tissue, apparently due to the fact that linoleic acid must elongate and desaturate to form arachidonic acid using the same enzymes than for the synthesis of eicosapentaenoic acid, starting from α-linolenic acid (Coyne et al., 2008).

There is evidence that during the prepartum period, lipid supplementation with 30% fatty acids as linoleic acid (*n*-6) increased uterine secretion of $PGF_{2\alpha}$ (Cullens, 2005). Increase in the synthesis of $PGF_{2\alpha}$ when cows are fed *n*-6 fatty acids during the transition period before calving or during the early postpartum (puerperium), can increase the potential of the uterus and of the immune system to secrete eicosanoids, which have influence in postpartum uterine health and in the inmunocompetence of the cow (Santos et al., 2008).

Childs et al. (2008b) fed heifers with a diet rich in *n*-6 fatty acids (entire soyabeans) or *n*-3 fatty acids (fish oil) and observed that on day 15 of the oestrous cycle, serum concentration of PGFM metabolite was higher than in the first group. These results are interesting if it is considered that by stimulating secretion of $PGF_{2\alpha}$ during early postpartum uterine involution can be favored (Mattos et al., 2004) and reproductive efficiency is improved, since when cows were supplemented before calving with calcium salts rich in *n*-6 fatty acids the occurrence of postpartum diseases such as membrane retention, metritis and mastitis, was reduced (Cullens, 2005). Thus, both arachidonic acid, but as well precursors of this fatty acid, such as linoleic acid increase the production of series 2 prostaglandin, while *n*-3 fatty acids compete with arachidonic acid and therefore reduce synthesis of such prostaglandin. In studies carried out *in vitro*, addition of eicosapentaenoic acid to the culture media of endometrial cells of cows, reduced production of endometrial $PGF_{2\alpha}$ from 88 to 40%, but this was reverted as the ratio of *n*-6:*n*-3 in the culture media was increased from 0 to 19% (Caldari-Torres et al., 2006). This observation is consistent with previous reports and suggest that the net inhibition of uterine $PGF_{2\alpha}$ synthesis by *n*-3 fatty acids may depend on the amount of *n*-6 fatty acids that reach the secretory tissue (Achard et al., 1997).

However, recent studies (Meier et al., 2009) showed that the bovine endometrial and trophoblastic tissues during short-term culture, incubated in a media supplemented with fatty acids: eicosapentaenoic (20:5-3; EPA), docosahexaenoic acids (22:6-3; DHA) or linoleic acids (C18:2-6; LIN), the release of PGE_2 from 'pregnant' endometrium was higher (P=0.094) than from 'non-pregnant' endometrium, while $PGF_{2\alpha}$ concentrations were similar. Treatment with fatty acids had no effect on $PGF_{2\alpha}$ or PGE_2 release from either pregnant or non-pregnant endometrium. The individual fatty acid treatments had no effect on the ratio of $PGF_{2\alpha}$ to PGE_2 from trophoblast tissues, but when the data from the three fatty acid treatments were combined (EPA, DHA and LIN treatment groups) the ratio of $PGF_{2\alpha}$ to PGE_2 was reduced (P=0.026) when compared to the medium only. This result indicated that the ability of exogenous fatty acids to modify embryonic prostaglandin release needs to be examined in the context of supplementing dairy cows with different sources of fats.

On other hand, the dynamics of bovine corpus luteum regression in response to exogenous $PGF_{2\alpha}$ can also be altered by dietary fish meal. In this respect, Burke et al., (1997) fed cows

(n=56) with fish meal at either 0 or 2.8% of ration dry matter from 24 to109 days postpartum. On day 58 postpartum, all cows were injected with a luteolytic dose of $PGF_{2\alpha}$. Two days after injection of $PGF_{2\alpha}$, the proportion of cows with plasma concentrations of progesterone that were >1 ng ml^{-1} was greater when fish meal was included in the ration than when a control ration was fed (29.0 *vs* 4%). Thus, it is possible that fatty acids present in fish oil reduce the sensitivity of the corpus luteum to $PGF_{2\alpha}$.

5. Lipids their effect on embryo development

Establishment of pregnancy in the ruminant requires the ovulation of a competent oocyte, of insemination at the appropriate time and of a correct pattern of secretion of oestradiol and progesterone during the follicular and luteal phase of oestrus. The embryo must develop in an appropriate way and avoid luteolysis producing enough interferon τ which stimulates the expression of genes in the endometrium to inhibit the synthesis of oxytocin receptors and consequently final production of $PGF_{2\alpha}$, allowing the establishment of a corpus luteum (Bott et al., 2010). In dairy cows there is a significant loss of embryos during this period, it is considered that only 40% of cows remain pregnant at day 28 after artificial insemination (Santos et al., 2008). There is evidence that such events can be influenced by PUFAs consumed in the ration (Wathes et al., 2007). Fatty acids play an important role in the modification of the biophysical properties and in the activity of biological membranes, including fluidity and cell proliferation (Bilby et al., 2006d). The competence and quality of the ovocyte and of the embryo are related to the type of fatty acid, specifically, with the content of particular fatty acids en the phospholipids of cell membrane which play a role in development and during and after fertilization (Santos et al., 2008).

The amount of lipids in the ovocyte of ruminants is about 76 ng approximately and has around 58% triglycerides, 20% phospholipids, 20% cholesterol and 10% free fatty acids (McEvoy et al., 2000). Fatty acids found in greater amounts in the phospholipid fraction of the membrane of cattle ovocyte are palmitic (16:0) and oleic (18:1) acids. PUFAs represent less than 20% of the total, being linoleic acid the most abundant of them (Santos et al., 2008). Marei et al. (2010) pointed out that linoleic acid (*n-6*) is the most abundant fatty acid in follicular fluid of cattle and has an important role in the regulation of the process of maturation of the ovocyte, since when the cell complex of the cumulus and ovocyte were treated with linoleic acid there was a delay in the growth of the latter. Some studies have shown the fatty acid profiles in follicular fluid are affected by the estrogenic activity of the follicle (Renaville et al., 2010). Table 4 shows saturated and unsaturated fatty acids in plasma and in some reproductive tissues.

Ratio of saturated fatty acids to PUFA in granulose cells (Adamiak et al., 2005) and in the ovocyte (Wonnacott et al., 2010) is greater than in plasma. This suggests the presence of a mechanism of selective uptake in the ovarian follicles or *de novo* synthesis of saturated fatty acids from acetate (Wonnacott et al., 2010). Fatty acids can be oxidized as an energy source during maturation of the ovocyte and during early embryo development before implantation, in such a way that cattle ovocytes exposed to metal palmoxirate to block oxidation of fatty acids, showed a lower ability to form blastocysts after *in vitro* fertilization (Ferguson & Leese, 2006). Cetica et al. (2002) reported a significant increment in the activity of the enzyme lipase during maturation of cattle ovocyte, which releases fatty acids from triglycerides for later oxidation. Apart from the role of fatty acids, particularly those saturated, as sources of energy, the content of PUFAs in the ovocyte may affect maturation,

Fatty acid group	Plasma (μg/ml)		Granulosa cell (μg/pellet)		Oocytes (ng/oocyte)	
	Dietary treatment [ab]					
	n-3	n-6	n-3	n-6	n-3	n-6
Saturated	30.9	42.1	39.1	39.7	75.7	71.1
Unsaturated	59.3	49.4	49.7	52.1	20.9	25.8
Monounsaturated fatty acids	21.5	18.0	20.9	23.9	7.8	12.9
Polyunsaturated fatty acids	37.8	31.4	28.9	28.2	13.0	12.9
n-6 PUFA	25.4	28.9	8.5[c]	24.1	5.2	10.9
n-3 PUFA	**12.4**	**2.5**	**20.4**	**4.1**	**7.8**	**2.1**
Ratio n6:n3	**2.1**	**11.5**	**0.4**	**6.2**	**0.7**	**8.3**

Table 4. Saturated and unsaturated fatty acids in plasma and some reproductive tissues. Adapted from Wonnacott et al. (2010) and Palmquist (2010). [a]6.4 % oil in the diet supplemented from linseed oil, [b]5.7% oil in the diet supplemented from sunflower oil. [c]Important effects due dietary fatty acids are in bold.

cryopreservation and its capacity for further development (Wathes et al., 2007). From the *n-3* fatty acids, linolenic acid has been implicated in the growth and differentiation of the ovocyte, regulation of meiotic arrest during the germinal vesicle stage and in avoiding the breaking of this structure (Kim et al., 2001).

In sheep, Zeron et al. (2002) showed that supplementation with Ca-LCFA from fish oil during 13 weeks, resulted in better quality ovocytes and better integrity of their membrane, compared to that of sheep which were not fed lipid supplements (74.3% and 57.0%, respectively), which increased the ratio of long chain fatty acids in plasma of cells from the cumulus, although these changes were not observed in the ovocytes, suggesting selective uptake by the ovocyte or a highly regulated uptake, which could limit potential impact of cow nutrition on the proportion of fatty acids in their gametes. While in beef cattle, Fouladi-Nashta et al. (2007) fed cows with 200 or 800 g per day of Ca-LCFA from palm oil, which resulted in a greater percentage of ovum which developed up to the blastocyst stage and had a greater amount of cells due to an increment in the number of cells of the trophectoderm. By influencing the molecular mechanisms which control nucleus maturation of the ovocyte, *in vitro* treatment of the cumulus-oocyte complex with linolenic acid (*n-3*), increased the percentage of gametes which reached the meiotic second division, increased the division of the embryo as well as the rate of blastocyst (Marei et al., 2009).

When a group of lactating superovulated cows were fed with rich sources of saturated fatty acids (*n*-6 or *n*-3), rate of fertilization and the number of transferable embryos was not different; however, embryo development was increased in cows which consumed unsaturated fatty acids, compared to the cows which consumed saturated fatty acids (Thangavelu et al., 2007). Cerri et al. (2009) supplemented dairy cows with Ca-LCFA from palm oil or linoleic + octadecaenoic acids between days 25 prepartum and 80 days postpartum observing in the second group a greater proportion of excellent and good quality embryos, apart from a higher number of blastomere.

In hair ewes, Herrera et al. (2008) showed that PUFAs in the ration increased superovulatory response, registering increased ($P<0.05$) numbers of corpus luteum (14.73±1.87 *vs* 10.73±1.42); total cells collected, including ova plus embryos (9.18±2.16 *vs* 4.18±1.36) and

embryos (6.72±1.78 *vs* 3.09±1.36) in the PUFAs treatment than in the control treatment, respectively.
On the contrary, Childs et al. (2008b) fed cows with a ration enriched with *n*-3 PUFAs and did not observe any effect on the number of normal embryos nor in the amount of good quality embryos (grade 1 and 2); however, these cows showed a lower number of degenerated embryos. Similarly, Bilby et al. (2006d) did not find an effect of fatty acids in the ration of dairy cows on the quality of embryos after maturation and *in vitro* fertilization. In a similar way, Thangavelu et al. (2007) did not establish a difference in the total number of transferable embryos of dairy cows supplemented with either PUFAs or saturated fat. Marques et al. (2007) did not observe any effect of the addition of arachidonic or eicosapentaenoic acids to the culture media for the *in vitro* maturation of ovocytes on the subsequent embryo development. This agrees with observations by Lawson et al. (2007) who added increasing amounts of eicosapentaenoic acid to the culture media for the maturation of ovocytes *in vitro*. In a recent study, Wakefield et al. (2007) suggested that contrary to the possible beneficial effects, supplementing a ration with *n*-3 PUFAs during the period just before or immediately after conception, may reduce normal development of the embryo, since this seems to disturb mitochondrial metabolism. Leroy et al. (2010) cultivated bovine zygotes in media supplemented with serum from heifers fed rations with a high content of lipids protected from rumen biohydrogenation and observed a lower production of blastocysts compared to a control treatment, noting that in the first there was a greater expression of genes related to apoptosis.
Even when *in vivo* and *in vitro* studies have shown a better embryo development with rations supplemented with lipids, results are not consistent and it is important to ascertain in particular, which fatty acids are the most beneficial for embryo survival (Santos et al., 2008). Oocytes of all mammals contain an endogenous lipid reserve. This feature reflects their common ancestral origin, the yolk-rich amniote egg. However, lipids are species-specific in terms of their apparent abundance and utilization. Despite the significant role of the lipid reserves in cell structure and function, very few studies have provided detailed descriptions of its nature and composition in mammalian oocytes. Table 5 gives the fatty acid composition of total lipid extracted from zone-intact oocytes of cattle and sheep.

6. Conclusion

Data reviewed shows that supplementation with different sources of lipids and fatty acids improve reproductive performance of the female ruminant. However, it is important to consider that the optimum response will be achieved when undernutrition status of the female is not extremely sever. A nutrient balance (protein:energy) in the ration consumed by the animal is fundamental to obtain maximum benefit from supplementation with fat, since fatty acids do not supply nitrogen for amino acid synthesis and consequently for the correct functioning of the hypothalamus-hypophysis axis. Improvements in reproductive performance may be a result of increased energy density of the ration or of the direct effects of specific fatty acids on reproductive processes. As is the case for any technology or management strategy that improves specific aspects of ovarian physiology and cyclic activity, actual improvements in pregnancy rate or total weight of calf weaned are dependent on a variety of management practices and environmental conditions. Until these interrelationships are better understood, livestock producers are recommended to attempt to formulate low cost/balanced rations. If a source of supplemental fat is available locally

		Mean (± SEM) distribution of fatty acids (%, w/w)[a]	
Name	Formula	Cattle (n = 3)[b]	Sheep (n = 2)
Lauric	12:0	0.23 ± 0.15	nd
Myristic	14:0	2.48 ± 1.02	0.39±0.032
Palmitic	16:0	32.0 ± 1.64	24.7±0.74
Palmitoleic	16:1 n-7	2.24 ± 0.45	4.38±0.20
Heptadecanoic	17:0	0.76 ± 0.14	0.41±0.407
Stearic	18:0	14.2±2.47	16.2±0.30
Oleic	18:1 n-9	25. ±1.75	26.2±0.23
Vaccenic	18:1 n-7	3.71± 0.12	3.64±0.32
Linoleic	18:2 n-6	5.17± 0.12	6.98±0.10
γ-Linolenic	18:3 n-6	0.75 ± 0.16	1.01±0.06
α-Linolenic	18:3 n-3	0.49±0.09	2.01±0.41
Stearidonic	18:4 n-3	nd	1.68±0.30
Arachidic	20:0	1.35±0.70	3.11±0.45
Eicosenoic	20:1 n-9	0.27±0.13	0.19±0.187
Eicosadienoic	20:2 n-6	0.54±0.20	0.91±0.476
Eicosatrienoic	20:3 n-6	0.27±0.15	0.52±0.070
Arachidonic	20:4 n-6	1.13±0.57	1.50±0.60
Eicosapentaenoic	20:5 n-3	1.15±1.15	3.03±1.09
Behenic	22:0	1.23±0.63	3.03±1.09
Erucic	22:1n-9	0.20±0.10	nd
Docosatetraenoic	22:4 n-6	0.27±0.15	nd
Docosapentaenoic	22:5 n-3	0.88±0.28	1.41±0.33
Docosahexaenoic	22:6 n-3	0.50±0.25	1.74±0.06
Lignoceric	24:0	2.30±1.21	nd

Table 5. Fatty acid composition of total lipid extracted from zone-intact oocytes of cattle and sheep (adapted from McEvoy et al., 2000). Each sample (n = 2–4) represents 1000 oocytes. [a]Percentage (w/w) of the total fatty acids in oocyte lipid. [b]One of the four original cattle oocyte samples was excluded because of uncertainty about the validity of the assay result involving cholesterol ester component of total lipid. nd: not detected.

and can be incorporated with little or no change in the cost of the ration, it would be wise for farmers to do so. Research studying the role of fat supplementation on reproductive responses has not been that consistent, therefore, adding fat to the ration would be advised when the risk of low reproductive performance (young, growing animals and limiting nutrients [protein, energy] in the basal ration) is the greatest.

7. References

Abayasekara, D.R.E. & Wathes, C.D. (1999). Effects of altering dietary fatty acid composition on prostaglandin synthesis and fertility. *Prostaglandins, Leukotrienes and Essential Fatty Acids*, Vol.61, No.5, (November 1999), pp. 275-287. ISSN 0952-3278

Achard, D.; Gilbert, M.; Benistant, C.; Slama, S.B.; DeWitt, D.L.; Smith, W.L. & Lagarde, M. (1997). Eicosapentaenoic and docosahexaenoic acids reduce PGH synthase 1 expression in bovine aortic endothelial cells. *Biochemical Biophysical Research Communications*, Vol.241, No.2, (December 1997), pp. 513-518. ISSN 0006-291X

Adamiak, S.J.; Mackie, K.;Watt, R.G.; Webb, R. & Sinclair, K.D. (2005). Impact of nutrition on oocyte quality: cumulative effects of body composition and diet leading to hyperinsulinemia in cattle. *Biology of Reproduction*, Vol.73, No.5, (November 2005), pp. 918-926. ISSN 0006-3363

Aguilar-Pérez, C.; Ku-Vera, J. & Garnsworthy C.P. (2009). Effects of bypass fat on energy balance, milk production and reproduction in grazing crossbred cows in the tropics. *Livestock Science*, Vol.121, No.1, (March 2009), pp64-71. ISSN: 1871-1413

Ambrose, D.J.; Estill, C.T.; Colazo, M.G.; Kastelic, J.P. & Corbett, R. (2006b). Conception rates and pregnancy losses in dairy cows fed a diet supplemented with rolled flaxseed. *Proceedings of the 7th International Ruminant Reproduction Symposium*, Wellington, New Zealand. Abstract 50.

Ambrose, D.K.; Kastelic, J.P.; Corbett, R.; Pitney, P.A.; Petit, H.V.; Small, J.A. & Zalkovic, P. (2006a). Lower pregnancy losses in lactating dairy cows fed a diet enriched in α-linolenic acid. *Journal of Dairy Science*, Vol.89, No.8, (August 2006), pp. 3066-3074. ISSN 1811-9751

Aranda-Ávila, I.; Herrera-Camacho J.; Aké-López J. R.; Delgado-León R.A. & Ku-Vera, J. C. (2010). Effect of supplementation with corn oil on postpartum ovarian activity, pregnancy rate, and serum concentration of progesterone and lipid metabolites in F1 (*Bos taurus* × *Bos indicus*) cows. *Tropical Animal Health and Production*, Vol.42, No.7 (October 2010), pp. 1435-1440. ISSN 1573-7438

Armstrong, J.D.; Goodall, E.A.; Gordon, F.J.; Rice, D.A. & McCaughey, W.J. (1990). The effects of levels of concentrate offered and inclusion of maize gluten or fish meal in the concentrate on reproductive performance and blood parameter of dairy cows. *Animal Production*, Vol.50, No.1, (September, 1990), pp. 1-10. ISSN 1357-7298

Bader, J.F.; Felton, E.E.D.; Kerley, M.S.; Simms, D.D. & Patterson, D.J. (2000). Effects of postpartum fat supplementation on reproduction in primiparous 2-year-old and mature cows. *Journal of Animal Science*, Vol.78, Suppl. No.1, (July 2000), pp. 224. ISSN 1525-3163. *Journal of Dairy Science*, Vol.83, Suppl. No.1, (July 2000), pp. 224. ISSN 0022-0302

Bernal SG.; O'Donnell, A. M.; Vicini, J. L.; Hartnell, G. F. & Bauman, D. E. (2010). Enhancing omega-3 fatty acids in milk fat of dairy cows by using stearidonic acid-enriched soybean oil from genetically modified soybeans. *Journal of Dairy Science*, Vol.93, No.1, (January 2010), pp. 32-37. ISSN 0022-0302

Bernal-Santos, G.; Perfield II, J.W.; Barbano, D. M.; Bauman, D.E. & Overton, T.R. (2003). Production responses of dairy cows to dietary supplementation with conjugated linoleic acid (CLA) during the transition period and early lactation. *Journal of Dairy Science*, Vol.86, No. 10, (October 2003), pp. 3218-3228. ISSN 0022-0302

Bilby, T.R.; Block, J.; do Amaral, B.C.; Sa Filho, O.; Silvestre, F.T.; Hansen, P.J.; Staples, C.R. & Thatcher, W.W. (2006d). Effects of dietary unsaturated fatty acids on oocyte quality and follicular development in lactating dairy cows in summer. *Journal of Dairy Science*, Vol.89, No.10 (October 2006), pp. 3891-3903. ISSN 0022-0302

Bilby, T.R.; Guzeloglu, A., MacLaren, L.A., Staples, C.R., Thatcher, W.W. (2006a). Pregnancy, bST and omega-3 fatty acids in lactating dairy cows: II. Gene expression related to maintenance of pregnancy. *Journal of Dairy Science*, Vol.89, No.9 (September 2006), pp. 3375-3385. ISSN 0022-0302

Bilby, T.R., Jenkins, T.; Staples, T.R. & Thatcher, W.W. (2006b). Pregnancy, bovine somatotropin, and dietary *n*-3 fatty acids in lactating dairy cows: III. Fatty acid distribution. *Journal of Dairy Science*, Vol.89, No.9, (September 2006), pp. 3386-3399. ISSN 0022-0302

Bilby, T.R.; Sozzi, A.; Lopez, M.M.; Silvestre, F.T.; Ealy, A.D.; Staples, C.R. & Thatcher, W.W. (2006c). Pregnancy, bovine somatotropin, and dietary *n*-3 fatty acids in lactating dairy cows: I. ovarian, conceptus, and growth hormone-insulin-like growth factor system responses. *Journal of Dairy Science*, Vol.89, No.9 (September 2006), pp. 3360-3374. ISSN 0022-0302

Binelli, M., Thatcher, W.W., Mattos, R., Baruselli, P.S. (2001). Antiluteolytic strategies to improve fertility in cattle. *Theriogenology*, Vol.56, No.9 (December 2001), pp. 1451-63. ISSN: 0093-691X

Bott, R.C.; Ashley, R.L.; Henkes, L.E.; Antoniazzi, A.Q.; Bruemmer, J.E.; Niswender, G.D.; Bazer, F.W.; Spencer, T.E.; Smirnova, N.P.; Anthony, R.V. & Hansen, T.R. (2010). Uterine vein infusion of interferon Tau (IFNT) extends luteal life span in ewes. *Biology of Reproduction*, Vol.82, No.4 (April 2010), pp. 725-735. ISSN 0006-3363

Bruckental, I.; Dori, D.; Kaim, M.; Lehrer. H. & Folman, Y. (1989). Effects of source and level of protein on milk yield and reproductive performance of high-producing primiparous and multiparous dairy cows. *Animal Production*, Vol.48, No.2 (April 1989), pp. 319-329. ISSN 1357-7298

Burke, J.M.; Staples, C.R.; Risco, C.A.; De La Sota, R.L. & Thatcher, W.W. (1997). Effect of ruminant grade menhaden fish meal on reproductive and productive performance of lactating dairy cows. *Journal of Dairy Science*, Vol.80, No.12 (December 1997), pp. 3386-3398. ISSN 0022-0302

Burns, P.D., Engle, T.E., Harris, M.A., Enns, R.M., Whittier, J.C. (2003). Effect of fish meal supplementation on plasma and endometrial fatty acid composition in nonlactating beef cows. *Journal of Animal Science*, Vol.81, No.11 (November 2003), pp. 2840-2846. ISSN 1525-3163

Burr, G.O. & Burr, M.M. (1930). On the nature and role of the fatty acids essential in nutrition. *Journal of Biological Chemistry*, Vol.86, No.2 (April 1930), pp. 587-621. ISSN 0021-9258

Caldari-Torres, C.; Rodriguez-Sallaberry, C.; Greene, E.S. & Badinga, L. (2006). Differential effects of *n*-3 and *n*-6 fatty acids on prostaglandin $F_{2\alpha}$ production by bovine endometrial cells. *Journal of Dairy Science*, Vol.89, No.3 (March 2006), pp 971-977. ISSN 0022-0302

Carroll, D.J.; Hossain, F.R. & Keller, M.R. (1994). Effect of supplemental fish meal on the lactation and reproductive performance of dairy cows. *Journal of Dairy Science*, Vol.77, No.10 (Octiber 1994), pp. 3058-3072. ISSN 0022-0302

Castañeda-Gutierrez, E.; Overton, T.R.; Butler, W.R. & Bauman, D.E. (2005). Dietary supplements of two doses of calcium salts of conjugated linoleic acid during the transition period and early lactation. *Journal of Dairy Science*, Vol.88, No.3 (March 2005), pp. 1078-1089. ISSN 0022-0302

Castellano CA, Audet, I. Bailey, J. L., Chouinard, P. Y., Laforest, J.P., Matte, J. J. (2010). Effect of dietary n-3 fatty acids (fish oils) on boar reproduction and semen quality. *Journal of Animal Science*, Vol.88, No7 (July 2010), pp. 2346-2355. ISSN 1525-3163

Cerri, R.L.A.; Juchem, S.O.; Chebel, R.C.; Rutgliano, H.; Bruno, R.G.S.; Galvaõ, K.N.; Thatcher, W.W. & Santos, J.E. (2009). Effect of fat source differing in fatty acid profile on metabolic parameters, fertilization, and embryo quality in high-producing dairy cows. *Journal of Dairy Science*, Vol.92, No.4 (April 2009), pp. 1520-1531. ISSN 0022-0302

Cetica, P.; Pintos, L.; Dalvit, G. & Beconi, M. (2002). Activity of key enzymes involved in glucose and triglyceride catabolism during bovine oocyte maturation in vitro. *Reproduction*, Vol.124, No5 (November 2002), pp. 675-681. ISSN 1741-7899

Childs, S.; Carter, F.; Lynch, C.O.; Sreenan, J.M.; Lonergan, P.; Hennessy, A.A. & Kenny, D.A. (2008b). Embryo yield and quality following dietary supplementation of beef heifers with *n*-3 polyunsaturated fatty acids (PUFA). *Theriogenology*, Vol.70, No.6 (October 2008), pp. 992-1003. ISSN 0093-691X

Childs, S.; Hennessy, A.A.; Sreenan, J.M.; Wathes, C.; Cheng, Z.; Stanton, C.; Diskin, M.G. & Kenny, D.A. (2008a). Effect of level of dietary *n*-3 polyunsaturated fatty acid supplementation on systemic and tissue fatty acid concentrations and on selected reproductive variables in cattle. *Theriogenology*, Vol.70, No.4 (September 2008), pp. 595-611. ISSN 0093-691X

Childs, S.; Lynch, C.O.; Hennessy, A.A.; Stanton, C.; Wathes, D.C.; Sreenan, J.M.; Diskin, M.G. & Kenny, D.A. (2008c). Effect of dietary enrichment with either *n*-3 or *n*-6 fatty acids on systemic metabolite and hormone concentration and ovarian function in heifers. *Animal*, Vol.2, No.6 (May 2008), pp. 883-893. ISSN 1751-7311

Coyne, G.S.; Kenny, D.A.; Childs, S.S.; Sreenan, J.M. & Waters, S.M. (2008). Dietary n-3 polyunsaturated fatty acids alter the expression of genes involved in prostaglandin biosynthesis in the bovine uterus. *Theriogenology*, Vol.70, No.5 (September 2008), pp. 772-782. ISSN 0093-691X

Cullens, F.M. (2005). *Effects of the timing of initiation of fat supplementation on productive and reproductive responses of periparturient dairy cows during summer*. MSc. Thesis. University of Florida, USA. Pp.146.

de Fries, C.A., Neuendorff, D.A., Randel, R.D. (1998). Fat supplementation influences postpartum reproductive performance in Brahman cows. *Journal of Animal Science*, Vol.76, No.3 (March 1998), pp. 864-870. ISSN 1525-3163

de Luna, C.J., Brown, W.H., Ray, D.E., Wegner, T.N. (1982). Effects of protected fat supplement on GnRH induced LH release in ovariectomized and early postpartum beef cow. *Journal of Animal Science*, Vol.55, No.Suppl. 1, pp. 348 (Abstr) ISSN 1525-3163

de Veth, M.J.; Bauman, D.E.; Koch, W.; Mann, G.E.; Pfeiffer, A.M. & Butler, W.R. (2009). Efficacy of conjugated linoleic acid for improving reproduction: A multi-study analysis in early-lactation dairy cows. *Journal of Dairy Science*, Vol.92, No.6 (June 2009), pp. 2662-2669. ISSN 0022-0302

Doreau, M.; Bauchart, D. & Chilliard, Y. (2011). Enhancing fatty acid composition of milk and meat through animal feeding. *Animal Production Science*, Vol.51, No.1 (December 2010), pp. 19-29. ISSN 1836-0939

El-Shahat, K.H. & Abo-El maaty, A.M. (2010). The effect of dietary supplementation with calcium salts of long chain fatty acids and/or l-carnitine on ovarian activity of Rahmani ewes. *Animal Reproduction Science*, Vol.117, No.1-2 (January 2010), pp. 78-82. ISSN: 0378-4320

Espinoza, J.L.; Ramírez-Godínez, J.A.; Jiménez, J.A. & Flores, A. (1995). Effects of calcium soaps of fatty acids on postpartum reproductive activity in beef cows and growth of calves. *Journal of Animal Science*, Vol.73, No.10 (October 1995), pp. 2888-2892. ISSN 1525-3163

Espinoza, J.L.; Ramirez-Godinez, J.A.; Simental, S.S.; Jiménez, J.; Ramirez, R.; Palacios, A., & de Luna, R. (1997). Effects of calcium soaps of fatty acids on serum hormones and lipid metabolites in Pelibuey ewes. *Small Ruminant Research*, Vol.26, No.1 (December 1997), pp. 61-68. ISSN: 0921-4488

Espinoza-Villavicencio, J.L.; Ortega-Pérez, R.; Palacios-Espinosa, A. & Guillén-Trujillo, A. (2010). Efecto de la suplementación de grasas sobre características productivas, tasas de preñez y algunos metabolitos de los lípidos en vacas para carne en pastoreo. *Archivos de Medicina Veterinaria*, Vol.42, No.1 (Enero 2010); pp. 25-32. ISSN 0301-732X

Ferguson, E.M. & Leese, H.J. (2006). A potential role for triglyceride as an energy source during bovine oocyte maturation and early embryo development. Molecular *Reproduction and Development*, Vol.73, No.9 (September 2006), pp. 1195-1201. ISSN 1040-452X

Ferguson, J.D.; Sklan, D.; Chalupa, W.V. & Kronfeld, D.S. (1990). Effects of hard fat on *in vitro* and *in vivo* rumen fermentation, milk production, and reproduction in dairy cows. *Journal of Dairy Science*; Vol.73, No.10 (October 1990), pp. 2864-2879. ISSN 0022-0302

Filley, S.J; Turner, H.A. & Stormshak F. (2000). Plasma fatty acids, prostaglandin F2*a* metabolite, and reproductive response in postpartum heifers fed rumen bypass fat. *Journal of Animal Science*, Vol.78, No.1 (January 2000), pp. 139-144. ISSN 1525-3163

Fouladi-Nashta, A.A.; Gutierrez, C.G.; Gong, J.G.; Garnsworthy, P.C. & Webb, R. (2007). Impact of dietary fatty acids on oocyte quality and development in lactating dairy cows. *Biology of Reproduction*, Vol.77, No. 1 (July 2007), pp. 9-17. ISSN: 0006-3363

Fuentes, M.C.; Calsamiglia, S.S.; Sánchez, C.; González, A.; Newbold, J.; Santos, J.E.P.; Rodríguez-Alcalá, L.M. & Fontecha, J. (2008). Effect of extruded linseed on productive and reproductive performance of lactating dairy cows. *Livestock Science*, Vol.113, No.2 (February 2008), pp. 144-154. ISSN: 1871-1413

Funston, R. & Filley, S. (2002). Effects of fat supplementation on reproduction in beef cattle. *Proceedings of The Applied Reproductive Strategies in Beef Cattle Workshop*, September 5-6, 2002, Manhattan, Kansas. USA. 1-8 p.

Funston, R.N. (2004). Fat supplementation and reproduction in beef females. *Journal of Animal Science*, Vol.82, No.13 (January 2004), pp. 154-161. E suppl. ISSN 1525-3163

Garcia-Bojalil, C.M.; Staples, C.R.; Risco, C.A.; Savio, J.D. & Thatcher, W.W. (1998). Protein degradability and calcium salts of long chain fatty acids in the diets of lactating dairy cows: productive responses. *Journal of Dairy Science*, Vol.81, No. 5 (May 1998), pp. 1374-1384. ISSN 0022-0302

Garnsworthy, P.C.; Lock, A.; Mann, G.E.; Sinclair, K.D. & Webb, R. (2008). Nutrition, metabolism, and fertility in dairy cows: 2. Dietary fatty acids and ovarian function. *Journal of Dairy Science*, Vol.91, No. 10 (October 2008), pp. 3824-3833. ISSN 0022-0302

Gray, C.A.; Taylor, K.M.; Ramsey, W.S.; Hill, J.R.; Bazer, F.W.; Bartol, F.F. & Spencer, T.E. (2001). Endometrial glands are required for preimplantation conceptus elongation and survival. *Biology of Reproduction* Vol.64, No.6 (June 2001), pp. 1608-1613. ISSN 0006-3363

Harris, M.A.; Hansen, R.A.; Vidsudhiphan, P.; Koslo, J.L.; Thomas, J.B.; Watkins, B.A. & Allen, K.G. (2001). Effects of conjugated linoleic acids and docosahexaenoic acid on rat liver and reproductive tissue fatty acids, prostaglandins and matrix metalloproteinase production. *Prostaglandins Leukotrienes and Essential Fatty Acids*, Vol.65, No.1 (July 2001), pp. 23-29. ISSN 0952-3278

Harrison J.H.; Kincaid, R.L.; McNamara, J.P.; Waltner, S.; Loney, K.A.; Riley, R.E. & Cronrath, J.D. (1995). Effect of whole cottonseeds and calcium salts of long-chain fatty acids on performance of lactating dairy cows. *Journal of Dairy Science*, Vol.78, No.1 (January 1995), pp. 181-193. ISSN 0022-0302

Heravi-Moussavi, A.R.; Gilbert, R.O.; Overton, T.R.; Bauman, D.E. & Butler, W.R. (2007). Effect of feeding fish meal and *n*-3 fatty acids on ovarian and uterine responses in early lactating dairy cows. *Journal of Dairy Science*, Vol.90, No.1 (January 2007), pp. 145-154. ISSN 0022-0302

Herrera-Camacho, J.; Aké-López, J.R.; Ku-Vera, J.C.; Williams, G.L. & Quintal-Franco, J.A. (2008). Respuesta ovulatoria, estado de desarrollo y calidad de embriones de ovejas Pelibuey superovuladas suplementadas con ácidos grasos poliinsaturados. *Tecnica Pecuaria en Mexico*, Vol.46, No.2 (Abril-Junio 2008), pp. 107-117. ISSN 0040-1889

Hightshoe, R.B., Cochran, R.C., Corah, L.R., Kiracofe, G.H., Harmon, D.L., Perry, R.C. (1991). Effects of calcium soaps of fatty acids on postpartum reproductive function in beef cows. *Journal of Animal Science*, Vol.69, No.10 (October 1991), pp. 4097-4103. ISSN 1525-3163

Hinckley, T., Clark, R.M., Bushmich, S.L. Milvae, R.A. (1996). Long chain polyunsaturated fatty acids and bovine luteal cell function. *Biology of Reproduction*, Vol.55, No.2 (August 1996), pp. 445-449. ISSN 0006-3363

Howard, J.J., Scott, R.G., Britt, J.H. (1990). Associations among progesterone, estradiol-17b, and prostaglandin in cattle treated with hCG during diestrus to extend corpus luteum function. *Prostaglandins*, Vol.40, No.1 (July 1990), pp. 51-70. ISSN1098-8823

Huante CR. (2010). *Efecto de la suplementación de dos tipos de ácidos grasos sobre el reinicio de la actividad ovárica y metabolitos de lípidos en vacas F1 (Bos taurus x Bos indicus) durante el posparto temprano*. Maestria Institucional en Ciencias Biológicas. Instituto de Investigaciones Agropecuarias y Forestales. Universidad Michoacana de San Nicolás de Hidalgo. Morelia, Michoacán, México.

Juchem, S.O. (2007). *Lipid Digestion and Metabolism in Dairy Cows: Effects on Production, Reproduction and Health*. PhD thesis, University of California Davis, USA.

Juchem, S.O.; Cerri, R.L.A.; Bruno, R.; Galvao, K.N.; Lemos, E.W.; Villasenor, M.; Coscioni, A.C.; Rutgliano, H.M.; Thatcher, W.W.; Luchini, D. & Santos, J.E.P. (2004). Effect of feeding Ca salts of palm oil (PO) or a blend of linoleic and monoenoic trans fatty acids (LTFA) on uterine involution and reproductive performance in Holstein cows. *Journal of Animal Science*, Vol.82 / *Journal of Dairy Science*, Vol.87 / *Poultry Science*, Vol.83, Suppl.1 pp. 310 (Abstract 633). ISSN 1525-3163 / ISSN 0022-0302 / ISSN: 0032-5791

Juchem, S.O.; Cerri, R.L.A.; Villaseñor, M.; Galvão, K.N.; Bruno, R.G.S.; Rutigliano, H.M.; DePeters, E.J.; Silvestre, F.T.; Thatcher, W.W. & Santos, J.E.P. (2010). Supplementation with calcium salts of linoleic and trans-octadecenoic acids improves fertility of lactating dairy cows. Reproduction in Domestic Animals, Vol.45, No.1 (February 2010), pp. 55-62. ISSN 1439-0531

Kim, J.Y.; Kinoshita, M.; Ohnishi, M. & Fukui, Y. (2001). Lipid and fatty acid analysis of fresh and frozen-thawed immature and *in vitro* matured bovine oocytes. *Reproduction*, Vol.122, No.1 (July 2001), pp. 131-138. ISSN 1470-1626.

Knickerbocker, J.J.; Thatcher, W.W.; Foster, D.B.; Wolfenson, D.; Bartol, F.F. & Caton, D. (1986). Uterine prostaglandin and blood flow responses to estradiol-17β in cyclic cattle. *Prostaglandins*, Vol.31, No.4 (April 1986), pp. 757-776. ISSN1098-8823

Lammoglia, M. A.; Willard, S. T.; Oldham, J. R. & Randel, R. D. (1996). Effects of dietary fat and season on steroid hormonal profiles before parturition and on hormonal, cholesterol, triglycerides, follicular patterns and postpartum reproduction in Brahman cows. *Journal of Animal Science*, Vol.74, No.9 (September 1996), pp. 2253-2262. ISSN 1525-3163

Lawson, C.; Wade, M.; Kenny, D.A. & Lonergan, P. (2007). Effect of addition of eicosapentaenoic acid (EPA) to culture medium on development of bovine embryos in vitro. In: *Annual Meeting of the European Embryo Transfer Association*. 190 p.

Lemley, C.O.; Butler, S.T.; Butler, W.R. & Wilson, M.E. (2008). Short communication: Insulin alters hepatic progesterone catabolic enzymes cytochrome P450 2C and 3A in dairy cows. *Journal of Dairy Science*, Vol.91, No.2 (February 2008), pp. 641-645. ISSN 0022-0302

Leroy, J.L.; Van Hoeck, V.; Clemente, M.; Rizoz, D.; Gutierrez-Adan, A.; Van Soom, A.; Uytterhoeven, M. & Bols, P.E. (2010). The effect of nutritionally induced hyperlipidemia on in vitro bovine embryo quality. *Human Reproduction*, Vol.25, No.3 (March 2010), pp. 768-778. ISSN 0268-1161

Lopes, N.; Scarpa, A.B.; Cappellozza, B.I.; Cooke, R.F. & Vasconcelos, J.L.M. (2009). Effects of rumen-protected polyunsaturated fatty acid supplementation on reproductive performance of *Bos indicus* beef cows. *Journal of Animal Science*, Vol.87, No.12 (December 2009), pp. 3935-3943. ISSN 1525-3163

Lucy, M.C.; De La Sota, R.L.; Staples, C.R. & Thatcher, W.W. (1993). Ovarian follicular populations in lactating dairy cows treated with recombinant bovine somatotropin (sometribove) or saline and fed diets differing in fat content and energy. *Journal of Dairy Science*; Vol.76, No.4 (April 1993), pp. 1014-1027. ISSN 0022-0302

Lucy, M.C.; Staples, C.R.; Michel, F.M. & Thatcher, W.W. (1991). Effect of feeding calcium soaps to early postpartum dairy cows on plasma prostaglandin F2α, Luteinizing hormone, and follicular growth. *Journal of Dairy Science,* Vol.74, No.2 (February 1991), pp. 483-489. ISSN 0022-0302

Lucy, M.C.; Thatcher, W.W.; Michel, F.J. & Staples, C.R. (1989). Effect of dietary calcium soaps of long chain fatty acids (Megalac) on plasma prostaglandin F metabolite (PGFM), LH, energy balance and follicular population in early postpartum dairy cattle. *Journal of Animal Science,* Vol.67, No. Suppl. 1 389 (Abstr). ISSN 1525-3163

Marei, F.W.; Wathes, D.C. & Fouladi-Nashta, A.A. (2010). Impact of linoleic acid on bovine oocyte maturation and embryo development. *Reproduction,* Vol.139, No.6 (June 2010), pp. 979-988. ISSN 1470-1626

Marei, W.F.; Wathes, D.C. & Fouladi-Nashta, A.A. (2009). The effect of linolenic acid on bovine oocyte maturation and development. *Biology of Reproduction,* Vol.81, No.6 (December 2009), pp. 1064-1072. ISSN 0006-3363

Marín-Aguilar, M.A.; Tinoco-Magaña, J.C.; Herrera-Camacho, J.; Sánchez-Gil, L.G.; Sánchez-Parra, V.M.; Solorio-Rivera, J.L. & García-Valladares, A. (2007). Reinicio de la actividad ovárica y nivel de metabolitos de lípidos en vacas lecheras suplementadas con aceite vegetal durante el posparto temprano. *Interciencia,* Vol.32, No.3, (March 21007), pp. 180-184. ISSN 0378-1844

Marques, C.C.; Baptista, M.C.; Vasques, M.I.; Horta, A.E.M. & Pereira, R.M. (2007). Effect of polyunsaturated fatty acids (PUFA) on bovine oocyte in vitro maturation and subsequent embryo development and freezability. *Reproduction in Domestic Animals,* Vol.109, No.Suppl. 2 (September 2007), pp. 116. ISSN: 0936-6768

Mattos, R.; Guzeloglu, A.; Badinga, L.; Staples, C.R. & Thatcher, W.W. (2003). Polyunsaturated fatty acids and bovine interferon-s modify phorbol ester-induced secretion of prostaglandin F2α and expression of prostaglandin endoperoxide synthase-2 and phospholipase-A2 in bovine endometrial cells. *Biology of Reproduction*, Vol.69, No.3 (September 2003), pp. 780-787. ISSN 0006-3363

Mattos, R.; Staples, C.R.; Arteche, A.; Wiltbank, M.C.; Diaz, F.J.; Jenkins, T.C. & Thatcher, W.W. (2004). The effects of feeding fish oil on uterine secretion of PGF2α, milk composition, and metabolic status of periparturient Holstein cows. *Journal of Dairy Science,* Vol.87, No.4 (April 2004), pp. 921-932. ISSN 0022-0302

Mattos, R.; Staples, C.R. & Thatcher, W.W. (2000). Effects of dietary fatty acids on reproduction in ruminants. *Reviews of Reproduction,* Vol.5, No.1 (January 2000), pp. 38-45. ISSN 1470-1626

McEvoy, T.G.; Coull, G.D.; Broadbent, P.J.; Hutchinson, J.S.M. & Speake, B.K. (2000). Fatty acid composition of lipids in immature cattle, pig and sheep oocytes with intact zona pellucida. *Journal of Reproduction and Fertility*, Vol.118, No.1 (January 2000), pp. 163-170. ISSN 0022-4251

McNamara, S.; Butler, T.; Ryan, D.P.; Mee, J.F.; Dillon, P.; O'Mara, F.P.; Butler, S.T.; Anglese, D.; Rath, M. & Murphy, J.J. (2003). Effect of offering rumen-protected fat supplements on fertility and performance in spring-calving Holstein-Friesian cows. *Animal Reproduction Science,* Vol.79, No.1-2; (November 2003); pp. 45-56. ISSN 0378-4320

Meier, S.; Ledgard, A.M.; Sato, T.A.; Peterson, A.J. & Mitchell, M.D. (2009). Polyunsaturated fatty acids differentially alter PGF2α and PGE_2 release from bovine trophoblast and endometrial tissues during short-term culture. *Animal Reproduction Science*, Vol.111, No.2-4 (April 2009), pp. 353-360. ISSN 0378-4320

Oldick, B.S.; Staples, C.R.; Thatcher, W.W. & Gyawu, P. (1997). Abomasal infusion of glucose and fat-effect on digestion, production, and ovarian and uterine function of cows. *Journal of Dairy Science*, Vol.80, No.7 (July 1997), pp. 1315-1328. ISSN 0022-0302

Palmquist, D.L. (2010). Essential fatty acids in ruminant diets. *Proceedings of the 21nd Annual Ruminant Nutrition Symposium*, February 2-3, 2010. Gainesville, Florida, USA. pp. 127-141

Piccinato, C.A.; Sartori, R.; Sangsritavong, S.; Souza, A.H.; Grummer, R.R.; Luchini, D. & Wiltbank, M.C. (2010). In vitro and in vivo analysis of fatty acid effects on metabolism of 17β-estradiol and progesterone in dairy cows. *Journal of Dairy Science*, Vol.93, No.5 (May 2010), pp. 1934-1943. ISSN 0022-0302

Rego, A.O.; Portugal, V.P.; Sousa B.M.; Rosa H.J.D.; Vozuela M.C.; Borba E.S.A. & Bessa R.J.B. (2004). Effect of diet on the fatty acid pattern of milk from dairy cows. *Animal Research*, Vol.53, No.3 (May-June 2004), pp. 213-220. ISSN 1627-3591

Renaville, B.; Bacciu, N.; Comin, A.; Motta, M.; Poli, I.; Vanini, G.; Prandi, A. (2010). Plasma and follicular fluid fatty acid profiles in dairy cows. *Reproduction in Domestic Animals*, Vol.45, No.1 (February 2010), pp. 118-121. ISSN 0936-6768

Robinson, R.S., Pushpakumara, P.G.A., Cheng, Z., Peters, A.R., Abayasekara, D-E-E., Wathes, D.C. (2002). Effects of dietary polyunsaturated fatty acids on ovarian and uterine function in lactating dairy cows. *Reproduction*, Vol.124, No.1 (July 2002); pp. 119-131. ISSN 1470-1626

Ryan, D. P.; Spoon, R.A.; Griffith, M.K. & Williams, G.L. (1994). Ovarian follicular recruitment, granulosa cell steroidogenic potential, and growth hormone/insulin-like growth factor-1 relationships in beef cows consuming high lipid diets: Effects of graded differences in body condition maintained during the puerperium. *Domestic Animal Endocrinology*, Vol.11, No.2 (April 1994), pp. 161-174. ISSN 0739-7240

Ryan, D.P.; Bao, B.; Griffith, M.K. & Williams, G.L. (1995). Metabolic and luteal sequelae to heightened dietary fat intake in postpartum beef cows. *Journal of Animal Science*, Vol.73, No.7 (July 1995), pp. 2086-2093. ISSN 1525-3163

Ryan, D.P.; Spoon, R.A. & Williams, G.L. (1992). Ovarian follicular characteristics, embryo recovery, and embryo viability in heifers fed high fat diets and treated with follicle-stimulating hormone. *Journal of Animal Science*, Vol.70, No.11 (November 1992); p. 3505-3513. ISSN 1525-3163

Salas-Razo, G.; Herrera-Camacho, J.; Gutiérrez-Vázquez, E.; Ku-Vera, J.C. & Aké-López J.R. (2011). Postpartum ovarian activity resumption and plasma concentration of lipid metabolites and progesterone in Indobrasil cows in the dry tropics of Michoacan supplemented with bypass fat. *Tropical and Subtropical Agroecosystems* (*in press*). ISSN 1870-0462

Santos, J.E.P.; Bilby, T.R.; Thatcher, W.W.; Staples, C.R. & Silvestre, F.T. (2008). Long chain fatty acids of diet as factors influencing reproduction in cattle. *Reproduction in Domestic Animals,* Vol.43, No. Suppl. 2 (July 2008), pp. 23-30. ISSN 1627-3591

Scott, T.A.; Shaver, R.D.; Zepeda, L.; Yandell, B. & Smith, T.R. (1995). Effects of rumen-inert fat on lactation, reproduction, and health of high producing Holstein herds. *Journal of Dairy Science,* Vol.78, No.11 (Novembre 1995), pp. 2435-2451. ISSN 0022-0302

Sklan, D.; Kaim, M.; Moallem, U. & Folman, Y. (1994). Effect of dietary calcium soaps on milk yield, body weight, reproductive hormones, and fertility in first parity and older cows. *Journal of Dairy Science,* Vol.77, No.6 (June 1994), pp. 1652-1660. ISSN 0022-0302

Sklan, D.; Moallem, U. & Folman, Y. (1991). Effect of feeding calcium soaps of fatty acids on production and reproductive responses in high producing lactating cows. *Journal of Dairy Science,* Vol.74, No.2 (February 1991), pp. 510-517. ISSN 0022-0302

Smith, S.S.; Neuringer, M. & Ojeda, S.R. (1989). Essential fatty acid deficiency delays the onset of puberty in the female rat. *Endocrinology,* 125:1650-1659. ISSN: 0013-7227.

Son, J.; Grant, R.J. & Larson, L.L. (1996). Effects of tallow and escape protein on lactational and reproductive performance of dairy cows. *Journal of Dairy Science,* Vol.79, No.5 (May 1996), pp. 822-830. ISSN 0022-0302

Sreenan, J.M.; Diskin, M.G. & Morris, D.G. (2001). Embryo survival rate in cattle: a major limitation to the achievement of high fertility. In: *Fertility in the high producing dairy cow.* BSAS Occasional Publication, Vol.1, pp. 93-105.

Stanko, R. L.; Fajersson, P.; Carver, L.A. & Williams, G.L. (1997). Follicular growth and metabolic changes in beef heifers fed incremental amounts of polyunsaturated fat. *Journal of Animal Science,* Vol.75, No. Suppl. 1 (July-August 1997), pp. 223 (Abstr 376). ISSN 1525-3163

Staples, C.R.; Burke, J.M. & Thatcher, W.W. (1998). Influence of supplemental fats on reproductive tissues and performance of lactating cows. *Journal of Dairy Science,* Vol.81, No.3 (March 1998), pp. 856-871. ISSN 0022-0302

Staples, C.R., Thatcher, W.W. (2005). Effects of fatty acids on reproduction of dairy cows. In: Garnsworthy PC, Wiseman, J. (Eds.), *Recent Advances in Animal Nutrition.* Nottingham University Press, Nottingham, UK, 229-256 p.

Stocco, D.M.; Wang, X.; Jo, Y. & Manna, P.R. (2005). Multiple signaling pathways regulating steroidogenesis and steroidogenic acute regulatory protein expression: more complicated than we thought. *Molecular Endocrinology,* Vol.19, No.11 (November 2005), pp. 2647-2659. ISSN 0888-8809

Talavera, F.; Park, C. S. & Williams, G. L. (1985). Relationships among dietary lipid intake, serum cholesterol and ovarian function in Holstein heifers. *Journal of Animal Science,* Vol.60, No.4 (April 1985); pp. 1045-1051. ISSN 1525-3163

Thangavelu, G.; Colazo, M.G.; Ambrose, D.J.; Oba, M.; Okine, E.K. & Dyck, M.K. (2007). Diets enriched in unsaturated fatty acids enhance early embryonic development in lactating Holstein cows. *Theriogenology* 68:949-957. ISSN 0093-691X

Thatcher, W.W.; Macmillan, K.L.; Hansen, P.J. & Bazer, F.W. (1994). Embryonic losses: causes and prevention. In: Fields, M.J.S., Sand, R.S. Editors. *Factors affecting calf crop.* Boca Raton, FL: CRC Press; 135-153 p.

Thatcher, W.W. & Staples, C.R. (2000). Effects of dietary fat supplementation on reproduction in lactating dairy cows. *Advanced in Dairy Technology*, Vol.12, No.12 (December 2000), pp. 213–232. ISSN 1184-0684.

Thatcher, W.W. & Staples, R.C. (2007). Using fats and fatty acids to enhance reproductive performance. *Proceedings of the 5th Mid-Atlantic Nutrition Conference*.. 115 Zimmermann, N.G., ed., University of Maryland, College Park, MD 20742. USA. 116-129 p.

Thomas, M.G. & Williams, G.L. (1996). Metabolic hormone secretion and FSH-induced superovulatory responses of beef heifers fed dietary fat supplements containing predominantly saturated or polyunsaturated fatty acids. *Theriogenology*, Vol.45 (January), pp. 451-458. ISSN 0093-691X

Thomas, M.G.; Bao, B. & Williams, G.L. (1997). Dietary fats varying in their fatty acid composition differentially influence follicular growth in cows fed isoenergetic diets. *Journal of Animal Science*, Vol.75, No.9 (September 1997), pp. 2512-2519. ISSN 1525-3163

Wakefield, S.L.; Lane, M.; Schulz, S.J.; Hebart, M.L.; Thompson, J.G. & Mitchell, M. (2007). Maternal supply of omega 3 polyunsaturated fatty acids alter mechanisms envolved in oocyte and early embryo development in the mouse. *American Journal of Physiology, Endocrinology and Metabolism*, Vol.294, No.2 (February 2008); pp. E425–E434. ISSN 0193-1849.

Wang, C.K.; Robinson, R.S.; Flint, A.P. & Mann, G.E. (2007). Quantitative analysis of changes in endometrial gland morphology during the bovine oestrous cycle and their association with progesterone levels. *Reproduction*, Vol.134, No.2 (August 2007); pp. 365-371. ISSN 1470-1626

Wathes, D.C.; Abayasekara, D.R. & Aitken, R.J. (2007). Polyunsaturated fatty acids in male and female reproduction. *Biology of Reproduction*, Vol.77, No.2 (August 2007), pp. 190-201. ISSN 0006-3363

Wehrman, M. E.; Welsh, T.H.Jr. & Williams, G.L. (1991). Diet-induced hyperlipidemia in cattle modifies the intrafollicular cholesterol environment, modulates ovarian follicular dynamics, and hastens the onset of postpartum luteal activity. *Biology of Reproduction*, Vol.45, No.3 (September 1991), pp. 514-522. ISSN 0006-3363

Williams, G.L.; Stanko, R.L. (2000). Dietary fats as reproductive nutraceuticals in cattle. Proceedings of the American Society for Animal Science 1998/1999. *Journal of Animal Science*, Vol.77, No.ESuppl (January 2000), pp. 1-12. ISSN 1525-3163

Williams, G.L. (1989). Modulation of luteal activity in postpartum beef cows through changes in dietary lipid. *Journal of Animal Science*, Vol.67, No.3 (March 1989); pp. 785-793. ISSN 1525-3163

Williams, G.L. & Amstalden, M. (2010). Understanding postpartum anestrus and puberty in the beef female. *Proceedings, Applied Reproductive Strategies in Beef Cattle*. January 28-29, 2010; San Antonio, TX. USA. 55-71 p.

Wonnacott, K.E.; Kwong, W.Y.; Hughes, J.; Salter, A.M.; Lea, R.G.; Garnsworthy, P.C. & Sinclair, K.D. (2010). Dietary omega-3 and -6 polyunsaturated fatty acids affect the composition and development of sheep granulosa cells, oocytes and embryos. *Reproduction*, Vol.139, No.1 (January 2010), pp. 57-69. ISSN 1470-1626

Wood, J.D.; Richardson, R.I.; Nute, G.R.; Fisher, A.V.; Campo, M.M.; Kasapidou, E.; Sheard, P.R. & Enser, M. (2003). Effects of fatty acids on meat quality: a review. *Meat Science*, Vol.66, No.1 (January 2004), pp. 21-32. ISSN 0309-1740

Zeron, Y.; Sklan, D. & Arav, A. (2002). Effect of polyunsaturated fatty acid supplementation on biophysical parameters and chilling sensitivity of ewe oocytes. *Molecular Reproduction and Development*, Vol.61, No.2 (February 2002), pp. 271-278. ISSN 1098-2795

14

Mechanical and Pharmacologic Applications of Artificial Insemination in Ewes

Faruk Aral[1], Füsun Temamoğulları[2] and Semra Sezen Aral[3]
[1]Nigde University, Bor Higher School for Business, Department of Veterinary, Nigde,
[2]Department of Pharmacology and Toxicology, Faculty of Veterinary Medicine, Harran University, Sanliurfa
[3]Agriculture and Rural Affairs Ministry, Konya
Turkey

1. Introduction

Artificial insemination (AI) is the keys to the efficient transfer of genetical knowledge from rams to ewes and to ensure proper productive traits of theirs. The efficient insemination of high-quality semen is very important in an artificial insemination of ewe. Artificial insemination is also part of the biotechnological studies. The insemination process itself may, in fact, cause of poor fertility or reduce of frozen semen quality.

Insemination process is regulated by a complex interplay of inseminator, semen, and genital tract structure of ewe. Although there is general agreement that cervix is of critical importance in the initiation and improvement of semen in mammals during insemination, the role of cervical canal in the regulation of frozen sperm transport in the ewes is stil problematic.

Because of the size and shape of the external os and the tortuous structure of the cervical canal, intrauterine insemination of ewes generally carries out with frozen sperm. Transcervical AI is applied using specially designed inseminating equipment and manipulation of the cervix using forceps. The number of reports in which transcervical deposition of semen has been achieved is relatively low and there are concerns about the potential trauma involved. The role of cervix in the transport of frozen sperm in the ewe is not entirely clear. Determination of the causes for the generally low fertility obtained following cervical deposition of frozen semen is still an important subject for AI procedure for achieving acceptable pregnancy rates in ewes.

A previous work observed that oxytocin treatment induced cervical dilation and decreased the difficulty of passing a catheter through the cervix and into the uterus. It decreases in fertility have been associated with cervical manipulation.

For a long time, the standard procedure with fresh semen when inseminating ewes has been to deposit the semen in the external os of the cervical canal. However, recently several groups have reported differences in pregnancy rates when ewes were bred with artificial insemination supported by air pomp, oxytocin, transcervical, etc.

There are many methods of artificial insemination of sheep. Specialization is concentrating or limiting one's focus to part of the whole methods of artificial insemination. Studies are guiding to the acquisition of new practice knowledge and skills. Artificial insemination is a powerful tool that provides common genetic information and deep insight into the insemination process that is at the heart of every embryo formation.

The earliest idea of artificial insemination definitely was a transfer of sperm from male to female. That is, based on the sperm form of fresh or chilled. In time, researchers observed that the fertility changes that produced physiologic reactions in ewes also are formed changes in the computable traits of sperm. Among these traits are the volume of a sperm, the number of sperm at a moment of fertilization, the physiological changes of a sperm in the female genitalia, and the transfer way of a sperm to female. Each of these traits can generate the basis for an effective action of an artificial insemination (Khalifa et al., 1992; Sayre and Lewis, 1996; Wulster-Radcliffe and Lewis, 2002; Candappa et al., 2009).

Donovan et al. (2004) reported higher pregnancy rates using fresh compared to frozen–thawed semen but found no differences in pregnancy rate following natural or synchronized estrus. The reason for the variation in fertility among ewe breeds following cervical AI with frozen–thawed semen may be due to differences in sperm transport through the cervix and uterus or due to early embryo mortality (Fair et al., 2005).

The place of deposition of frozen–thawed semen has a key effect on fertilization rate. In consequence, considerably advanced fertility is usually achieved with laparoscopic AI via frozen– thawed ram semen after transcervical or cervical insemination (Fair et al., 2005).

There are two obvious methods for struggle with the physical characteristics of the ovine cervix: set straight the servix and increase the diameter of the cervical lumen; or redesign TCAI (Trans-Cervical Artificial Insemination) equipment, or modify of embryo transfer catheter to invent the tight, convolute configuration of the cervix. Methods for straightening (such as, attaching a hemostat to the external cervical os and retracting the cervix) and dilating the cervix (chemically with PGE2 or oxytocin, etc., or mechanically) are effective (Khalifa et al., 1992; Sayre and Lewis, 1996; Wulster-Radcliffe et al., 1999; Wulster-Radcliffe and Lewis, 2002; Candappa et al., 2009; Gunduz et al., 2010).

Thus it is tried to give information about the last development of artificial insemination in the ewes.

2. Cervix antomy and function

The ewe cervix is a long and fibrous tubular organ. It contains connective tissue with an outer serosal layer and inner luminal epithelium. Because the lumen is the presence of 4-7 cervical rings that caudal opening of its provide a physical barrier to external contaminants and convolute and tortuous structure catheter entrance is somewhat more difficult than in the cow. These cervical rings constitute the greatest obstacle against TCA. The first, second and third ring in lumens does not take place in same line, ensuing in the inseminating pipette being misdirected apart from the central lumen. In addition, the first ring is the most difficult will be further than 1 cm, can practically insemination pipette. Cervical canal length ranges between 2.5 and 10.5 cm according to breed, age, parity and physiological state. These major changes in length of the channel affect the success of in TCAI. The mean number of cervical rings is approximately 5 with a range of two–seven rings per cervix. (Halbert et al., 1990; Campbell et al., 1996; Wulster-Radcliffe and Lewis, 2002; Kaabi et al., 2006).

The external cervical os between ewes has in different location in the vagina. The cervical os in sheep makes to protrude into the vagina and in some animals completely obscure

Five types of external os were identified in the vagina (Halbert et al., 1990). (Fig. 1):

1. The Duckbill: two opposing folds of cervical tissue protruding into the vagina with a central horizontal slit like external os.
2. The Slit: no protrusions into the anterior vagina with a slit like opening at the os of the cervix giving entry to the cervical canal.

3. The Rose: a cluster of cervical folds protruding into the anterior vagina obscuring the external os.
4. The Papilla: a papilla protruding into the anterior vagina with the external os at its apex
5. The Flap: one-fold of cervical tissue protruding into the anterior vagina and completely or partially overlaying the external os creating the appearance of a flap.

Kershaw et al. (2005) a found that the spreading of external os types differed with age. In particular, the rose type os is more common in adult ewes than ewe lambs and the reverse is true for the papilla type os.

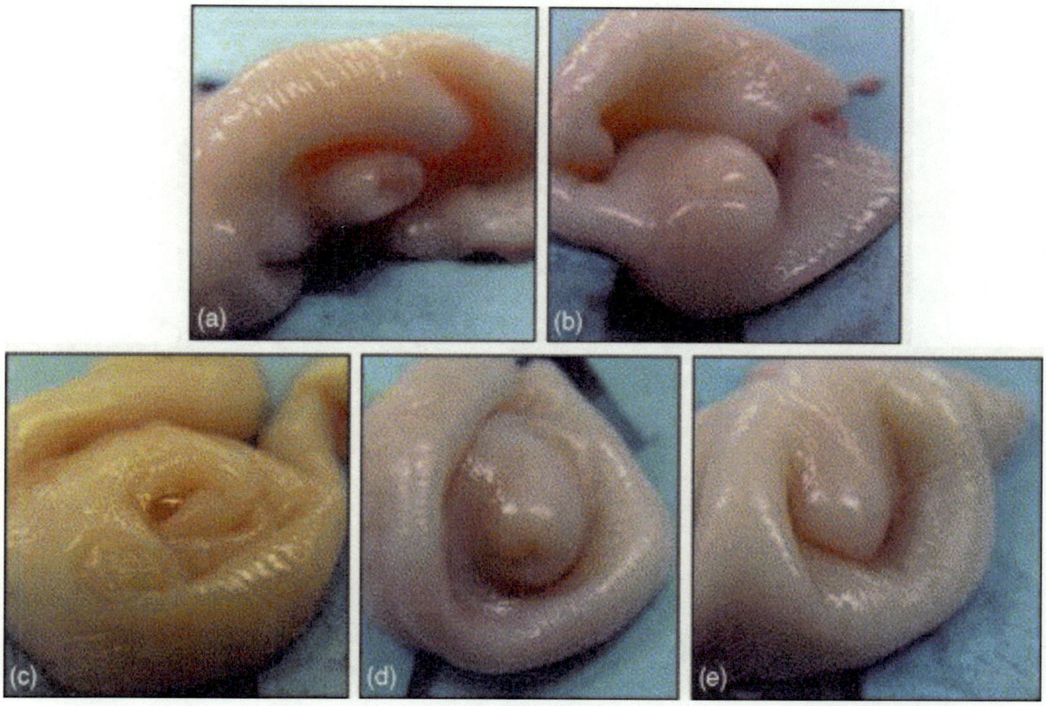

Fig. 1. The classification of the appearance of the external os of the ewe (a) duckbill, (b) slit, (c) rose, (d) papilla, and (e) flap. from Kershaw et al., 2005 .

Cervical penetration measuring is evaluated the penetration of the insemination pipette as shallow, middle and deep without being informed about the group to which the inseminated ewe belonged (shallow: <10mm; mid: 10-20mm; or deep: >20mm, using the colored tip of the plastic sheath as reference (Gunduz et al., 2010).

3. Transcervical AI method

There generally are 3 AI techniques 1) vaginal insemination, 2) the laparoscopic intrauterine insemination 3) cervical insemination that have been used in the sheep industry and newly developed fourth technique, trans-cervical artificial insemination (Leethongdee, 2010).
Transcervical AI (TCAI) is seemed as a potential alternative to laparoscopic AI. The basis of this technique, a AI catheter is passed through cervix for sperm to leave the uterus. This technique is used in other animals, but they are not used due to the difference of the sheep cervix. There is as a degree of natural cervical relaxation in oestrus and trans-cervical

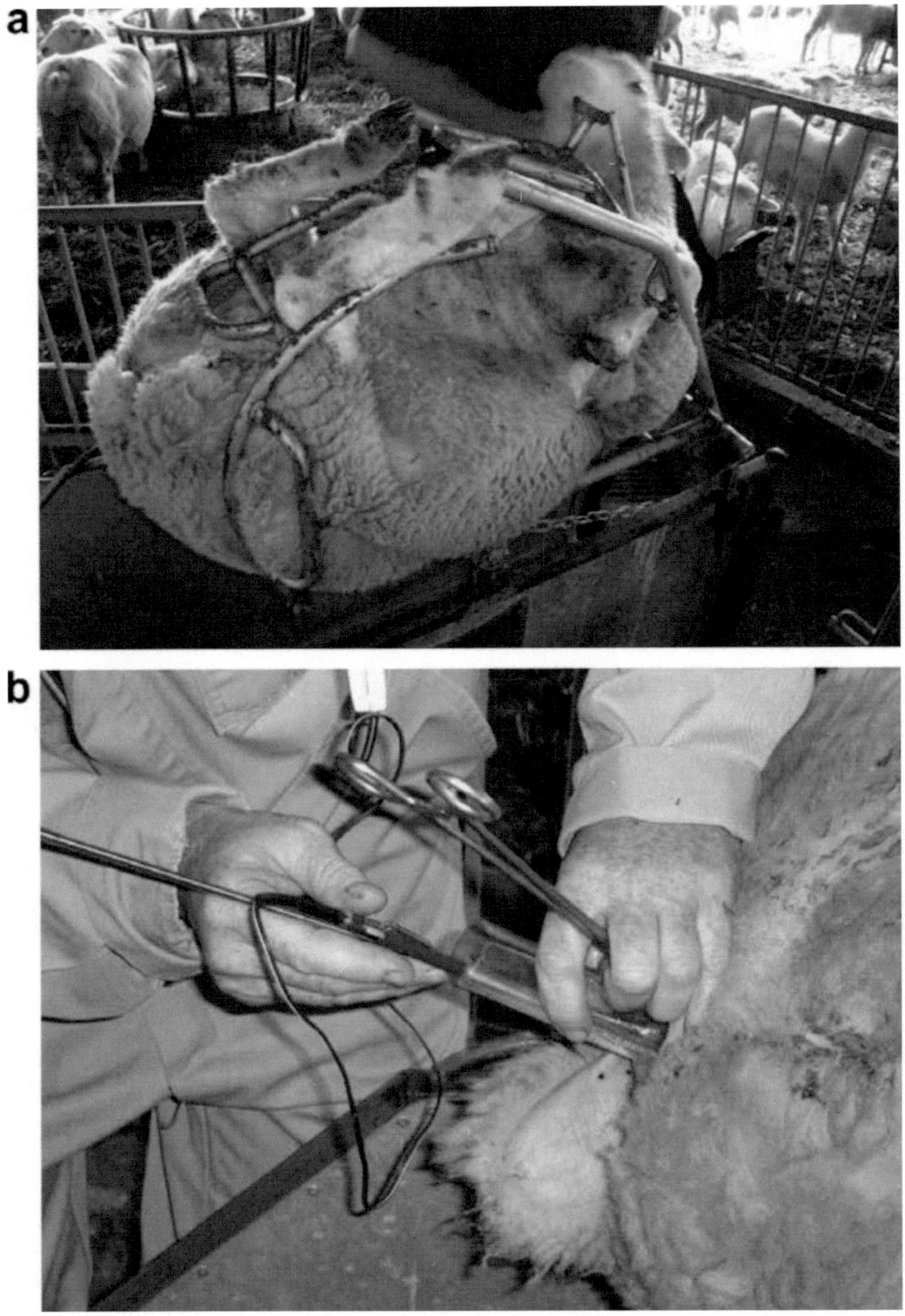

Fig. 2. The Guelph TCAI System: (a) fetal-like positioning of ewes in dorsal recumbency; (b) a plexiglass speculum with light source is inserted into the vagina and forceps are used to grab the cervix near the os and retract it. Subsequently, a bent-tipped and preloaded insemination gun is introduced and manipulated through the cervix to deposit semen. From Candappa et al., 2009.

penetration in low rate in multiparous ewes seems to be possible. The cervical relaxation is due to affect of peri-ovulatory hormones such as oxytocin, estradiol and progesterone on the cervix. In Cows, the potential effect of oxytocin on cervical relaxation, leads to local growth of cyclooxygenase-2 (COX-2) after that, COX-2 causes an increase in the synthesis of prostaglandin E2 (PGE2) (Zhang et al., 2007).

3.1 The Guelph System for TCAI

The Guelph System of AI equipment fetal-like positioning of ewes in dorsal recumbency (Fig. 2). A speculum with light source is inserted into the vagina, and upon apparition of the cervix. A bent-tipped and preloaded insemination gun is lead into the cervix to deposit semen (Wulster- Radcliffe and Lewis, 2002; Candappa et al., 2009).

3.2 Application of TCAI catheter

Some studies were used an insemination catheter with a blunt and angled end, some flexibility, and a diameter that is smaller than the narrowest point of the cervical lumen in the ewe (Halbert et al., 1990; Campbell et al., 1996; Wulster-Radcliffe Lewis, 2002; Kaabi et al., 2006; Candappa et al., 2009).

The catheter used for embryo transfer. Later, he modified for sheep transcervical AI. The catheter is depicted as the actual size (17.5 cm long, 1.47 mm o.d, 1.07 mm i.d.) (Wulster-Radcliffe et al., 1999).

Ewes are held back in a chute used for sheep in a dorsal recumbent position. The perineal area is cleaned with an antiseptic soap and rinsed with water. Excess water and antiseptic are removed with paper towel. A outside layer of obstetrics lubricant is applied to a speculum, and the speculum is inserted into the vagina and pressed against tissue nearby the cervix. The TC-AI catheter is located at the external cervical os and manually control from beginning to end of the cervix. A TC-AI catheter used for cervical manipulation in transcervical AI (Fig 3) is equal to the TC embryo transfer apparatus described previously (Wulster-Radcliffe et al., 1999).

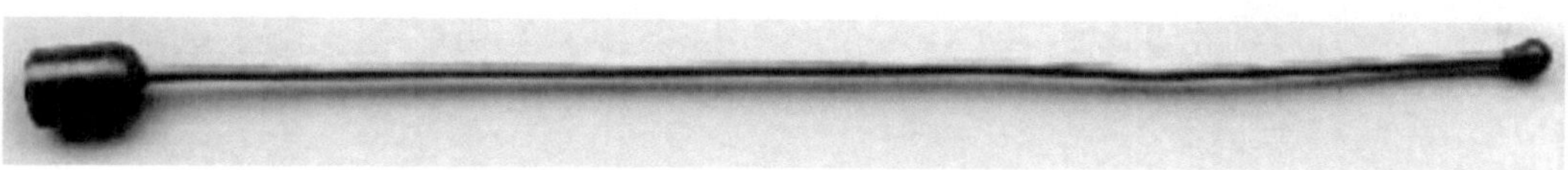

Fig. 3. Modified embryo transfer catheter. A machined brass zero-volume fitting was used to secure the catheter. From Wulster-Radcliffee al., 1999.

During penetration of a pipette through the cervix the sheep position affects the success of the transition. Pipette passage is more easily with the standing ewe than over-the rail ewe. Rear side of the light (approximately 15 cm) elevated ewe with standing is stated as in a very convenient position (leethongdee, 2010). In this position, uterine penetration is achieved in 82.0 %.

Transcervical AI is applied using specially designed inseminating equipment (Wulster-Radcliffe et al., 2002; Wulster-Radcliffe et al., 2004) and manipulation of the cervix using forceps (Halbert et al., 1990). The number of reports in which position of semen has been achieved is relatively low and there are concerns about the potential trauma involved.

4. Application of Air Pressure with Cervical Artificial Insemination (APCAI)

Cervical artificial insemination (CAI) is a less expensive and invasive method in comparison to the transcervical and intrauterine methods, and has been widely used for the artificial insemination of ewes. The site of deposition of frozen-thawed semen in ewes has a major effect on fertilization rate (Fair et al., 2005).

Whilst pregnancy rates in excess of 60% can be achieved with a single artificial insemination of fresh semen deposited at the external cervical opening , corresponding rates for frozen-thawed semen occasionally exceed 45%, with values less than 17% not rare (O'Meara et a1., 2005).

The insemination device in Air Pressure with Cervical Artificial Insemination method (APCAI) is modified from a stainless steel outer pipette sheath of a cattle AI pipette. The air pump (2 liter/min capacity; aerator, portable battery pump) is attached to the blunt rounded end of the pipette by means of a rubber pipe with an internal diameter of 2.6 mm (Fig 4). A speculum was introduced into the vagina so that the external opening of the cervix could be seen in the light of the speculum lamp. Subsequently, 0.1 ml of semen is drawn into the pipette sheath through a plastic syringe, and the pipette sheath is connected to the air pump. The pipette tip is placed at the external opening of the cervix and the air pump is run to spray semen into the cervical canal. For each ewe, a different pipette sheath is used (Aral et al., 2010).

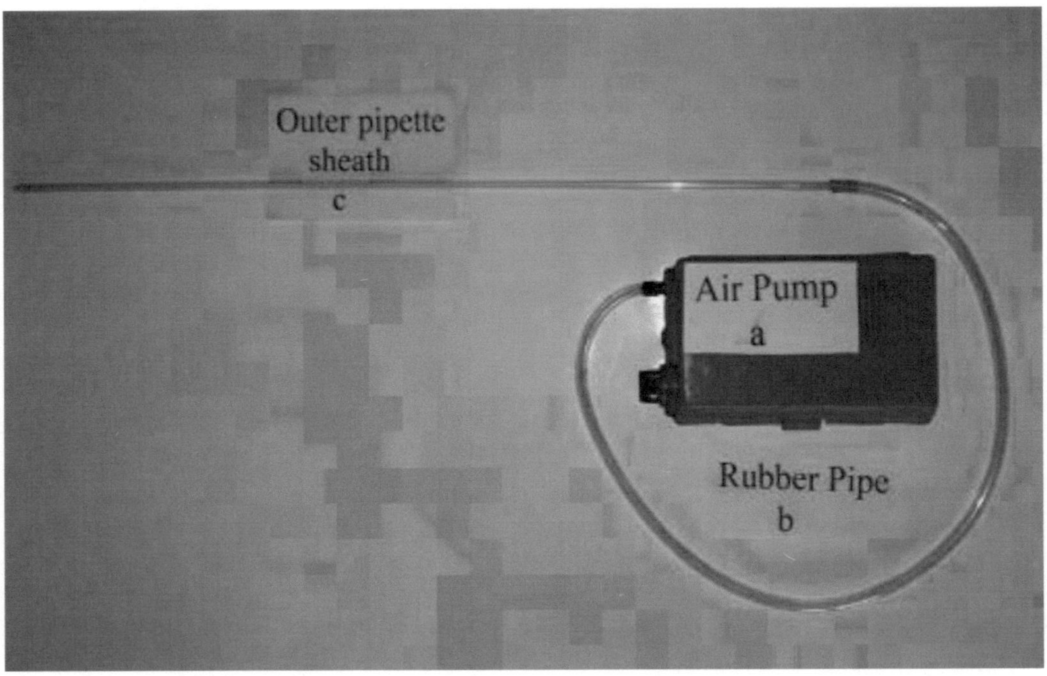

Fig. 4. Artificial insemination equipment of APCAI method; (A) Air pump, (B) Rubber pipe, (C) a stainless steel outer pipette sheath used in cattle AI. From Aral et al., 2010.

The pregnancy rate in this method was found to be significantly high the APCAI group than in the CAI group (80.0% versus 46.7%) Table 1.

Parameters Number of ewes		CAI (n=30)	APCAI (n=30)
Pregnancy rate	(n/n) %	(14/30) 46.7 a	(24/30) 80.0 b
Lambing rate	(n/n) %	(14/30) 46.7 c	(21/30) 70.0 d
Prolificacy	(n/n)	(16/14) 1.14	(23/21) 1.09

Table 1. Pregnancy, lambing rate, prolificacy, following different AI methods in Awassi ewes. From Aral et al., 2010.

5. Pharmacologic cervical dilatation

5.1 Prostaglandin E analogues

5.1.1 Cervidil

Cervical ripening involves enzymatic corruption of the connective tissues. It causes a relaxation of its smooth muscle fibers. Cervical ripening encourage with chemical matter. Thus, penetration of the cervix during TCAI may be achieved with effortlessness (Candappa et al., 2009). Cervidil® contains 10 mg of dinoprostone and have a vaginal form. Hormone releases a constant rate of 0.3 mg/h over a 12-h period in a women vagina. For cervical ripening and induction of labour in women is a safe agent (Sánchez-Partida et al., 1999; Lambers et al., 2001). Adapting the use of Cervidil® to sheep was performed by Candappa et al., 2009.

Cervidil® is inserted 12 h prior to insemination in ewes. Cervidil®, containing 10 mg dinoprostone (prostaglandin E2), introduce into the vagina in the immediacy of the cervix. After the 12-h priming with Cervidil, transcervical semen deposition is possible in all ewes (Candappa et al., 2009).

5.1.2 Ovagen and misoprostol

Cervical relaxation and penetration were examined in Ovagen and misoprostol-treated sheep in a previous study. Ovine FSH (2 mg; Ovagen; 1 CP bio (UK) limited, Wiltshire, UK) was administered at a dose of 2 mg dissolved in 0.5 ml of 50 % Gum acacia (Sigma-Aldrich Co.,). A prostaglandin E_1 analogue, Misoprostol (1 mg; Misoprostol; Sigma-Aldrich Co., Dorset England) was administered at a dose of 1 mg dissolved in 0,5 ml of 30 % gelatine (Sigma-Aldrich Co.,). External opening of the cervix treated sheep Ovagen and misoprostol significantly loosened. It is easier penetration of the cervix in these sheep (Leethongdee et al., 2007).

5.2 Hyaluronan

The cervix is relatively relaxed at oestrus. These are both a high-hyaluronan (HA) content of the cervix and the related increase in its water content. When aqueous 0.5 ml of the HA suspension (2 mg low molecular weight (LMW) HA) and (25 mg high molecular weight (HMW) HA) is applied to an intra-cervical, it promotes cervical relaxation in oestrus ewes.

LMW HA has the greatest impact on vascularization, leading to the collection of leukocytes. In addition, it stimulates the biochemical changes in the cervix during softening (Perry et al., 2010).

5.3 Oxytocin

Oxytocin treatment caused relaxation of cervix and uterine catheter through the cervix have demonstrated that reduced the difficulty of the transition (Khalifa et al., 1992; Sayre and Lewis, 1996). The effect of oxytocin as a cervical dilator is different on the reproductive outcome in ewe. Sayre and Lewis (1997) observed no undesirable effect of oxytocin on ovum fertilisation rate. Stellflug et al., (2001) show a negative effect of oxytocin but not of the transcervical insemination procedure. Fertilization rate decreases in the treatment of oxytocin-cervical manipulations. However, the oxytocin treatment does not affect ovulation rate. Atraumatic cervical manipulation, does not affect the time of ovulation, fertilization rate, early embryonic development and rate of lambing. Thus, oxytocin is used to softening the cervix decreases the ease of transition to a transcervical AI instrument, the fertilization rate, pregnancy rate and lambing rate.

For transcervical AI, different (50 to 400 USP units in Table 2 and 3; 10 IU of oxytocin) dose of oxytocin can be given to ewes via intravenously 30 min. before AI to dilate the cervix. When oxytocin is given intramuscularly 15–30 min before insemination with frozen/thawed semen, it produced an impressive reduction (10% versus 42%) in the lambing rate of ewes inseminated cervically. However, oxytocin makes possible intrauterine insemination via the cervix, its undesirable effect on lambing rate may be less significant oxytocin has a small and non-significant damaging outcome on litter size (King et al., 2004; Table 2, 3).

	oxytocin. USP units					
Item	0	200	400	600	SE	Overall oxytocine
Cervical penetration, cm						
Before oxytocin	2.6	2.2d	1.0d	.9d	.3	1.5d
After oxytocin	2.9	5.6e	6.1e	5.1e	.3	5.7e
Time to deepest cervical penetrationf, min	10.0g	6.9h	5.6h	6.2h	.4	6.4
Uterine entries/no. Of ewes	0/15g	15/19h	10/12h	8/12h	-	33/43
(%)	0	79	83	67		77

*Values are means or proportions.
bSE are standard errors from analyses of variance models used to analyze the data.
Values with different superscripts differ (P < .01).

Table 2. Effects of intravenous oxytocin injection 52 hours after removal of progestogenated pessaries from ewes. From Khalifa et al., 1992.

Oxytocin injections dilate the cervix in some ewes. However, oxytocin administration 12 h after 100 or 200 pg of estradiol-17β ((0, 100, or 200 pg in 5 mL of 1:1 saline ethanol) are the majority successful at dilating the cervix and permitting acceptance of a stainless steel rod into the uterus. The 100-μg dose of estradiol-17β seem to be as a valuable dose (Khalifa et al., 1992; Wulster-Radcliffe et al., 1999).

Item	laparoscopic		Cervical		Significance of treatment effects	
	Control	Oxytocin	Control	Oxytocin		
Number of ewes	49	50	100	99		
Number lambing (%)	34(69a)	29(58 c)	42(42 b)	10 (10 d)	a>b**	c>d***
Mean litter size	1.91 a	1.83 c	1.52 b	1.40 d	a>b*	c>dz

Z: $P < 0.10$.
* $P < 0.05$.
** $P < 0.01$.
*** $P < 0.001$.

Table 3. Data for lambing rates and litter sizes in relation to treatments and week of insemination. From King et al., 2004.

These observations, together with those from the present experiment, suggest that any adverse effect of oxytocin on lamb production when ewes are subjected to laparoscopic intrauterine insemination with frozen/thawed semen is likely to be small. Thus, had the oxytocin in the present experiment. Oxytocin make possible intrauterine insemination via the cervix, its undesirable effect on lambing rate may have been less significant.
The cervical manipulation seems to unfavorable an effect on fertility after AI, because the oxytocin treatment is not harmful. It likely to affect the sperm survival in the reproductive tract of sheep, or some issues of sperm capacitation (Stellflug et al., 2001). Perhaps, manipulation of the cervix may affect sperm transport within the reproductive tract, or a stressed cervix may produce a spermicidal compound (Hawk et al., 1981).

5.4 Human interleukin 8 (huIL-8)

Human interleukin 8 (huIL-8) was applied to use in sheep to stimulate the cervical relaxation. This cytokine causes a neutrophil recruitment and an increase in collagenases in the cervix during the peripartum period in mammals. However, its administration is failed to induce cervical dilatation in ewes
After estrus synchronization protocol is applied, and a wax suppository (Witepsol as the wax formulation, mm x 3 mm in size) containing either 5 pg huIL-8a (derived from large scale human fibroblast cell culture) with an estimated total release of 0.6 pg huIL-8 is inserted into the anterior vagina near the cervical os (Croy et al., 1999).

5.5 Carazolol

When animals are exposed to stress during artificial insemination, their bodies react by raising the adrenaline amount. The beta 2 adrenoreceptors in the myometrium is affected by adrenalin. After that, uterine contractions occurred by oxytocin is destroyed by it, which in turn produce a long time to get ahead of the genital canal for the spermatozoa. Thus, artificial insemination with aged spermatozoa leads to decrease of fertility in ewes (Kırsan et al., 1998; Gunduz et al., 2010).

It eliminates the effect of oxytocin, stimulating uterine contractions. Carazolol (Suacron, Divasa, Farmavic, Spain) intramuscularly for each sheep is 0.5 mg administered 30 minutes before insemination. It increases the number of ewes inseminated with deep. In contrast, it does not have a significant effect on the pregnancy rate (85% for control, 95% for carazolol) (Gündüz et al., 2010). The middle and deep penetration rates are high but was found non-significant (for control 82 % and carazolol 85%).

6. References

[1] Aral F, Yavuzer U, Zonturlu AK. 2010. The effect of air pressure with cervical artificial insemination on the fertility of Awassi ewes synchronized with PGF2α . Kafkas Univ Vet Fak Derg., 16 (1), 37-41.

[2] Campbell JW, Harvey TJ, McDonald MF, Sparksman RI. 1996. Transcervical insemination in sheep: an anatomical and histological evaluation. Theriogenology, 45, 1535–1544.

[3] Candappa IBR, Bainbridge HC, Price NT, Hourigan KR, Bartlewski PMA. 2009. Preliminary study on the suitability of Cervidil to induce cervical dilation for artificial insemination in ewes. Research in Veterinary Science, 87, 204–206.

[4] Croy BA, Prudencio J, Minhas K, Ashkar AA, Galligan C, Foster RA, Buckrell B, Coomber BL. 1999. A preliminary study on the usefulness of huIL-8 in cervical relaxation of the ewe for artificial insemination and for embryo transfer. Theriogenology, 52, 271–287.

[5] Donovan A, Hanrahan JP, Kummen E, Duffy P, Boland MP. 2004. Fertility in the ewe following cervical insemination with fresh or frozen–thawed semen at a natural or synchronised oestrus. Anim Reprod Sci, 84, 359–68.

[6] Fair S, Hanrahan JP, O'Meara CM, Duffy P, Rizos D, Wade M, Donovan A, Boland MP, Lonergan P, Evans AC. 2005. Differences between Belclare and Suffolk ewes in fertilization rate, embryo quality and accessory sperm number after cervical or laparoscopic artificial insemination.Theriogenology, 63, 1995–2005.

[7] Gunduz MC, Turna Ö, Cirit Ü, Uçmak M, Tek Ç, Sabuncu A, Bacınoğlu S. 2010. Lambing rates and litter size following carazolol administration prior to insemination in Kivircik ewes. Animal Reproduction Science, 118, 32–36.

[8] Halbert G, Dobson H, Walton J, Buckrell B. 1990. The structure of the cervical canal of the ewe. Theriogenology, 33, 977–992.

[9] Hawk HW, Cooper BS, Pursel VG. 1981. Increased sperm death in the cervix and uterus of estrous ewes after synchronization of estrus with prostaglandin or progestagen. J Anim Sci, 52, 601-610.

[10] Kaabi M, Alvarez M, Anel E, Chamorro CA, Boixo JC, de Paz P, Anel L. 2006. Influence of breed and age on morphometry and depth of inseminating catheter penetration in the ewe cervix: a postmortem study. Theriogenology, 66, 1876– 1883.

[11] Kershaw CM, Khalid M, McGowan MR, Ingram K, Leethongdee S, Wax G, Scaramuzzi RJ. 2005. The anatomy of the sheep cervix and its influence on the transcervical passage of an inseminating pipette into the uterine lumen. Theriogenology, 64(5), 1225-1235.

[12] Khalifa RME, Sayre BL, Lewis GS. 1992. Exogenous oxytocin dilates the cervix in ewes. J Anim Sci, 70(1), 38–42.

[13] Kırsan I, Alkan S, Baran A, Ozturkler Y, Senunver A, Ileri K. 1998. Sıgırlarda suni tohumlama anında uygulanan beta-2 blokoru carazololun uterus tonusu ve gebe kalma oranı üzerine etkisi. I U Veteriner Fakultesi Dergisi, 24 (1), 89–97.

[14] King ME, McKelvey WAC, Dingwall WS, Matthews KP, Gebbie FE, Mylne MJA, Stewart E, Robinson JJ. 2004.Lambing rates and litter sizes following intrauterine or cervical insemination of frozen/thawed semen with or without oxytocin administration. Theriogenology, 62, 1236–1244.

[15] Lambers D, Khoury J, Ventolini G. 2001. A meta-analysis of the safety and efficacy of Cervidil (dinoprostone): a vaginal insert for cervical ripening. American Journal of Obstetrics and Gynecology, 185, 203.

[16] Leethongdee S, Khalid M, Bhatti A, Ponglowhapan S, Kershaw CM, Scaramuzzi RJ.2007.The effects of the prostaglandin E analogue Misoprostol and follicle-stimulating hormone on cervical penetrability in ewes during the peri-ovulatory period. Theriogenology, 67(4), 767-777.

[17] Leethongdee S. 2010. Development of trans-cervical artificial Insemination in sheep with special reference to anatomy of cervix. Suranaree J Sci Technol, 17, 157-169.

[18] O'Meara CM, Hanrahan JP, Donovan A, Fair S, Rizos D, Wade M, Boland MP, Evans ACO, Lonergan P. 2005. Relationship between in vitro fertilization of ewe oocytes and the fertility of ewes following cervical artificial insemination with frozen-thawed ram semen. Theriogenology, 64, 1797-1808.

[19] Perry K, Haresign W, Wathes DC, Khalid M. 2010. Intracervical application of hyaluronan improves cervical relaxation in the ewe. Theriogenology , 1685-1690.

[20] Sánchez-Partida LG, Windsor DP, Eppleston J, Setchell BP, Maxwell WMC. 1999. Fertility and its relationship to motility characteristics of spermatozoa in ewes after cervical, transcervical, and intrauterine insemination with frozenthawed ram semen. Journal of Andrology, 20, 280–288.

[21] Sayre BL, Lewis GS.1997. Fertility and ovum fertilization rate after laparoscopic or transcervical intrauterine artificial insemination of oxytocin-treated ewes. Theriogenology, 48,267–275.

[22] Sayre BL, Lewis GS. 1996. Cervical dilation with exogenous oxytocin does not affect sperm movement into the oviducts in ewes. Theriogenology, 45, 1523-1533.

[23] Stellflug JN, Wulster-Radcliffe MC, Hensley EL, Cowardin EA, Seals RC and Lewis GS. 2001. Oxytocin-induced cervical dilation and cervical manipulation in sheep: effects on laparoscopic artificial insemination. J Anim Sci, 79, 568-573.

[24] Zhang Q, Collins V, Chakrabarty K, Rose JC, Wu WX.2007. Regulation of the prostaglandin enzymatic system by estradiol and progesterone in nonpregnant sheep cervix. Reproduction,133, 1027–1034.

[25] Wulster-Radcliffe MC, Wang S, Lewis GS. 2004.Transcervical artificial insemination in sheep: effects of a new transcervical artificial insemination instrument and traversing the cervix on pregnancy and lambing rates. Theriogenology, 62,990–1002.

[26] Wulster-Radcliffe MC, Costine BA, Lewis GS. 1999. Estradiol- 17β-oxytocin-induced cervical dilation in sheep: Application to transcervical embryo transfer. J. Anim. Sci, 77, 2587–2593.

[27] Wulster-Radcliffe MC, Lewis GS. 2002. Development of a new transcervical artificial insemination method for sheep: effects of a new transcervical artificial insemination catheter and traversing the cervix on semen quality and fertility. Theriogenology, 58, 1361–1371.

15

Relationship between IFN-τ Production by Bovines Embryos Derived *Ex Vivo* and Completely Produced *In Vitro*

Jorge Alberto Neira[1,2], Daniel Tainturier[2],
René L'Haridon[3] and Jacques Martal[4]
[1]Laboratoire de Pathologie de la Reproduction et Biotechnologie animale, Ecole Nationale Vétérinaire, Agroalimentaire et de l'Alimentation Nantes-Atlantique: ONIRIS
[2]Centro de Reproducción animal CRIA de la Corporación Colombiana de Investigación Agropecuaria CORPOICA, Grupo Biología del Desarrollo, Bogotá DC,
[3]Laboratoire de Virologie et Immunologie Moléculaire, INRA Jouy-en-Josas cedex
[4]Station de Physiologie Animale, UMR-BDR, INRA. Jouy-en-Josas cedex
[1,3,4]France
[2]Colombia

1. Introduction

Interferon-tau (IFN-τ) is secreted by the mononuclear cells of the primitive extra-embryonic trophoblast (Farin et al. 1989; Guillomot et al. 1990) which will become the main part of the future placenta, in ruminants. This cytokine is constitutively produced during the short period of the conceptus periimplantation (Martal et al. 1979; Godkin et al. 1982; Hansen et al. 1988; Charlier et al. 1989). It plays an essential role for maternal recognition of pregnancy, particularly allowing the maintenance of the *corpus luteum* and its progesterone secretion (Spencer et al. 2004). Indeed, intrauterine injections of recombinant IFN-τ extend the progesterone secretion by inhibiting pulsatile uterine secretion of luteolytic prostaglandin F-2α (Martal et al. 1990, 1998; Ott et al. 1993; Meyer et al. 1995). IFN-τ downregulates the expression of endometrial oxytocin receptors concentrations (Spencer and Bazer 1996; Mann et al. 1999). In early pregnancy, IFN-τ constitutes therefore a major signal in ruminants. Thus, it plays a role of both cytokine and reproductive paracrine hormone (Roberts et al. 1992; Bazer et al. 1994; Martal et al. 1997). In addition, IFN-τ exhibits potent antiviral and antiproliferative activities (Fillon et al. 1991; Pontzer et al. 1991, 1997; Bazer et al. 1994; Derreuddre et al. 1996).

The regulation of IFN-τ secretion remains poorly understood (Martal et al. 1998; Yamagushi et al. 2001; Demmers et al. 2001; Ezashi et al. 2001; Stewart et al. 2002; Spencer and Bazer 2002). Some growth factors and cytokines are implicated in the positive control of IFN-τ secretion such as Insulin-like Growth Factor (IGF-I) and IGF-II (Ko et al. 1991), Granulocyte-Macrophage Colony Stimulating Factor (GM-CSF) and Interleukine-3 (Imakawa et al. 1993, 1995; Emond et al. 2004). Indeed, these factors are secreted by trophoblast and endometrium in early pregnancy (Mathialagan et al. 1992; Vogiagis et al. 1997; Martal et al. 1997, 2002).

The induction of IFN-τ expression appeared genetically determined because IFN-τ secretion has been evidenced from hatched blastocysts completely produced *in vitro* (Hernández-Ledezma et al. 1992, 1993; Stojkovic et al. 1995). Therefore, the uterine environment is not necessary for the induction of IFN-τ expression but it could play an essential role in the control of IFN-τ secretion. Paternal genotype was a significant determinant of the embryo's ability to develop the blastocyst stage and of subsequent IFN-τ secretion (Kubish et al. 2001a). Besides, there is some evidence that the presence of other blastocysts could increase IFN-τ secretion (Larson and Kubish 1999).

Generally, the evaluation of the development potential of embryos today still depends on subjective morphological examination (Lindner and Wright, 1983; Buttler and Biggers 1989; Shamsuddin et al. 1992, Massip et al. 1995). However, the development stage and quality of the embryos significantly influence the IFN-τ secretion. Some authors have proposed that the produced amount of IFN-τ could be a useful objective indicator of embryo quality (Hernandez-Ledezma et al. 1992, 1993). But others, considering that the age of blastocysts formation *in vitro* exhibits significant effects on the IFN-τ production, have suggested a negative relationship between early IFN-τ production and blastocysts competence for embryonic development (Kubish et al. 1998, 2004).

The aim of this study was therefore to compare the IFN-τ secretion after hatching in bovine blastocysts of good homogeneous quality wether they are produced *in vivo* or completely *in vitro.*

2. Materials and methods

2.1 Production of *in vitro* bovine blastocysts

2.1.1 *In vitro* maturation of oocytes

Unless otherwise indicated, all chemicals in this study were purchased from Sigma-Aldrich, (Saint Quentin. Fallavier, France). Ovaries from Prim Holstein cows were quickly collected after death in a local slaughter-house and transferred to the laboratory into a saline solution with 0.9% (w/v) NaCl at approximately 35°C. The largest interval between animal killing and oocyte conditioning was 3 hours. Cumulus-oocyte complexes (COCs) were recovered by aspiration of follicles of 2-8 mm in diameter using a 18 gauge needle under vacuum pressure of approximately 50 mm Hg. The COCs were collected into Hepes-buffered tissue culture medium 199 (TCM 199 ref. M-7528) supplemented with 0.4% (w/v) BSA (Cohn Fraction V, ref. 9647). Before *in vitro* maturation, COCs were assessed morphologically: only those which displaid a compact and non-atretic *cumulus oophorus-corona radiata* with an oocyte exhibiting homogeneous cytoplasm were chosen for further *in vitro* culture. Selected COCs were washed thoroughly in TCM 199 (ref. M-4530) plus 10% (v/v) fetal calf serum (FCS, Life Technologies, Inc., Grand Island, NY USA). The maturation of about 60 COCs batches were achieved in 500μl TCM199 (ref. M-4530) supplemented with 10% FCS, and 10ng per ml EGF (ref. E-4127) with 100 μg/ml gentamicin (ref. G-1264), for 24 h at 39°C under humidified 5% CO_2 in air.

2.1.2 *In vitro* fertilization

Spermatozoa were prepared from frozen-thawed semen of a sole bull (Prim Holstein breed, electronic number: 44 13 835058) that had been characterized as suitable for *in vitro* fertilization in our laboratory. The contents of two 0.25 ml straws (each containing approximately 10^6 *spermatozoa* per ml) were layered upon a Percoll discontinuous gradient

(Hasler et al. 1995). Motile *spermatozoa* were collected after centrifugation at approximately 700g for 30 min, at room temperature. Then they washed in Hepes-buffered Tyrode's albumin lactate pyruvate medium (Talp) (Parrish et al. 1986) and pelleted by centrifugation at approximately 200g for 10 min at room temperature. Meanwhile, COCs were transferred to another four-wells dish containing 250µl of *in vitro* fertilization Talp supplemented with 0.01 mmol/l heparin (ref. H-3149), 0.2 mmol/l penicillamine (ref. P-4875), 0.1 mmol/l hypotaurine, 0.1 mmol/l epinephrine (ref. E-4250) and 6mg/ml fatty acid-free BSA. (ref. A-8806) Insemination was performed to get the final concentration of 2×10^6 *spermatozoa*/ml to fertilize the oocytes. Plates were incubated 5% CO_2 in humidified air at 39°C.

2.1.3 *In vitro* culture

After 20 hours, the *cumulus* cells were removed from the presumptive zygotes by intermittent gentle shaking for 2 min. Presumptive zygotes were then washed 4 times in synthetic oviduct fluid medium SOF (Tervit et al. 1972) according to Holm et al. (1999) containing 0.7 mM Na-pyruvate, 4.2 mM Na-lactate, 2.8 mM myo-inositol, 0.2 mM glutamine, 0.3 mM citrate, 30 ml/l essential amino acids mixture, 10 ml/l non-essential amino acids, 50 µg/ml gentamycin and 10% (v/v) fetal calf serum (SOF-FCS). All media were passed through a 0.2 µm membrane filter and were equilibrated overnight in an incubator at 39°C in 5% O_2 in humidified air. Presumptive zygotes were cultured in groups of 10-12 in 20µl droplets of SOF-FCS, culture was performed in a humidified atmosphere of 5% CO_2, 5% O_2 and 90% N_2 at 39 C. Cleavage was examined once between days 2 and 3, embryo development rate was evaluated on day 7 post insemination. On day 7, excellent and good quality blastocysts of grade 1 (according to the International Embryo Transfer Society standards-IETS, Stringfellow and Seidel, 1990) were selected for this study.

2.2 Production of *in vivo* bovine blastocysts

The oestrous cycles of french Prim Holstein donor cows were synchronised with an implant of 3mg Norgestomet-3.8 mg valerate oestradiol (Crestar® INTERVET S.A.- Holland) for 9 days. The oestrous reference was observed 48-68 hours after removing the implant. The cows were superovulated 8 to 12 days after oestrous with p-FSH (Stimufol® Merial SAS - France). A total dose of 450µg p-FSH was administered (8 i.m. injections with decreasing doses for 4 days) and an analogue of $PGF_{2\alpha}$ (500 µg i.m.; Cloprostenol Estrumate® Schering Plough Vet. S.A.) was injected at the moment of the 5th p-FSH injection. Two artificial inseminations (IA) were performed 12 and 24 hours after starting oestrous (day 0). The frozen-thawed semen for IA of embryos donor cows was the same that used for the production of *in vitro* bovine blastocysts. Generally, the *in vivo* embryos have a small chronological delay in their development in comparison with the *in vitro* produced embryos, because of the lack of precision in the moment of fertilization. For this reason the cows were collected at day seven and a half after IA. Embryos were recovered by uterine flushing with PBS (phosphate buffer saline) supplemented with 0.04% (w/v) BSA fraction V (same previous reference). Then embryos were washed 4 times in PBS supplemented with 0.4% (w/v) BSA fraction V. The viability of embryos was estimated according to IETS. Only excellent and good quality blastocysts grade I were selected for this study.

2.3 Determination of IFN-τ antiviral activity

Embryo culture media were assayed for antiviral activity by use of a cytopathic effect titration assay that used a bovine kidney cell line designated Madin and Darby Bovine

Kidney (MDBK cells) challenged with vesicular stomatitis virus. The extent of cell protection against viral lysis was compared with that of a diluted human INF-α (Alpha therapeutics Corporation Los Angeles, CA) used as a standard. This standard possesses 8.8 International Reference Units of activity per laboratory unit (u) when compared to human INF-α (Leukocyte IFN standard: GA-23-902-530 reference sample, obtained from NIH Bethesda MD, USA.)
The sensitivity of the IFN-τ assay was 0.012 u /100µl. Titrated IFN were expressed in laboratory units/embryo/24h, where one unit was equivalent to that amount of IFN that protected 50% of the MDBK cells monolayer from lysis upon exposure to the cytopathic effects of the virus. Immunoneutralization assays were performed with polyclonal antisera raised against IFN-τ. Briefly, IFN samples were serially diluted in a given dilution of anti-INF antisera (L'Haridon 1991). The excess of immunoneutralization results was determined from the IFN-τ activity compared with that of untreated controls.

2.4 Determination of the numbers of inner mass (ICM) and trophectoderm (TE) cells of blastocysts produced *in vitro* and *ex vivo*.

Equal numbers of hatched blastocysts (per treatment group, completely *in vitro* and *ex vivo* origin's) on day 10 after fertilizations (72h-cultured in individual droplets), were subjected to differential cell staining with fluorocrome using a modification of the procedure described by Stojkovic et al. (1997). Briefly, hatched blastocysts were washed several times in 0.1M phosphate-buffered saline (PBS, pH 7.2) containing 0,2% BSA. Hatched blastocysts were incubated in a 1:10 dilution in PBS of antiserum raised in rabbit against recombinant ovine IFN-τ (Martal et al. 1998) for 45 min at 39°C in a humidified atmosphere of 5% CO_2 in air. Subsequently, embryos were washed five times in PBS supplemented with 5% (v/v) guinea-pig complement (ref. 72122 Bio-Mérieux S.A.) and 50µg/ml propidium iodide (ref. P4170) for 45 min at 39°C in a humidified atmosphere of 5% CO_2. Blastocysts were then washed in PBS and placed in cold absolute ethanol containing 25µg/ml fluorochrome bisbenzimide (ref. B-2883) 30 min at 4°C. Finally embryos were washed in absolute ethanol, mounted in undiluted glycerol. Specific fluorescence was examined by confocal microscope (Zeiss, Paris, France) with mercury lamp under transmittance illumination and an UV exitation filter of 365 nm and a barrier filter of 420nm.

2.5 Experimental design

The aim of this experiment was to compare IFN-τ production of blastocysts *in vitro* culture from days 7 to 12 according to their origin (from completely *in vitro* and *in vivo*) and their quality. For this purpose, excellent and good quality blastocysts, developed over a stage of 7 days of *in vitro* and *in vivo* origin were sorted and cultured in individual droppers in 50µl of SOF- FCS for 5 days under paraffin oil. Plates were incubated in 5% CO_2, 5% O_2 and 90% N_2 at 39 °C in humidified air at 39°C. During the time of *in vitro* culture each equal volume of fresh medium was then added back to each culture every 24 hours and kept refrigerated at 4°C, and the blastocysts morphologically evaluated as indicated by Lindner and Wright (1983). Briefly, embryos were evaluated and graded by morphological criteria as follows: excellent (spherical, symmetrical with cells of uniform size, color and texture), good (a few imperfections such as few extruded blastomeres, irregular shape and presence of vesicles, >50% of extruded dark cells, cells of different size), fair (several imperfections, several extruded blastomeres, high percentage of extruded dark cells, too many cells of different size.)

2.6 Statistical analysis

Data on embryos origin (*in vitro* and *ex vivo*) and the quantity of IFN-τ released in a 24-h culture period and quality embryos, from day 7(Day 1 was the day of insemination) today 12, were evaluated in a 3 X 3 factorial arrangement in a complete randomized block design. The general linear models procedure (SAS Institute Inc.) was used by analysis of variance and regression coefficient least squares means. Differences were considered significant at $p<0.05$ (Little et al. 1996).

3. Results

3.1 Obtaining homogeneous expanded blastocysts of *in vitro* and *in vivo* origins on day 7

The results of the processes to obtain derived *ex vivo* and completely produced *in vitro* embryos are described in table 1. In five replicates, a total of 559 oocytes was chosen for production of completely *in vitro* bovine blastocysts. The average percentage of cleavage was 83% and the average blastocyst per oocyte rate of these trials was 43% (range 29-53%). Only day 7 grade I (excellent and good quality) blastocysts (n=46, about 29% of the total blastocysts on day 7) were removed and cultured in individual droppers. For production of *in vivo* bovine blastocysts, a total of 11 cows were treated. An average of 7.9 embryos were recovered per cow on day 7, only grade I (excellent and good quality) blastocysts (n=40 about 46% of total embryos) were recovered and cultured in individual droplets.

			Day 7				Day 8			
In vitro	Oocytes n	Cleavage day 2 % (n)	Blastocysts % (n)	Expanded Blastocysts % (n)	Total % (n)	**Embryos quality I used**	Blastocysts % (n)	Expanded Blastocysts % (n)	Total % (n)	Total % (n)
	559	83 (464)	17 (98)	8 (44)	25 (142)	**44**	6 (32)	17 (94)	23 (126)	48 (268)

			Recovered embryos on day 7				
In vivo	Superovulated cows n	Recovere d embryos % (n)	Morulas % (n)	Blastocysts % (n)	Expanded Blastocysts % (n)	Degenerated Embryos % (n)	**Embryos quality I used**
	11	100 (87)	18 (16)	28 (24)	32 (28)	22 (I9)	**40**

Table 1. Description of the processes to obtain bovine *ex vivo* and completely produced *in vitro* embryos.

3.2 Effect of embryos origin on the IFN-τ production (Table 2).

On day 8, after 24h-culture,96% blastocysts (n=46) completely produced *in vitro* (group A) and 100% *ex vivo* blastocysts (group B) (n=40) secreted <54 pM IFN-τ. After 48h-culture, 41% group A (n=19) had an average IFN-τ production of 143 ± 24 pM versus 85 ± 12 pM for group B (53%, n= 21) ($p< 0.01$). The rest of group A (57%, n=26) and those of group B (47%, n= 19) both produced <54 pM IFN-τ.

On day 10, after 72 h-culture 63% group A (n=29) exhibits an average IFN-τ production of 491 ± 128 pM versus 216 ± 37 pM for group B (58%, n=23) (NS). The rest of group A (19%

n=9) and those of group B (13%, n=5) both secreted <54 pM IFN-τ. After 96 h-culture 57% group A (n= 26) had an average IFN-τ production of 499 ± 135 pM versus 353 ± 93 pM for group B (53%, n=21) (NS). The rest of group A (6% n=3) and those of group B (8%, n=3) both produced <54 pM IFN-τ.

Time culture (hours)	*In vitro* (Group A)		*Ex vivo* (Group B)	
	% (n)	IFN-τ concentration mean ± sem (pM)	% (n)	IFN-τ concentration mean ± sem (pM)
24	96(44) 4 (2)	< 54 93 ± 0	100 (40)	<54
48	41 (19) 57 (26)	143 ± 24 b < 54	53 (21) 47(19)	85 ± 12 a < 54
72	63 (29) 19 (9)	491 ± 128 a <54	58 (23) 13 (5)	216 ± 37 a < 54
96	57 (26) 6 (3)	499 ± 135 a < 54	53 (21) 8 (3)	353 ± 93 a < 54
120	48 (22) 13 (6)	559 ± 136 a < 54	50 (20) 10 (4)	333 ± 75 a < 54

Table 2. Comparative secretion of IFN-τ by bovine hatched blastocysts derived *ex vivo* and completely produced in vitro after 24h of individual culture in medium droplets from days 7 to 12.
Different superscripts within columns (a vs b) indicate significant differences ($p<0.05$).

The average of accumulated IFN-τ production per embryo from days 7 to 10 (72 hours) of group A was 550±129 pM IFN-τ (n=38) versus group B 277±41pM IFN-τ (n=28) ($p<0.05$) figure 1. At this stage of culture, on day 10 after fertilization, the morphological aspects of completely produced *in vitro* and *ex vivo* embryos were comparable as it is illustrated in the photographies 1 and 2 after examination by confocal microscope. The cellular counts of the group A embryos showed 50±17 cells (n=6) for inner cell mass(ICM) and 62±14 (n=4) for those of group B. The trophoblast cells were 369±135 (n=6) for group A and 393±98 (n=4) for group B, respectively. At this stage, the number of total embryonic cells were 418±152 for group A and 455±112 for group B, respectively. No statistically significant difference of the cells number between the groups A and B were observed, suggesting that the difference of IFN-τ production between them did not come from difference of embryonic cells growth.

Between days 7 to 11 (96 hours), the production of IFN-τ increased in 1100±20 pM IFN-τ (n=29) for group A versus 670±117 pM IFN-τ (n=24) for group B, (p<0.05). Between days 7 to 12 (120 hours) of *in vitro* culture, it exhibits 1691±290 pM IFN-τ (n=28) for group A versus 982±182 pM IFN-τ (n=24) for group B (p<0.05), figure 1.
According to the linear regression analysis, the IFN-τ production increases during the time of culture independently of the embryos origins (r = 0.13 for group A, r = 0.23 for group B; p > 0.05).

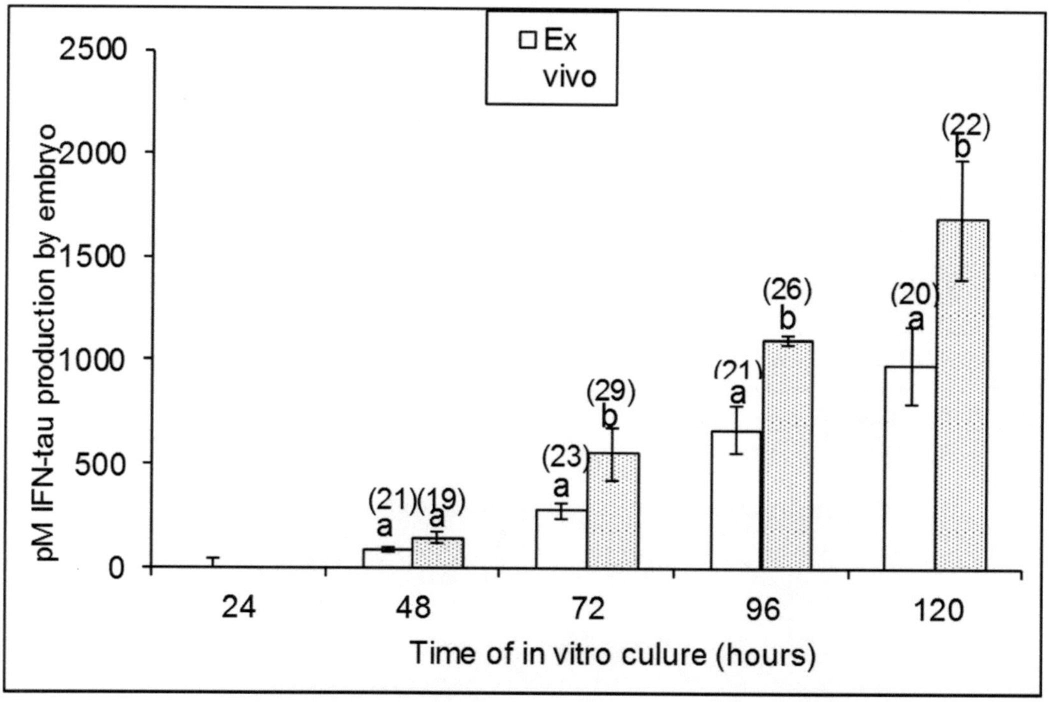

Fig. 1. Compared means of accumulated IFN-τ productions per blastocyst derived completely produced in vitro(group A) and *ex vivo* (group B), cultured individually from days 7 to12.
Least Squares Means indicate values with different superscripts (a vs b) are significantly different (p<0.05). (n): number of embryos.

3.3 Relationship between embryo quality and accumulated IFN-τ production by embryo, independently of its origin

The average IFN-τ production from days 7 to 10 (72h-culture) in relationship with embryo quality did not show significant differences, (p>0.05): for quality I (excellent) the average IFN-τ production was 534±138 pM IFN-τ (n=21), for quality I (good) 389±101 pM IFN-τ (n=29) and for quality II (fair) 328±108 pM (n=5). The average IFN-τ production from days 7 to 11 (96h-culture) in relationship with embryo quality did not show significant differences (p>0.05); 1040±216 pM IFN-τ (n=17); 870±158 pM (n=33) and 507±262 pM (n=5),respectively. But the average IFN-τ production from days 7 to 12 (120h-culture) in relationship with embryo quality shows significant differences between excellent quality (1815±453 pM, n=10) or good quality (1356±200 pM , n=29) with fair quality (360±188 pM, n=4), (p<0.02), Table 3.

The logistic regression analysis of the relationship between the embryo quality and IFN-τ production showed predicted probabilities from observed responses: Concordance: 60.3% and Discordance: 23.9%.

Embryo quality	Time of culture (hours)						
	0 h	72 h.		96 h.		120 h.	
	n (%)	n (%)	IFN-τ concentration mean ± sem (pM)	n (%)	IFN-τ concentration mean ± sem (pM)	n (%)	IFN-τ concentration mean ± sem (pM)
Q1(Ex.)	81 (70)	24 (21)	534 ± 138a	20 (17)	1040 ± 216a	10 (12)	1815 ± 453 a
Q1(G.)	19 (16)	34 (29)	389 ± 101a	38 (33)	870 ± 158a	29 (34)	1356 ± 200ab
Q II	-	6 (5)	328 ± 108a	6 (5)	507± 262a	4 (5)	360 ± 188 b

QI (Ex.): excellent quality grade I; QI (G.): good quality grade I; QII: fair quality grade II. Least Squares Means indicate values with different superscripts (a vs b) are significantly different ($p<0.05$).

Table 3. Relationship between embryo quality with accumulated IFN-τ production after culture individually of blastocysts whatever their *in vitro* or *in vivo* origins, from days 7 to 12.

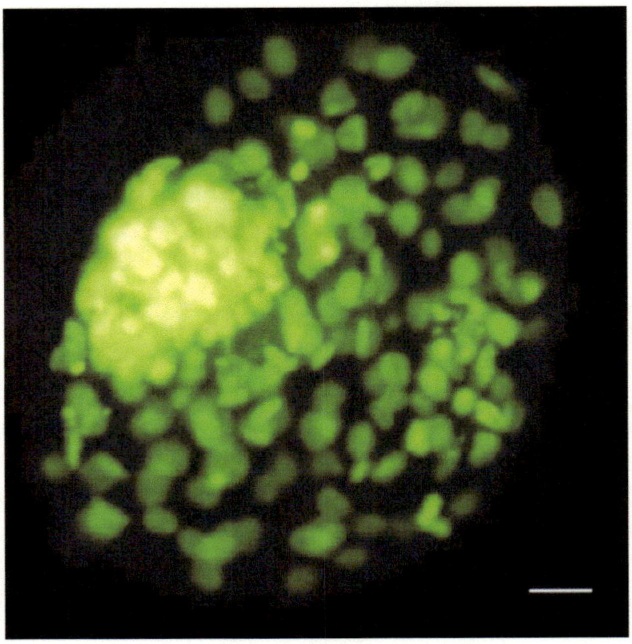

Bar corresponds to 50μm.

Photograph 1. Blastocyst of ex vivo origin on day 10 (from day 7 and cultured during 3 days individually in droplet). Staining was by immunochemistry with ainti-IFN-τ immmunserum and propidium iodide - bisbenzimide. The nuclei of ICM and TE cells are fluorescent.

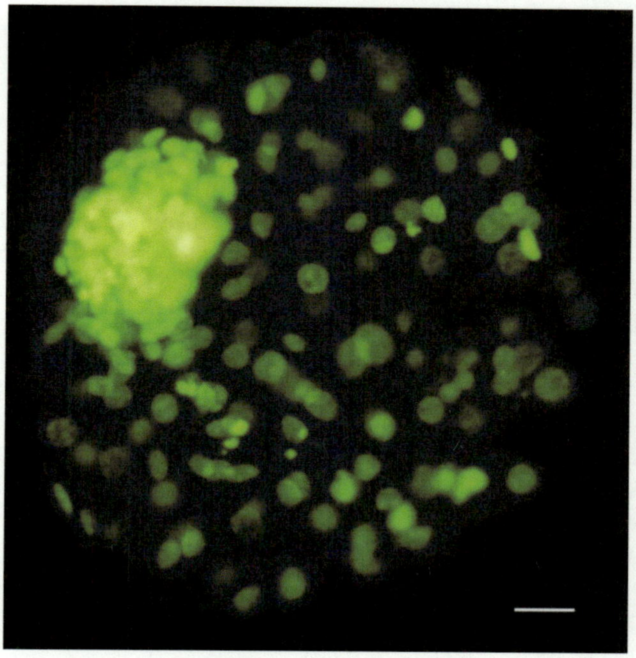

Bar corresponds to 50μm.

Photograph 2. Blastocyst of completely in vitro origin, was cultured 10 days 7 individually in droplet. Staining was by immunochemistry is like in photograph 1.

4. Discussion and conclusion

Our average results for producing bovine blastocysts *in vitro* can be compared with different reports, (Greve et al, 1993 Brackett and Zuelke 1993; Holm et al, 1999; Thompson 1997). Nowadays, after years of development, these techniques have reached a level of stability. The analysis of IFN-τ production by *in vitro* blastocysts confirms earlier studies (Kubish et al. 2004, 1998; Hernández-Ledezma et al. 1993; Stojkovic et al. 1995, 1999) and strongly suggests that expression of IFN-τ is constitutive and partly non dependent on factors from the uterine environment. Nevertheless, it is known that IFN-τ expression and secretion level might be modulated *in vivo* by growth factors and cytokines (Ko et al. 1991; Imakawa et al. 1993; Martal et al. 1998; Spencer and Bazer 2002; Miyazaki et al. 2002; Emond et al. 2004).
The IFN-τ production on day 8, after 24 hours of *in vitro* culture, was below 54pM and therefore undetectable in both *ex vivo* and completely produced *in vitro*; The IFN-τ is first produced by bovine conceptuses soon after the blastocysts expand and just prior to the time that the zona pellucida ruptures and hatching occurs (Hernández –Ledezma et al. 1992). It was only detectable from day 9 in both cases. These results have no relationship with the results reported by Kubish et al. (1998). In our study we only used very homogeneous blastocysts of good quality. We reported the production generated every 24 hours from day 7 to 12. Nevertheless, the accumulated production for each embryo agrees with values obtained by Kubish et al., (1998, 2004); Stojkovic et al., (1999); Hernandez- Ledezma et al., (1993).
To compare well the IFN-τ production of *ex vivo* and completely produced *in vitro* embryos in *in vitro* culture from day 7 to 12, in the present study only excellent and good quality

expanded blastocysts were chosen on day 7 after fertilization. Thus, a homogeneous production would be expected, however, significant differences in the average production of IFN-τ were found in relationship with embryo origin, *ex vivo* and completely produced *in vitro,* between day 8 and 9, after 48h of culture and in IFN-τ production for embryo accumulated, which showed that the IFN-τ production was greater for completely produced *in vitro* embryos even on day 9.

In vitro, modulation of the IFN-τ production could be induced on one hand by the conditions of the culture associated to the presence of biological factors contained in the fetal calf serum, and in the other hand by intrinsic causes of the embryo. Those reasons could explain the individual variability of IFN-τ production between the embryos. Our data showed high ranges of standard deviation for *in vitro* and *ex vivo* embryos and were in agreement with the results of Kubish et al. (1998) who also obtained ample ranges in the standard deviation; they also observed that the amount of IFN-τ produced was independent of the quality score of embryos received. Larson and Kubisch (1999) report that the presence of more blastocysts in the same medium can increase the IFN-τ secretion, nevertheless the nature of most of these factors of variation are badly known. In *in-vivo* conditions, the production of IFN-τ is modulated by the uterine environment. This production seems to be strongly correlated to the progesterone seric concentration, which would suggest that more elevated rates of progesterone would be favorable to the conceptus environment (Kerbler et al. 1997; Spencer et al. 2004). Indeed, progesterone stimulates the production of many others uterine factors than the IFN (Mann et al. 1999; Martal, 2002.). Several growth factors or citokynes have been involved in the secretion of IFN: IGF-I and IGF II (Ko et al. 1991), GM-CSF (Imakawa et al. 1995; Emond et al. 2004), this one is known as a powerful growth factor for the trophoblastic cells. It is possible that the variations in IFN-τ production between blastocysts at any of the stages of development is the result of genetic factors; others have previously reported that the fact sire genotype appears to influence IFN-τ secretion (Kubish et al. 2001); for this study, the frozen-thawed semen for IA of donor cows was the same as production of *in vitro* bovine. More over, according to Kubish et al. (2001), the batch of ovaries for production of *in vitro* bovine blastocysts, does not take into account the composition of breeds or ages of cows slaughter, these conditions may influence the variation in IFN-τ production.

However, their early-forming blastocysts were generally considered more developmentally competent than those which formed late, and these last authors suggested a possible negative relationship between early IFN-τ production and competence. In fact, this hypothesis has not been verified in the present study, possibly because of the homogeneity of the embryos chosen on the good appearance on day 7 according to the usual morphological criteria. Embryo quality is usually based on series of subjective visual assessments of morphologic parameters evaluation which may include embryo shape, size, cellular integrity, appearance of the cytoplasm and nucleus and other often intangible criteria (Lindner and Wright, 1983; Shamsuddin et al. 1992, Massip et al. 1995). In this study, the embryos which maintained in good and excellent quality had a better production of IFN-τ compared with those which turned to fair quality. This can be explained by a higher number of degenerating cells; in others the present study shows that the embryo quality is associated with IFN-τ production and confirms earlier studies (Kubish et al. 1998; Hernández-Ledezma et al; 1993; Stojkovic et al. 1995 and 1999).

Finally this study leads to the conclusion that significant differences in the production of IFN-τ were found in relationship with embryo origin, *ex vivo* and completely produced *in vitro*. The detectable interferon production in the precocious stage on days 7 to 8 reflects the degree of embryonic development, but the amount of produced interferon has neither a positive nor negative effect on the future of the embryo viability

9. References

[1] Brackett B. and Zuelke K.A. (1993) Analysis of factors involved in the in vitro production of bovine embryos. Theriogenology 39, pp 43-64.

[2] Bazer F.W., Ot T.L., and Spencer TE, (1994) Analysis Pregnancy recognition in ruminants, pigs and horses: signals from the trophoblast. Theriogenology 41, pp. 79-94.

[3] Butler J.E. and Biggers J.D. (1989) Assessing the viability of preimplantation embryos in vitro. Theriogenology 3, pp. 115-126.

[4] Chalier M., Hue D., Boisnasr M., Martal J. and Gaye P. (1989) Cloning and expression of cDNA encoding ovine trophoblastin: its idently with a class-II alpha interferon. Gene 77, pp. 341-348.

[5] Derreuddre-Bosquet N., Clayette P., Martin M., Mabondzo A., Frétier P., Gas G., Martal J. , and Dormon D. (1996) Anti-HIV potential of a new interferon, interferon-τ (trophoblastin). J. AIDS Human Retrovi. vol. 11, pp. 241-246,.

[6] Demmers, K. Derecka K. and Flint A. (2001) Trophoblast interferon and pregnancy. Reproduction vol. 121, pp. 41-49.

[7] Emond V., MacLaren L.A., Kimminis S., Arosh J.A., Fortie M.A. and R.D. (2004) Expression of cyclooxygenase-2 and granulocyte-macrophage-colony-stimulating factor in the endometrial epithelium of the cow is up-regulated during early pregnancy and in response to intrauterine infusions of interferon-tau. Biol. Reprod. vol. 70, pp. 54-64,.

[8] Ezashi T., Ghosh D. and Roberts R.M. (2001) Repression of Ets-2-induced transactivation of the tau interferon promoter by Oct-4. Mol Cell Biology vol. 21, pp. 7883-7891.

[9] Farin C.E., Imakawa K. and Roberts R.M. (1989) In situ localization of mRNA for the interferon, ovine trophoblast protein-1 during early embryonic development of the sheep. Mol Endocrinology vol. 3, pp. 1099-1107.

[10] Fillon C., Chauat G., Reianud P., Charpigny G., and Martal J. (1991) Immunoregulatory effects of trophoblastin (oTP): all 5 isoforms are immunosuppressive of PHA driven lymphocyte proliferation. J Reprod Immunol vol. 19, pp. 237-249,.

[11] Guillomot M., Michel C., Gaye P., Charlier M., Thojan J., and Martal J. (1990) Cellular localization of an embryonic interferon, ovine trophoblastin and its in-rna in sheep embryos during early pregnancy. Biol Cell vol. 68, pp. 205-211.

[12] Godkin J.D., Bazer F.W., Moffat J., Session F. and Roberts M. (1982) Purification and properties of a major, low molecular weight protein released by the trophoblaste of sheep blastocysts at day 13-21 J Reprod Fertil vol. 65, pp. 141-150,.

[13] Greve T., Avery B. and Callesen H. (1993) Viability of in vivo and in vitro produced bovine embryos. Reprod Dom Anim vol. 28, pp. 645-654.

[14] Hasler J.F., Henderson W.B., Hurtgen P.J., Jin Z.Q, McCauley A.D., Mower S.A., Neely B., Shuey L.S., Stokes J.E. and Trimmer S.A. (1995) Production, freezing and transfer of bovine IVF embryos and subsequent calving results. Theriogenology vol. 33, pp. 644-645,.

[15] Hansen T.R., Imakawa K., Polites H.G., Marotti, K.R. Anthony R.V. and Roberts RM, (1988) Interferon RNA of embryonic origin is expressed transiently during early pregnancy in the ewe. J Biol Chem vol. 263, pp. 12801-12804.
[16] Hernández-Ledezma J.J., Mathialagan N., Villanueva C., Sikes J.D. and Roberts R.M., (1993) Expression of bovine trophoblast interferons by in vitro-derived blastocysts is correlated with their morphological quality and stage of development. Mol Reprod Dev vol. 36, pp. 1-6.
[17] Holm P., Booth P.I., Schmidt M.H., Greve T. and Callesen H. (1999) High bovine blastocyst development in a static in vitro production system using SOFaa medium supplemented with sodium citrate and myo-inositol with or without serum-proteins. Theriogenology vol. 52, pp. 683-700.
[18] Imakawa K., Helmer S.D., Nephew K.P., Meka C.S.R. and Christenson R.K.A. (1993) Novel role for GM-CSF:enhancement of pregnancy specific interferon production,ovine trophoblast protein-1. Endocrinology, vol. 3, pp. 1869-1871.
[19] Imakawa K., Taruma K., McGuire W.J., Khan S., Harbinson I.A., Stanga J.P, Helmer S.D. and Christenson R.K.A. (1995) Effect of interleukin-3 on ovine trophoblast interferon during early conceptus development. Endocrinology, vol. 3, pp. 511-517.
[20] Kerbler T.L., Buhr M.M., Jordan L.T., Leslie K.E. and Walton J.S. (1997) Relationship between maternal plasma progesterone concentration and interferon-tau synthesis by the conceptus in cattle, Theriogenology vol. 47, pp. 703-714.
[21] Kerbler T.L., Buhr M.M., Jordan L.T., Leslie K.E. and Walton J.S. (1997) Relationship between maternal plasma progesterone concentration and interferon-tau synthesis by the conceptus in cattle, Theriogenology vol. 47, pp. 703-714.
[22] Ko Y., Lee C.Y., Ott T.L., Davis M.A., Simmen R.C., Bazer F.W. and Simmen F.A. (1991) Insulin-like growth factors in sheep uterine fluids: concentrations and relationship to ovine trophoblast protein-1production during early pregnancy. Biol Reprod vol. 45, pp. 135-142.
[23] Kubisch H.M., Sirisathien S., Bosc h P., Hernandez-Fonseca H., Clements G., Liukkonen J. and Brackett B. (2004) Effects of developmental stage, embryonic interferon-tau and recipient synchrony on pregnancy rate after transfer of in vitro produced bovine blastocysts. Reprod Domest Anim. vol. 39, pp. 120-124,.
[24] Kubisch H.M., Larson M.A., Ealy A.D., Murphy C.N. and Roberts R.M., (2001a) Genetic and environmental determinants of interferon-τ secretion by in vivo-and in vitro-derived bovine blastocysts. Anim Reprod Sci vol. 66, pp. 1-13.
[25] Kubisch H.M., Larson M.A. and Roberts R.M.(1998) Relationship between age of blastocyst formation and interferon-τ secretion by in vitro-derived bovine embryos. Mol Reprod Dev vol. 49, pp. 254-260.
[26] Larson M.A. and Kubisch H.M. (1999) The effects of group size on development and IFN-τ secretion by in vitro fertilized and cultured bovine blastocysts. Hum Reprod vol. 14, pp. 254-260.
[27] L'Haridon RM, (1991) Immunosorbent binding bioassy: a solid phase biological immunoassay for the titration of antisera to alpha interferons. J Immunoassay vol. 12, pp. 99-112.
[28] Little R., Milliken G., Stroup W. and Wolfinger R. (1996) System for Mixed Models SAS Institute Inc Cary, NC.
[29] Lindner G.M. and Wright R.W. (1983) Bovine embryo morphology and evaluation. Theriogenology, vol. 20, pp. 407-416.

[30] Mann G.E., Lamming G.E., Robinson R.S. and Wathes DC. (1999) The regulation of interferon- τ production and uterine hormone receptors during early pregnancy. J Reprod Fertil suppl vol. 54, pp. 317-328.

[31] Mathialagan N., Bixby J.A. and Roberts R.M. (1992) Expression of interleukin-6 in porcine ovine, and bovine preimplantation conceptuses. Mol Reprod Dev. vol. 32, pp. 324-330.

[32] Martal J., Lacroix M.C., Loudes C., Saunier M. and Wintenberg-Torres S. (1979) Trophoblastin, an antiluteolytic protein present in early pregnancy in sheep. J Reprod Fert vol. 56, pp. 63-73.

[33] Martal, Degryse E., Charpigny G., Assal N., Reinaud P., Charlier M., Gaye P. and Lecocq J.P. (1990) Evidence for extended maintenance of the corpus luteum by uterine infusion of a recombinant trophoblast α-interferon (trophoblastin) in sheep. J Endocrin, 127, R5-R8.

[34] Martal J., N. Chêne, Camous S., Huynh L., F. Lantier, Hermier P., L'Haridon R., Charpigny G., Charlier M. and Chaouat G. (1997) Recent developments and potentialities for reducing embyo mortality in ruminants: the role of IFN-τ and other cytokines in early pregnancy. Mol Reprod Dev vol. 9, pp. 355-380.

[35] Martal J., Chêne N., Huynh L., L'Haridon R., Charpigny G., Reinaud P., Guillomot M. and Charlier M. (1998) IFN-tau: A novel subtype I IFN1. Structural characteristics, non-ubiquitous expression, structure-function relationships, a pregnancy hormonal embryonic signal and cross-species therapeutic potentialities. Rev Biochimie. Vol. 80, pp. 755-777.

[36] Martal J., Chene N., Huynh L., Zourbas S., Rogez C., Charpentier N., Hermier P., L'haridon R., Charlier M., Chaoua G.t and Germain G. (2002) Les interactions immuno-endocrines entre la mère et l'embryon. Dans L'embryon Chez L'homme et l'animal. INSERM–INRA, Paris, 159-201.

[37] Massip, P. Mermillod P. and Dinnyes A. (1995) Morphology and biochemistry of in vitro produced bovine embryos: implications for their cryopreservation. Hum Reprod, Vol. 10, pp. 3004-3011.

[38] Meyer M.D., Hansen P.J., Thatcher W.W., Drost M. and Badinga L. (1995) Extension of corpus luteum lifespan and reduction of uterine secretion of prostaglandin F_2 of cows in response to recombinant interferon-τ. J Dairy Sci.,Vol. 78, pp. 1921-1931.

[39] Miyazaki H., Imai M., Hirayama T., Saburi S., Tanaka M., Maruyama M., Matsuo C., Meguro H., Nishibashi K., Inoue F., Djiane J., Gertler A., Tachi S., Imakawa K. and Tachi C. (2002) Establishment of feeder-independent cloned caprine trophoblast cell line expresses placental lactogen and interferon tau. Placenta,Vol. 23, pp. 613-630.

[40] Ott T.L., Van Heeke G., Hostetler C.E., Schalue T.K., Olmsted J.J., Johnson H.M. and Bazer F.W. (1993) Intrauterine injection of recombinant ovine interferon-tau extends the interestrous interval in sheep. Theriogenology. Vol. 40, pp. 757-769.

[41] Parrish J.J., Susko-Parrish J.L., Leibfried-Rutledge M.L., Cristser E.S., Eyestone W.H. and First N.L. (1986) Bovine in vitro fertilization with frozen-thawed semen. Theriogenology Vol. 25, pp. 591-600.

[42] Pontzer C.P., Bazer F.W. and Johnson H.M. (1991) Antiproliferative activity of pregnancy recognition hormone, ovine trophoblast protein-1. Cancer Res Vol. 51, pp. 5304-5307.

[43] Pontzer C.P., Yamamoto J.K., Bazer F.W., Ott T.L., and Johnson H.M. (1997) Potent anti-feline immunodeficiency virus and anti-human immunodeficiency virus effect of IFN-τ. J. Immunol. Vol. 158, pp. 4351-4357.
[44] Roberts R.M., Cross J.C. and Leaman D.W. (1992) Interferons as hormone of pregnancy. Endocrinology Revue Vol. 13, pp. 432-452.
[45] Spencer T.E., Burghardt R.C., Johnson G.A. and Bazer F.W., (2004) Conceptus signals for establishment and maintenance of pregnancy. Anim Reprod Sci Vol. 82, pp. 535-550.
[46] Spencer T.E., and Bazer F.W. (2002) Biology of progesterone action during pregnancy recognition and maintenance of pregnancy. Frontier Bioscience Vol. 7, pp. 1879-1898.
[47] Spencer T.E., and Bazer F.W. (1996) Ovine interferon-tau suppress transcription of the estrogen receptor and oxytocin receptor genes in the ovine endometrium. Endocrinology Vol. 137, pp. 1144-1147.
[48] Stewart MD, Choi Y, Johnson GA, Yu-Lee L, Bazer FW, Spencer TE. (2002) Roles of Stat 1, Stat 2, and Interferon Regulatory Factor-9 (IRF-9) in Interferon tau regulation of IRF-1. Biol Reprod Vol. 66, pp. 393-400.
[49] Stojkovic M., Wolf E., Buttner M., Berg U., Charpigny G., Schmitt A. and Brem G. (1995)Secretion of biologically active interferon tau by in vitro-Derived bovine trophoblastic Tissue. Biol Reprod Vol. 53, pp. 1500-1507.
[50] Stojkovic M., Wolf E., Van Langendonckt, Vansteenbrugge G., Charpigny G., Reinaud P., Gandolfi F., Brevini T.A., Mermillod P., Terqui M., Brem G. and Massip A. (1997) Correlations between chemical parameters, mitogenic activity and embryotrophic activity of oviduct-conditioned medium. Theriogenology, Vol. 48, pp. 659-673.
[51] Stojkovic M., Wolf E., Buttner M., Zakhartchenko V., Riedl J., Reichenbach H., Wenigerkind H. and Brem G. (1999) Secretion of interferon-τ bovine embryos in long-term culture: comparison of in vivo-derived, invitro-produced, nuclear transfer and demi-embryos. Anim Reprod Sci, Vol. 55, pp. 151-162.
[52] Shamsuddin M., Larsson B., Gustafsson H., Gustari S. and Rodríguez-Martínez H, (1992) Comparative morphological evaluation of in vivo and in vitro produced bovine embryos. In: Proc. 12th Con. Anim Reprod vol. 3, pp. 1333-1335.
[53] Stringfellow D.S. and Seidel S.M. (1990) Manual of the I.E.T.S., vol 79 2° Ed., I.E.T.S. Champaign, I 11. U.S.A.
[54] Thompson J.G. (1997) Comparison between in vivo-derived and in vitro-produced pre-elongation embryos from domestic ruminants. Mol Reprod Dev vol 9, 341-354.
[55] Tervi H.R., Whittingham D.G. and Rowson L.E.A. (1972) Successful culture in vitro of sheep and cattle ova. J Reprod Fertil vol 30, 493-497.
[56] Vogiagis D., Fry R.C., Sandeman R.M., and Salamonsen L.A. (1997)Leukaemia inhibitory factor in endometrium during the estrous cycle, early pregnancy and in ovariectomized steroid-treatment ewes. J Reprod Fertil vol 109, 279-288.
[57] Yamagushi H., Nagaoka K., Imakawa K., Sakai S. and Christenson R.K. (2001) Enhancer regions of ovine interferon-τ gene that confer PMA response or cell type specific transcription. Mol. Cel. Endocrin vol. 173, 147-155

16

Reproductive Endocrinology Diseases: Hormone Replacement and Therapy for Peri/Menopause

Zoe Roupa[1], Greta Wozniak[2], Konstantinos Tsipras[3] and Penelope Sotiropoulou[4]
[1]European University, Nicosia,
[2]Medical School, University of Thessaly, Larissa,
[3]Endocrinology Primary Health Care Center, Athens
[4]Technological Education Institute of Athens,
[1]Cyprus
[2,3,4]Greece

1. Introduction

There are many female causes for infertility but the incidence of infertility increases with advancing age. Colombat de L'Isere in a chapter on 'Change of Life' in his "Treatise on the diseases and special hygiene of females" (1845) stated: Compelled to yield to the power of time, women now cease to exist for the species, and hence forward live only for themselves" (Colombat de L'Isere M., 1945). Fortunately, this pessimistic outlook on life after menopause has become outdated. Aiming to standardize terminology The World Health Organization (WHO) assembled in 1996 and the Council of Affiliated Menopause Societies (CAMS) in 1999 (WHO Scientific Group: Research on Menopause in the 1990s, Utian WH, 1999). Commonly accepted terms, including pre-menopause, peri-menopause, menopausal transition, and climacteric, were thought to be too vague to be useful. In July of 2001, the Stages of Reproductive Aging Workshop (STRAW) was held to address the absence of a relevant staging system for female reproductive aging, and to discuss the confusing current nomenclature for the pre-menopause (Soules MR, et al., 2001).

The average age of menopause is 51 and less than 1% of women experience it before the age of 40. Some women undergo premature menopause at a very early age affecting their ability to have children. As more and more women delay child bearing, this life altering condition has become more prevalent. Population aging must be added to population growth as very important social problems. Women in our society get married and have children later in life. Therefore, evaluation of ovarian reserve is critical to understanding a patient's reproductive potential.

Ovulatory disorders are a common cause of infertility. Ovulation is controlled by complex interactions between numerous endocrine hormones including FSH, LH, estradiol, progesterone and others. Menopause is the cessation of the primary functions of the human ovaries, with associated changes in pituitary gonadotropin secretion occurring secondary to the decline in ovarian sex steroid and protein production. However, increasing evidence suggests that aging is associated with dynamic changes in the hypothalamic and pituitary components of the reproductive axis that are independent of changes in gonadal hormone secretion (Hall JE, et al., 2000). Imbalances in these hormones, or alterations in the "feedback mechanism", can prevent ovulation, or cause it to be irregular.

2. Epidemiology of menopause

Most estimates of age at natural menopause are based on samples of Caucasian women in Western societies. In one large, comprehensive, prospective cohort study of mid-aged, Caucasian U.S. women (the Massachusetts Women's Health Study [MWHS]) the age at natural menopause occurred at 51.3 years, (Gold EB, et al., 2001) confirming prior reports. The Study of Women's Health Across the Nation (SWAN), a multicenter, multiethnic, community-based cohort study of women and the menopausal transition, reported the overall median age at natural menopause to be 51.4 years, after adjustment for other factors (Gold EB, et al., 2001). Studies performed outside the United States suggest that Africans, African Americans, (Bromberger JT, et al., 1997) and Hispanics of Mexican descent experience menopause at an earlier age than Caucasian women, as opposed to Japanese (Tamada T & Iwasake H., 1995) and Malaysian (Ismael NN., 1994) women, who report a similar median age of menopause to women of European descent.

Lower educational attainment and unemployment have been independently associated with earlier age at menopause (Gold EB, et al., 2001; Cramer DW, 1994 et al) and may be markers for elevated bio-psychosocial stress. Women who are separated, divorced, or widowed have been shown to have an earlier menopause than women who are married (Gold EB, et al., 2001). Age at natural menopause for parous women has been reported to occur significantly later than for nulliparous women. (Gold EB, et al., 2001; Anasti JN., 1998; Tibilette MG, et al., 1999; Weel AE, , et al., 1999). Gold et al. and Cramer et al. observed a trend of increasing age at menopause with increasing number of life births, and that prior use of oral contraceptives was associated with earlier age at natural menopause however, a slight prolongation of the reproductive life-span has been associated with oral contraceptive use (Cramer DW, et al., 1994).

The proposed mechanism by which parity and use of oral contraceptives may result in later age at natural menopause involves reducing ovulatory cycles earlier in life and thus preserving oocytes longer, resulting in later menopause (Gold EB, et al., 2001). Some studies show that women with a lower body mass index (BMI) experience an earlier menopause; other studies have not confirmed this finding (Zapantis G & Santoro N., 2002). Environmental toxicants may play a role in early menopause. A large body of literature shows that current smokers tend to experience menopause at an earlier age (1 to 2 years) than non-smokers (Reynaud K,, et al, 2001, Hreinsson JG, et al., 2002, Loffler KA, et al., 2003, Burger HG, et al., 2002) and may have a shorter menopausal transition (Gold EB, 2001, et al).

It has been shown that polycyclic hydrocarbons in cigarette smoke are toxic to ovarian follicles and may lead to their loss and thus an earlier menopause in smokers. Harlow et al. observed that women with a history of medically treated depression had a 20% increased rate of entering peri-menopause sooner than women with no depression history, after adjustment for age, parity, age at menarche, education, cigarette smoking, and BMI. Epidemiology gives answers about populations, whereas clinical medicine deals with patient samples and individuals. For example, in population-based studies, (Gold EB, et al., 2001) no global increased prevalence of depression has been associated with the menopause transition, whereas in clinical samples, depression around menopause has reportedly increased. Furthermore, symptoms vary among women, and the distinction between populations versus individuals must be made when one is evaluating epidemiologic factors related to menopause.

3. Menopause pathogenesis

The basis of reproductive senescence in women is oocyte/follicle depletion in the ovary. Developmentally, a woman attains her peak oocyte complement at 20 weeks' gestational age. Between 20 and 40 weeks' gestation, two thirds of a woman's oocyte complement is lost, and total oocyte counts drop from a mean of about 6 to 8 million to 1 to 2 million (Zapantis G & Santoro N., 2002).

The most massive wave of atresia (rate of follicle loss) that a woman ever experiences happens before she is born. At the onset of puberty, germ cell mass has been reduced to 300,000 to 500,000 units. Subsequent reproductive aging consists of a steady loss of oocytes through atresia or ovulation and does not necessarily occur at a constant rate. Atresia is an apoptotic process. During the 35 to 40 years of reproductive life, 400 to 500 oocytes will be selected for ovulation. By menopause, only a few hundred follicles remain (Speroff L, et al., 1999).

The relatively wide age range (42 to 58 years) for menopause in normal women seems to indicate that women may be endowed with a highly variable number of oocytes, or that the rate of oocyte loss varies greatly (Soules MR, et al., 2001). Concurrent with the loss of ovarian follicles as a woman transitions to menopause are hormonal changes in the hypothalamic-pituitary-ovarian axis. Follicle-stimulating hormone (FSH) is an established indirect marker of follicular activity; as follicle numbers decline, FSH levels increase (Burger HG, et al., 2002). An elevated level is often the first clinically measurable sign of reproductive aging. Large cross-sectional studies have reported a progressive, quantitative rise in FSH with age (Ahmed-Ebbiary NA, et al., 1994). In the late reproductive years, initial elevations in FSH are most prominent in the early follicular phase of the menstrual cycle but are intermittent and do not occur in every cycle (Klein NA, Soules MR., 1998). This increase is first detectable some years before any clinical indications of approaching menopause are evident (Burger HG, et al., 2002).

The rise in FSH appears to be the result of a decline in inhibin -B, a dimeric protein that reflects the fall in ovarian follicle numbers. Is a small pleomorphic peptide made within the ovarian granulosa and luteinized granulosa cells, which, although assay specificity and sensitivity in ovarian physiology (Burger HG 1993). Inhibin may be an intraovarian regulator although other peptides such as activin and follistatin are more likely paracrine factors (Findlay JK, et al., 1990) but one of its more important functions appears to be feedback suppression of FSH production (Seifer DB, et al., 1996). In reproductive life, inhibin serves to selectively inhibit FSH by binding to receptors on the anterior pituitary (Robertson DM & Burger HG., 2002). Estradiol is stable or even elevated during the earlier menopause transition; closer to the final menstrual period, a decline is clearly observed (Longscope C, et al., 1986).

Findings from the Melbourne Women's Midlife Health Project, a cohort of women followed through the menopause transition, confirm that a decline in inhibin B precedes the increase in FSH and the decline in estradiol that occur later in the transition (Burger HG, et al., 2007).

The remaining follicles are less likely to function normally, which may lead to erratic follicular development and dysregulation of folliculogenesis (Whiteman MK, et al., 2003, Schwingl PJ, et al., 1994). Although FSH and estradiol vary near menopause, steroidogenic enzymes appear to be completely absent in the postmenopausal ovary after all functional follicles are lost (Couzinet B, et al., 2001). Between the ages of 20 and 40 years, concentrations of total testosterone have been reported to fall by about 50% (Zumoff B, et al., 1995). This age-related decline does not change further during the transition years (Burger HG, et al., 2000). Similarly, dehydroepiandosterone (DHEA) and its sulphate, DHEAS, decline with age (Rossmanith W et al., 1991., Santoro N, et al., 1998). Because circulating sex hormone-binding globulin (SHBG) decreases across the menopausal transition, free androgen levels actually rise, as indicated by a small increase in free androgen index (T ÷ SHBG × 100) (Burger HG, et al., 2000). Androstenedione, which remains relatively stable during the transition, is converted to estrone in extra-glandular tissue. This accounts for almost all the estrogen in circulation after menopause.

When ovulation stops, concurrent with a woman's FMP, serum progesterone levels are invariably low (Rannevik G, et al., 1995). Luteinizing hormone (LH) eventually increases, although at a slower rate than FSH. Despite the epidemiologic trend toward elevated FSH and decreased estradiol with progression through the transition, measurement of FSH, inhibin, and estradiol provides at best an unreliable guide to the menopausal status of an individual woman (El-Hage G, et al., 2007; Braunstein GD, et al., 2005). A more rational approach to diagnosing menopause would include an assessment of the longitudinal symptoms of a woman who presents with peri-menopausal complaints (Lobo RA., 1999). Hormone profiles correlate well with symptoms and cycle features (Burger HD, et al., 1995). Thus, if a woman is >45 years old and has had a recent disruption in her menstrual pattern and symptoms suggestive of transient hypo-estrogenemia, it is likely that she has entered her menopausal transition (Santoro N., 2002). That being said, the clinician should take care to rule out other pathologies that can be masked by common complaints associated with the menopausal transition. At minimum, a screening TSH level should be performed, as menstrual irregularity may be the only manifestation of thyroid dysfunction.

4. Regulation of gonadotropins and control of ovarian steroid production

Pituitary gonadotropes synthesize and secrete both LH and FSH. They account for 7% to 15% of anterior pituitary cells. Gonadotropin subunit gene expression is regulated by the frequency of GnRH signal input to pituitary gonadotropes (Haisenleder DJ, et al., 1991). During the menstrual cycle, LH pulse frequency is approximately every 90 minutes in the early follicular phase, 60 to 70 minutes during the late follicular phase, 100 minutes during the early luteal phase, and 200 minutes during the late luteal phase. This variation reflects changes in GnRH pulse frequency, which regulates relative FSH and LH secretion; this, in turn, determines follicle recruitment, development, and ovulation. More rapid GnRH pulse frequencies promote LH secretion, and slower frequencies promote FSH secretion. Although good evidence indicates that changes in GnRH pulse frequency determines differential LH and FSH secretion (Marshall JC, et al., 1993) it is apparent that ovarian steroids and peptide hormones have a major role. Women with hypothalamic stalk section regain their characteristic cycle length when administered an unchanging frequency of exogenous GnRH pulses every 90 minutes.

This indicates that intrinsic rates of follicle development and regression of the corpus luteum, along with their phasing of steroid and peptide hormone production, are major determinants of LH and FSH responses to GnRH. Gonadotropins control the growth and differentiation of the steroid hormone–secreting cells of the ovary, intrinsically linking form and function. A defined sequence of gonadotropin action propels the growth of follicles and the production of steroid hormones. Positive feedback on the pituitary by high concentrations of estrogens leads to the ovulatory surge of LH, which in turn triggers a dramatic differentiation event, resulting in structural reorganization of the pre-ovulatory follicle, release of the ovum, and striking changes in the steroidogenic capacity of the luteinizing cells. Follicular growth, which culminates in ovulation and corpus luteum formation, requires both FSH and LH. Steroidogenic competence of the ovarian follicle is not achieved in the absence of FSH, even if LH is present in abundance. FSH promotes proliferation of the granulosa cells and induces the expression of genes involved in estradiol biosynthesis (Haisenleder DJ, et al., 1991; Kaiser UB, et al., 1997). During the last phase of follicular maturation, when granulosa cells acquire LH receptors, LH is then able to sustain follicular estradiol synthesis. This LH substitution is thought to compensate for the diminished levels of FSH of the late follicular phase consequent to negative-feedback action of estradiol and inhibin. LH action on the granulosa thus rescues the dominant LH-expressing follicle from the fate of atresia. LH stimulation is indispensable for normal ovarian hormone production not only before but also after ovulation. Suppression of LH release leads to a prompt decline in progesterone levels that precede changes in the abundance of mRNAs encoding steroidogenic enzymes or structural changes in the corpus luteum (King JA & Millar RP., 1982).

This acute regulation of ovarian progesterone secretion is controlled by LH via the expression of steroidogenic acute regulatory protein (StAR) messenger RNA (mRNA) and protein, present in both theca-lutein and granulosa-lutein cells throughout the luteal phase are highly expressed in early and midluteal phase, whereas declining StAR mRNA and protein levels are characteristic of late luteal phase. Moreover, StAR protein levels in the corpus luteum are highly correlated with plasma progesterone levels; suppression of LH levels during the midluteal phase markedly decreases plasma progesterone levels and abundance of StAR mRNA transcripts in the corpus luteum (Millar RP, et al., 2004).

4.1 Intra-ovarian control mechanisms

The growth of follicles and the function of the corpus luteum, while under the primary direction of the pituitary, are highly influenced by intra-ovarian factors that modulate the action of gonadotropins. These intra-ovarian factors most likely account for gonadotropin-independent follicular growth, observed differences in the rate and extent of development of ovarian follicles, arrest and initiation of meiosis, dominant follicle selection, and luteolysis. The list of potential paracrine factors that can influence steroid production by theca and granulosa cells is long and diverse. The previous theca cells lacked the aromatase enzyme that is necessary to produce estrogen (Schwanzel-Fukuda M, & Pfaff DW, 1984) so the production of estrogen in granulosa cells indicates presence of aromatase. It includes various growth factors, cytokines, peptide hormones, and steroids such as epidermal growth factor, transforming growth factor β (TGF-β), platelet-derived growth factor, fibroblast growth factors, transforming growth factor α (TGF-α), activins, inhibins, Anti-Müllerian hormone, insulin-like growth factors, estradiol, progesterone, and GnRH (Millar R: 2005; King JA, et al., 2002)

5. The peri-menopausal transition

There is only one marker, menstrual irregularity that can be used to objectively define and establish what is called the peri-menopausal transition. This irregularity will be perceived by patients as skipped menstrual periods or longer durations (about 40 to 60 days) between periods (Harlow SD, et al., 2008) There is no universal pattern; each woman will perceive a change that is her own individual characteristic alteration. Literally means "about or around the menopause." Generally speaking, the term "menopausal transition" is preferred over peri-menopause and climacteric.

The menopause is that point in time when permanent cessation of menstruation occurs following the loss of ovarian activity. Menopause is derived from the Greek words men (month) and pausis (cessation). The years prior to menopause that encompass the change from normal ovulatory cycles to cessation of menses are known as the peri-menopausal transitional years, marked by irregularity of menstrual cycles. Climacteric, an older, more general, and less precise term, indicates the period of time when a woman passes from the reproductive stage of life through the peri-menopausal transition and the menopause to the postmenopausal years (Treloar AE, et al., 1967). Menarche is followed by approximately 5–7 years of relatively long cycles at first, and then there is increasing regularity as cycles shorten to reach the usual reproductive age pattern. In the 40s, cycles begin to lengthen again. The highest incidence of anovulatory cycles is under age 20 and over age 40 (Collett ME, et al., 1954). At age 25, over 40% of cycles are between 25 and 28 days in length; from 25 to 35, over 60% are between 25 and 28 days. The perfect 28-day cycle is indeed the most common mode, but it totalled only 12.4% of Vollman's study cycles. Overall, approximately 15% of reproductive-age cycles are 28 days in length. Only 0.5% of women experience a cycle less than 21 days long, and only 0.9% a cycle greater than 35 days (Munster K, et al., 1992).

Most women have cycles that last from 24 to 35 days, but at least 20% of women experience irregular cycles (Belsey EM & Pinol APY, 1997). When women are in their 40s, anovulation becomes more prevalent, and prior to anovulation, menstrual cycle length increases, beginning 2 to 8 years before menopause (Treloar AE, et al., 1967). Cycles greater than 40 days in length are prevalent in the year before menopause (Ferrell RJ, et al) The duration of the follicular phase is the major determinant of cycle length (Sherman BM, et al) This menstrual cycle change prior to menopause is marked by elevated follicle-stimulating hormone (FSH) levels and decreased levels of inhibin, but normal levels of luteinizing hormone (LH) and slightly elevated levels of estradiol (Buckler HM, et al., 1991; MacNaughton J, et al., 1992; Hee J, et al., 1993; Burger HG, et al., 2000,2008). In the average woman, continuing follicular depletion and declining fertility begin at age 37–38, and menopause follows approximately 13 years later (average age 51). However, in epidemiologic studies approximately 10% of women in the general population become menopausal by the age of 45, probably because they were born with a smaller than normal ovarian follicular pool that is functionally depleted at an earlier age. Menopause occurs when the number of remaining follicles falls below a critical threshold, about 1,000, regardless of age (Treloar AE, 1981).

Recent longitudinal studies of women as they pass through the peri-menopausal transition reveal that estrogen levels do not begin a major decline until about a year before menopause. (Burger HG, et al., 2008; Lasley BL, et al., 2002). Indeed, women experiencing the peri-menopausal transition actually have higher overall estrogen levels, a response that is logically explained by an increased ovarian follicular reaction to the increase in FSH secretion during these years (Santoro N, et al). Variability in estrogen levels is characteristic of the peri-menopausal transition, with greater variability observed in menstrual cycles that display greater irregularity (Meyer PM, et al). As noted, most women experience a 2- to 8-year period of time prior to menopause when anovulation becomes common (Treloar AE, et al., 1996). During this period of time ovarian follicles continue their rate of loss until eventually the supply of follicles is finally depleted (Gougeon A, et al., 1994). The age-related changes in the endocrine characteristics of the menstrual cycle that result from progressive follicular depletion correlate with a measurable decrease in ovarian volume and in the number of antral follicles observed by trans-vaginal ultrasonography during the early follicular phase (Lass A, et al., 1997; Yong PY, et al., 2003; Frattarelli JL, et al., 2000; Dumesic DA, et al., 2001; Bancsi LF, et al., 2002; Kupesic S, et., 2003). The inverse and tight relationship between FSH and inhibin indicates that inhibin is a sensitive marker of ovarian follicular competence and, in turn, that FSH measurement is a clinical assessment of inhibin (MacNaughton J, et al., 1992; Hee J, et al., 1993). The decrease in inhibin secretion by the ovarian follicles begins early (around age 35), but accelerates after 40 years of age. This is reflected in the decrease in fecundity that occurs with aging. The major decrease in estradiol levels began about 2 years before menopause (Sowers MR, , et al., 2008). Declining levels of inhibin-B and Anti-Müllerian Hormone (AMH) reached a low to non-detectable point about 5 years before menopause (Sowers MR, et al., 2008).

Although the inhibin-B and AMH results are in general agreement with other reports, the exactness of the timing is limited by the fact that the blood samples were obtained from only 50 women in the study. Nevertheless, the Michigan study confirms the validity of AMH as a marker for the ovarian reserve of follicles. Unlike inhibin-B, AMH is not a participant in the feedback relationship between the ovary and the pituitary gonadotropins, rather AMH, a product of granulosa cells, reflects the number of follicles present in the ovaries awaiting FSH stimulation (Visser JA, et al). The variability in these measurements from individual to individual, however, precludes the practical use of these tests to predict with accuracy the future rate of menopause.The peri-menopausal years are a time period during which postmenopausal levels of FSH (greater than 20 IU/L) can be seen despite continued menstrual bleeding, while LH levels still remain in the normal range. Occasionally, corpus luteum formation and function occur, and the peri-menopausal woman is not safely beyond the risk of an unplanned and unexpected pregnancy until elevated levels of both FSH (>20 IU/L) and LH (>30 IU/L) can be demonstrated. The median age for the onset of this transition was 47.5 years. Only 10% of women ceased men-struating abruptly with no period of prolonged irregularity. The peri-menopausal transition from reproductive to post-reproductive status was, for most women, approximately 4 years in duration. In the study by Treloar, the average age for entry into the peri-menopausal transition was 45.1, and the age range that included 95% of the women was 39–51 (Treloar AE, 1996). The mean duration of the peri-menopausal transition was 5.0 years, with a range of 2 to 8 years.

5.1 Endocrine activity of the peri and post-menopausal ovary

As reviewed above, mean estradiol levels are normal or high in peri-menopausal women, and FSH levels are often not suppressed despite these high estradiol levels. These aspects of pituitary-ovarian relationships are contrary to expected physiology. It is proposed that, decreasing ovarian production of inhibin plays a role in the high average estrogen levels documented during the peri-menopause. More specifically, the B subtype of inhibin, a small peptide made in ovarian granulosa cells, which is known to be stimulated by FSH and, in turn, to suppress FSH, may play a role in the altered physiology of the peri-menopause (Klein NA, et al., 1996, 1998). Increasing evidence suggests that ovarian inhibin plays a role in ovarian folliculogenesis (McLachlan RI, et al., 1986; Hughes EG,,et al., 1992), therefore, new information about inhibin levels and their functional relationships in women in there forties and fifties becomes important.

The peri and post-menopausal ovary contains two different populations of cells with steroidogenic capacity: hilar cells and cortico stromal cells that may represent residual thecal elements (De Roux N, et al., 1999). In vitro studies suggest that the post-menopausal ovary has some steroidogenic potential. Incubation of post-menopausal ovarian stromal slices with pregnenolone yielded progesterone, dehydroepiandrosterone, and testosterone. Incubation of strips of ovarian hilar tissue from postmenopausal women revealed a steroidogenic pattern similar to that of the postmenopausal ovarian stroma. However, the overall amount of steroids produced was substantially greater compared with stroma. Measurable in vitro formation of estradiol by postmenopausal cortical stroma and hilar cells has also been reported (Bertherat J 1998: Ulloa-Aguirre A, et al., 1998).

With increasing age, the adrenal contribution of precursors for estrogen production proves inadequate. In this final stage of estrogen availability, levels are insufficient to sustain secondary sex tissues. Estrogens in peri and post-menopausal women appear to arise almost exclusively from extra-glandular aromatization of androstenedione (Arora KK, et al., 1997). Oophorectomy results in no significant reduction in urinary estrogen excretion by post-menopausal women. However, adrenalectomy after oophorectomy virtually eliminates measurable estrogens from the urine. In vitro studies concluded that the postmenopausal ovarian stroma is unable to aromatize androgens (Everest HM, et al., 2001). However, others have suggested that the post-menopausal ovary may synthesize limited amounts of estrogens, because the concentrations of estradiol and estrone are two times higher in ovarian venous blood than in peripheral blood of post-menopausal women (Illing N, et al., 1999).

There is some evidence that ovarian androgen production in post-menopausal women can be gonadotropin dependent. Administration of hCG to postmenopausal women results in a small increase in the circulating levels of testosterone (Sun YM, et al). Daily injection of hCG causes hyperplasia of the ovarian hilar cells and histochemical evidence suggestive of active steroidogenesis (Tensen C, et al., 1997). Administration of hCG, but not ACTH, resulted in increased androgen but not estrogen production by the ovaries (Wang L, et al., 2001). Binding sites for both LH and FSH were identified in the cortical stroma and in hilar cells (Davidson JS, et al., 1994). Addition of hCG to hilar cells results in increased cAMP formation and steroid biosynthesis, indicating preserved responsiveness to gonadotropins. Taken together, these observations suggest that ovarian androgen biosynthesis of the post-reproductive ovary is at least partially gonadotropin dependent.

The post-menopausal ovary is occasionally involved in pathologic endocrine activity. Stromal hyperplasia can occur, with the ovary enlarging with hyperplastic stromal nodules consisting of lipid-rich luteinized cells that resemble theca interna. The ovaries with stromal hyperplasia produce large amounts of androstenedione, resulting in hirsutism and virilisation (Vrecl M, et al., 1998). Hilar cells can give rise to functional hilar cell tumors, which produce excess amounts of androgens, leading to virilisation (Pawson AJ, et al., 1998; Blomenrohr M, et al., 1999; Heding A, et al., 2000). Signs and symptoms of estrogen excess may also be evident in circumstances of significant peripheral aromatization.

6. Treatment of anovulation

If no primary pathology is apparent, or if the primary pathology has been treated appropriately without restoration of normal endocrinology, treatment options lie between estrogen replacement (or the oral contraceptive in a younger woman) to prevent osteoporosis and ovulation induction to restore fertility. Estrogen antagonists usually are ineffective in inducing ovulation in progestogen-negative women, and treatment with pulsatile GnRH or gonadotropin treatment is normally required. (Elizur SE, et al., 2005). Treatment with pulsatile GnRH involves the woman carrying a small portable pump but has the important advantage of a lower multiple pregnancy rates than is seen with gonadotropin treatment. Women with a low LH concentration (<4 IU/L) require treatment with combined gonadotropin treatment regimens that include both FSH and LH bioactivity. The older urinary gonadotropin preparations have sufficient LH bioactivity, but when a recombinant FSH is used, it must be supplemented with recombinant LH or with a low dosage of urinary hCG.

6.1 Ovulation inductions and assisted reproduction

The reproductive period in women is characterized by their ability to ovulate. Ovulation, the release of an oocyte within the peritoneal cavity, follows rupture of a dominant follicle, developed in response to stimulation by endogenous gonadotropins. In the presence of normal fallopian tubes, the released oocyte will be able to interact with spermatozoa ascending the female genital tract. This may lead to production of the zygote and establishment of pregnancy if implantation occurs. When ovarian activity is disrupted, no ovulation takes place and, as a consequence, achievement of pregnancy is not feasible.

Ovulation induction refers to exogenous direct or indirect stimulation of the ovary with the aim of alleviating sub-fertility due to anovulation. Ovulation induction should be differentiated from *reestablishment of ovulation,* which occurs after treatment of conditions interfering with the normal function of the hypothalamic-pituitary-ovarian (HPO) axis. These include weight and eating disorders, thyroid dysfunction, hyper-prolactinemia, and excess exercise. It should also be differentiated from *enhancement of ovulation.* This is usually performed in ovulatory women with unexplained infertility in the hope of increasing the probability of pregnancy. More important, ovulation induction must be differentiated from superovulation for in vitro fertilization (IVF), in which the aim of ovarian stimulation is to induce multi-follicular development. This leads to the retrieval of multiple oocytes and thus allows the selection of the morphologically best embryo(s) for replacement. In IVF, follicular rupture is not necessary, because oocytes are collected by trans-vaginal aspiration (Pelinck MJ, et al., 2001; Castelo-Branco A, et al., 2004; Kolibianakis E, et al., 2002,2003).

6.2 Ovarian stimulation regimens

The ideal ovarian stimulation regimen for IVF should have a low cancellation rate, minimize drug costs, risks and side effects, require limited monitoring for practical convenience, and maximize singleton pregnancy rates. Numerous regimens have been described, ranging from no stimulation (natural cycles), to minimal stimulation (clomiphene citrate) or mild stimulation (sequential treatment with clomiphene citrate and low dose exogenous gonadotropins), to aggressive stimulation (high dose exogenous gonadotropins, alone or in combination with a gonadotropin-releasing hormone agonist or antagonist). Ovarian stimulation has been a basic element of IVF for more than 25 years, but concerns about multiple pregnancies and the costs of IVF have sparked renewed interest in natural cycle IVF and mild stimulation regimens (Nargund G, et al., 2001)

7. Natural cycle

The first birth resulting from IVF derived from a single oocyte collected in a natural ovulatory cycle (Steptoe PC, & Edwards RG, 1978). Compared to stimulated IVF cycles, natural cycle IVF offers a number of attractive advantages. Natural cycle IVF involves only monitoring the spontaneous cycle and retrieving a single oocyte before the midcycle LH surge occurs. It is physically less demanding, requires little or no medication, decreases costs by 75–80%, (Aboulghar MA, et al., 1995; Nargund G, et al., 2001) and all but eliminates risks for multiple pregnancy and ovarian hyper-stimulation syndrome (OHSS). The chief disadvantages of natural cycle IVF are high cancellation rates due to premature LH surges and ovulation, and the comparatively low success rate, which is approximately 7% (Pelinck MJ, et al., 2002). When oocyte retrieval is based on detection of the mid-cycle rise in LH, careful and frequent monitoring is required and procedures are difficult to schedule efficiently.

Alternatively, exogenous human chorionic gonadotropin (hCG) can be administered when the lead follicle reaches a size consistent with maturity, thereby better defining the optimum time for oocyte retrieval (Nargund G, et al., 2001). Adjuvant treatment with a GnRH antagonist also can be used to prevent a premature LH surge, but requires "add-back" treatment with exogenous FSH, and success rates are still quite low, ranging up to 14% per cycle in non-randomized trials (Castelo-Branco A, et al., 2004; Kolibianakis E, et al., 2002, 2003; Weghofer A, et al., 2004; Elizur SE, et al., 2005). In one large cohort study involving 844 treatment cycles in 350 good prognosis patients, the cancellation rate was 13%, the pregnancy rate was 8% per cycle and the cumulative pregnancy rate after three "modified natural IVF cycles" was 21% (Pelinck MJ, et al., 2002). In a cohort of infertile couples with male factor infertility, success rates in modified natural cycles have reached as high as 13% per cycle, with a cumulative pregnancy rate of 44% after six treatment cycles (Verberg MF, et al., 2006).

8. Clomiphene citrate

Clomiphene citrate (CC) was the first method of ovarian stimulation used in IVF, (Quigley MM, et al., 1984) but now has been almost entirely replaced by more effective stimulation regimens using human menopausal gonadotropins (hMG) or FSH, in combination with a GnRH agonist or antagonist (Macklon NS, et al., 2006). Clomiphene (100 mg daily) usually is administered for 5–8 days, beginning on cycle day 3, and induces development of two or more follicles in most normally ovulating women, (Dickey RP, et al., 1998; Messinis IE & Milingos SD 1998; Ingerslev HJ, et al., 2001) although egg yields 1–3, are only slightly greater than in un-stimulated cycles and substantially lower than in cycles stimulated with exogenous gonadotropins (Ingerslev HJ, et al., 2001; Branigan EF & Estes MA 2000; MacDougall MJ, Tan SL, Hall V, et al., 1996).

Cycle cancellation rates are somewhat lower than in natural cycles and the numbers of oocytes retrieved, embryos transferred, and pregnancy rates are greater. As in natural stimulates multi-follicular development more effectively than treatment with Clomiphene alone (Corfman RS, et al., 1993; Dor J, et al., 1992). Drug costs and monitoring requirements are moderately cycles, exogenous hCG is administered when the lead follicle reaches mature size and a GnRH antagonist can be used to prevent a premature endogenous LH surge. Sequential treatment with clomiphene (100 mg daily for 5 days) and modest doses of exogenous gonadotropins (150–225 IU daily beginning on the last day of clomiphene treatment or the day after) higher, but still substantially less than in standard stimulation regimens involving higher dose gonadotropin treatment after down-regulation with a long-acting GnRH agonist (described below) (Weigert M, et al., 2002; Dhont M, et al., 1995). In one comparative trial, higher cancellation rates and lower pregnancy rates were observed in sequential clomiphene/gonadotropin cycles (Dhont M, et al., 1995). In another, the sequential stimulation regimen yielded fewer oocytes and embryos, but pregnancy rates were similar and the risks of ovarian hyper-stimulation syndrome (OHSS) were lower (Weigert M, et al., 2002).

In a randomized trial, sequential clomiphene/gonadotropin stimulation and GnRH antagonist treatment yielded a pregnancy rate comparable to that achieved with a more aggressive standard treatment protocol, (Lin YH, et al., 2006) confirming the results of two earlier retrospective studies, (Fiedler K & Ludwig M 2003; Williams SC, et al., 2002), but contrasting with those of another observing lower pregnancy rates (Mansour R, et al., 2003).

9. GnRH agonist "flare" gonadotropins stimulation protocol

The "short" or "flare" protocol is an alternative stimulation regimen designed to exploit both the brief initial agonistic phase of response to a GnRH agonist and the suppression that results from longer-term treatment (Padilla SL, et al., 1996; Garcia JE, et al., 1990). In a typical standard short protocol, leuprolide acetate (1.0 mg daily) is administered on cycle days 2–4, continuing thereafter at a reduced dose (0.5 mg daily), and gonadotropin stimulation (225–450 IU daily) begins on cycle day 3. Later adjustments in the dose of gonadotropin stimulation, if needed, are based on response and indications for hCG administration are the same as in the long protocol (described above). An early meta-analysis including seven clinical trials comparing the short and long GnRH agonist treatment regimens determined that the two protocols yielded similar cancellation and pregnancy rates: (Hughes EG, et al., 1992).

A 2000 systematic review including 22 trials concluded that pregnancy rates achieved with the long protocol were superior to those using the flare regimen (OR=1.27, CI=1.04–1.56) overall, (Daya S., 2000), but the analysis did not control for diagnosis and other prognostic factors and results may not apply to all women, or to poor responders in particular. Whereas some have observed improved follicular response and lower cycle cancellation rates in poor responders treated with a flare protocol, pregnancy and live birth rates remained low (Karande V, et al., 1997; Karacan M, et al., 2001). Decreased scheduling flare exibility is a distinct disadvantage of the flare is protocol, unless the onset of menses is controlled by preliminary treatment with an OC. The regimen also can result in a significant increase in serum progesterone and androgen levels, presumably resulting from late corpus luteum rescue, (San Roman GA, et al., 1992) which may adversely affect oocyte quality and fertilization and pregnancy rates (Loumaye E, et al., 1989). The "OC micro-dose GnRH agonist flare" stimulation regimen is a variation of the standard short protocol involving 14–21 days of preliminary ovarian suppression with an OC (one pill daily), followed by micro-dose leuprolide treatment (40 µg twice daily) beginning 3 days after discontinuation of OC treatment, and high-dose gonadotropin stimulation (300–450 IU daily) starting on day 3 of leuprolide therapy. Indications for later gonadotropin dose adjustments and hCG administration are the same as in other stimulation regimens. Its primary advantage over the standard short protocol is that it does not induce any increases in serum progesterone or androgen concentrations, possibly because the doses of GnRH agonist administered are much lower, but likely also because preliminary OC treatment all but eliminates the possibility there may be a corpus luteum left to respond (Gonen Y, et al., 1990; Cedrin-Durnerin et al., 1996). The OC-micro-dose GnRH agonist flare protocol may be useful in previous poor responders, in whom it can stimulate increased endogenous FSH release and may yield lower cancellation rates and higher peak serum estradiol levels, transfer rates and pregnancy rates (Surrey ES, et al., 1998; Scott RT et al., 1994) GnRH Antagonist Gonadotropin Stimulation Protocol.

The introduction of GnRH antagonists into clinical practice provided another option for ovarian stimulation in ART. In contrast to the long-acting agonists, which first stimulate and later inhibit pituitary gonadotropin secretion by desensitizing gonadotropes to GnRH via receptor down-regulation, the antagonists block the GnRH receptor in a dose-dependent competitive fashion and have no similar flare effect (Matikainen T, et al., 1992; Reissmann T, et al., 1974,1995) gonadotropin suppression is almost immediate. GnRH antagonists offer several potential advantages over agonists. First, the duration of treatment for an antagonist is substantially shorter than for an agonist. Since its only purpose is to prevent a premature endogenous LH surge and its effects are immediate, antagonist treatment can be postponed until later in follicular development (after 5-6 days of gonadotropin stimulation), after estradiol levels are already elevated, thereby eliminating the estrogen deficiency symptoms that may emerge in women treated with an agonist (Olivennes F, et al., 2002).

Second, because any suppressive effects that agonists may exert on the ovarian response to gonadotropin stimulation also are eliminated, the total dose and duration of gonadotropin stimulation required is decreased (Olivennes F, et al., 2002; Albano C, et al., 2000). For the same reason, GnRH antagonist stimulation protocols may benefit women who are poor responders when treated with a standard long protocol (Olivennes F, et al., 2003; Akman MA, et al., 2001). Third, by eliminating the flare effect of agonists; GnRH antagonists avoid the risk of stimulating development of a follicular cyst. Finally, the risk of severe OHSS associated with use of antagonists also appears lower than with agonists. GnRH antagonists have some potential disadvantages. When administered in small daily doses, strict compliance with the prescribed treatment regimen is essential (Olivennes F, et al., 2002).

Antagonists suppress endogenous gonadotropin secretion more completely than agonists. Whereas the low levels of LH observed during agonist treatment are usually sufficient to support normal follicular steroid-genesis during stimulation with uFSH or rFSH, the even lower concentrations in women treated with an antagonist may not be. Indeed, serum estradiol levels may plateau or fall when antagonist treatment begins (Olivennes F, et al 2002;, de Jong D, et al., 2001). Although follicular growth appears unaffected, most prefer to add or substitute a low dose of hMG (75 IU) at the same time if it was not already part of the stimulation regimen. Evidence also suggests that pregnancy rates in antagonist treatment cycles may be modestly lower than in cycles using agonists in the long protocol (Al-Inany et al., 2006).

The two GnRH antagonists available for clinical use, ganirelix and cetrorelix, are equally potent and effective. For both, the minimum effective dose to prevent a premature LH surge is 0.25 mg daily, administered sub-cutaneously (Albano C, et al., 1997). Either can be administered in a series of small daily doses (0.25 mg). The treatment protocol may be fixed and begin after 5–6 days of gonadotropin stimulation, (Albano C, et al., 1997; Diedrich K, et al., 1994), or tailored to the response of the individual, starting treatment when the lead follicle reaches approximately 13–14 mm in diameter. The individualized treatment regimen generally requires fewer total doses and may yield better overall results (Ludwig M, et al., 2002). Alternatively, a single larger dose of cetrorelix (3.0 mg) will effectively prevent an LH surge for 96 hours. If given on day 6-7 of stimulation, the interval of effective suppression will encompass the day of hCG administration in most women (75–90%); the remainder may receive additional daily doses (0.25 mg) as needed, ending on the day of hCG treatment (Olivennes F, et al 1995; Olivennes F, et al., 2000; Olivennes F, et al., 2003). The single dose antagonist treatment regimen also can be withheld until the lead follicle reaches 13–14 mm in diameter (Fanchin R, et al., 2003,2005).

A common variation of the antagonist stimulation regimen uses preliminary treatment with an OC to control the onset of menses, typically ending approximately 5 days before the scheduled start, which also may help to synchronize the follicular cohort before stimulation begins. Another variation advocated for poor responders uses micronized estradiol (2 mg twice daily, administered orally, beginning on day 21 of the preceding cycle) to suppress FSH during the late luteal phase for the same purpose, ending on the day before gonadotropins stimulation begins, (Fanchin R, et al 2003, 2005), or continuing through the first 3 days of gonadotropin stimulation (Hill MJ, et al., 2009). The improved follicular dynamics observed are similar to those achieved by down-regulation with a GnRH agonist in the long protocol. The rebound increase in endogenous FSH levels that follows the discontinuation of estradiol treatment also may synergize with exogenous gonadotropins to promote multi-follicular development (de Ziegler D, et al., 1998; Fanchin R, et al., 2003). Results of a number of early trials comparing a fixed antagonist treatment protocol to the standard long protocol suggested that the two stimulation regimens yielded similar pregnancy rates (Albano C, et al., 2000; Olivennes F, et al., 2000); The European Middle East Orgalutran Study Group, 2001; Fluker M, et al., 2001). However, a 2006 systematic review and meta-analysis including 27 trials comparing different antagonist stimulation protocols with the long GnRH agonist protocol observed a significantly lower clinical pregnancy rate (OR=0.84, CI=0.72–0.97) and ongoing pregnancy/live birth rate (OR=0.82, CI=0.69–0.98). Overall, the total dose and duration of gonadotropin stimulation required, peak serum estradiol levels, and the number of follicles and oocytes were lower in antagonist cycles.

The explanation for the modestly lower pregnancy rates observed in antagonist treatment cycles is not clear. It is possible, but unlikely, that GnRH antagonists may have adverse effects on oocytes, embryos, or the endometrium (Hernandez ER 200; Ortmann O, et al., 2001). It is far more likely that early results reflected inexperience and improved with time and further refinements in the treatment regimen like those described above. Many of the advantages originally envisioned for GnRH antagonists already have been realized. Whether antagonists ultimately will replace agonists and become the standard ovarian stimulation regimen in ART cycles remains to be seen, but their place in the therapeutic arsenal already is firmly established. Whereas a single bolus injection of an agonist (leuprolide 0.5 mg, triptorelin 0.2 mg) triggers a physiologic LH surge that lasts less than 24 hours, hCG levels remain elevated for several days and stimulate markedly higher estradiol and progesterone concentrations (Fauser BC, et al., 2002).

The antagonist treatment regimens currently in use have potential disadvantages for women with PCOS. Their tonically elevated LH levels will remain high until antagonist treatment begins. Consequently, LH levels may rise prematurely, particularly if antagonist treatment is withheld until the lead follicle reaches 14 mm or more. Moreover, evidence indicates that increased LH exposure during early follicular development may be detrimental and predispose to lower pregnancy rates (Kolibianakis E, et al., 2002; Kolibianakis EM, et al., 2003; Kolibianakis EM, et al., 2003; Kolibianakis E, et al., 2003). In theory, pre-treatment with an OC might prove quite useful by suppressing LH and androgen levels before stimulation begins, decreasing exposure during early follicular development and the risk of rising LH levels before antagonist treatment starts. Preliminary OC suppression and later antagonist treatment may help to limit the follicular response to gonadotropin stimulation while preserving the option to use an agonist to trigger final oocyte maturation. These considerations simply serve to illustrate that GnRH antagonists are not a panacea and are not necessarily the best choice even for women with PCOS. Antagonist stimulation protocols are advocated for poor responders, primarily because they avoid the suppressive effects that agonists can have on follicular response and can prevent the premature LH surges observed commonly in women stimulated with gonadotropins alone (Surrey ES & Schoolcraft WB., 2000). However, evidence is insufficient to indicate they yield results consistently better than other stimulation regimens (Pandian Z, et al., 2010; Centers for Disease Control and Prevention, Atlanta, GA, 2009).

10. Ovarian reserve

The concept of ovarian reserve, generally defined as the size and quality of the remaining ovarian follicular pool, and the various methods for its measurement. The total number of oocytes in any given women is genetically determined and inexorably declines throughout life, from approximately 1-2 million at birth, to about 300,000 at puberty, 25,000 at age 40, and fewer than 1,000 at menopause (Battaglia DE, et al., 1996; Faddy MJ & Gosden RG, 1996). The rate of follicular depletion is not constant, but increases gradually as the number of follicles remaining decreases (Nilsson E, et al., 2007; Adhikari D & Liu K, 2009; Da Silva-Buttkus P, et al., 2009; Coxworth JE, & Hawkes K, 2010). As the size of the remaining follicular pool decreases, circulating inhibin-B levels (derived primarily from smaller antral follicles) decrease, resulting in lower levels of feedback inhibition and a progressive increase in serum follicle-stimulating hormone (FSH) levels, most noticeably during the early follicular phase (Klein NA, et al., 1996; Welt CK, McNicholl DJ, Taylor AE, et al; Hale GE, et al., 2007 ; Knauff EA, et al., 2009; Burger HG, et al., 2008). Increasing inter-cycle FSH concentrations stimulate earlier follicular recruitment, resulting in advanced follicular development early in the cycle, an earlier rise in serum estradiol levels, a shorter follicular phase, and decreasing overall cycle length (Klein NA, et al., 2002; de Koning CH, et al., 2008).

The physiology of reproductive aging provides the foundation for all contemporary tests of ovarian reserve. In clinical practice, the basal early follicular phase (cycle day 2-4) FSH level is the most common test, but antimüllerian hormone (AMH) and antral follicle count are alternatives having significant potential advantages. As basal FSH levels increase, peak estradiol levels during stimulation, the number of oocytes retrieved, and the probability for pregnancy or live birth decline steadily (Pearlstone AC, et al., 1992; Scott Jr RT & Hofmann GE, 1995; Bukman A, & Heineman MJ, 2001). With current assays (using IRP 78/549), FSH levels greater than 10 IU/L (10-20 IU/L) have high specificity (80-100%) for predicting poor response to stimulation, but their sensitivity for identifying such women is generally low (10-30%) and decreases with the threshold value (Broekmans FJ, et al., 2006) . Although most women who are tested have a normal result, including those with a diminished ovarian reserve (DOR), the test is still useful because those with abnormal results are very likely to have DOR. In a 2008 study, an FSH concentration above 18 IU/L had 100% specificity for failure to achieve a live birth (Scott Jr RT, et al., 2008). The basal serum estradiol concentration, by itself, has little value as an ovarian reserve test (Hazout A, et al., 2004; Eldar-Geva T, et al., 2005; McIlveen M, et al., 2007), but can provide additional information that helps in the interpretation of the basal FSH level. An early elevation in serum estradiol reflects advanced follicular development and early selection of a dominant follicle (as classically observed in women with advanced reproductive aging), and will suppress FSH concentrations, thereby possibly masking an otherwise obviously high FSH level indicating DOR. When the basal FSH is normal and the estradiol concentration is elevated (>60–80 pg/mL), the likelihood of poor response to stimulation is increased and the chance for pregnancy is decreased (Evers JL, et al., 1998; Buyalos RP, al., 1997). When both FSH and estradiol are elevated, ovarian response to stimulation is likely to be very poor. Antimüllerian hormone (AMH) derives from pre-antral and small antral follicles. Levels are gonadotropin-independent and vary little within and between cycles (Fanchin R, et al., 2005; Tsepelidis S, et al., 2007; Hehenkamp WJ, et al., 2006). The number of small antral follicles correlates with the size of the residual follicular pool and AMH levels decline progressively with age, becoming undetectable near the menopause (Sowers MR, et al., 2008; van Rooij IA, et al., 2004; van Rooij IA, et al., 2005).

10.1 Oocyte and ovarian tissue cryopreservation

Each year, cancer occurs in approximately 100 per 100,000 women under age 50 in the United States. Chemotherapy and radiation therapy for malignant and non-malignant systemic disease very often results in ovarian failure. Women with cancer and other serious illnesses requiring treatments that pose a serious threat to their future fertility have relatively few options. In some cases, the ovaries may be moved out of the radiation field. Treatment with GnRH agonists has been suggested as a way to protect the gonads from the insult of chemotherapy, but there is no convincing evidence for its efficacy. Although embryo banking is effective, the time required for stimulation and retrieval are often prohibitive. With recent advances in cryobiology, oocyte and ovarian tissue cryopreservation hold promise as methods to preserve reproductive potential (Shaw JM, et al., 2000).

10.2 Oocyte cryopreservation

Although the first pregnancy resulting from oocyte cryopreservation was reported in 1986, (Chen C, 1986), success rates achieved with the technology were historically very low, and only recently improving. The primary obstacle was the poor survival of oocytes, which are fragile due to their size, high water content, and chromosomal arrangement; the meiotic spindle is easily damaged by intracellular ice formation during freezing or thawing (Shaw JM, et al., 2000). Germinal vesicle stage oocytes are hardier, (Boiso I, et al., 2002), but progress with in vitro maturation of immature oocytes has been slow. Another obstacle was hardening of the zona pellucida, which interfered with normal fertilization. The improved survival of cryopreserved oocytes today relates primarily to modifications in the sucrose and sodium concentrations in traditional "slow-freeze" protocols, (Fabbri R, et al., 2001; Stachecki JJ & Willadsen SM, 2000; Bianchi V, et al., 2007; De Santis L, et al., 2007), changes.,

in the initial temperature of the cryoprotectant, and-seeding temperature (Trad FS, et al., 1999). Survival rates have been further improved with vitrification, a technique that uses high concentrations of cryoprotectant and rapid freezing by immersion in liquid nitrogen, preserving oocytes in a solid glass-like state without ice formation (Loutradi KE, et al., 2008; Oktay K, et al., 1997). With the use of intra-cytoplasmic sperm injection (ICSI), the hardened zona is not a barrier to fertilization (Polak de Fried E, et al., 1998). Survival, fertilization, and pregnancy rates achieved with cryopreserved oocytes are rap-idly improving and approaching those achieved with fresh oocytes (Grifo JA, & Noyes N, 2010; Nagy ZP, et al., 2009). A randomized comparison of results achieved with slow-freeze and vitrification observed that vitrification resulted in better oocyte survival (81% vs. 67%), fertilization (77% vs. 67%), and clinical pregnancy rates per thawed oocyte (5.2% vs. 1.7%).
A study examining outcomes achieved with vitrified donor oocytes observed 87% thaw survival, 87% fertilization, and 68% blastocyst formation, with 15/20 recipients (75%) achieving pregnancy after embryo transfer (Cobo A, Kuwayama M, Perez S, et al). Another using both slow-frozen and vitrified oocytes observed 92% survival, 79% fertilization, 42% implantation, and a 57% on going pregnancy rate (Grifo JA & Noyes N, 2010). Although the number of pregnancies and deliveries resulting from oocyte cryopreservation is still somewhat small, the number is rapidly increasing, and early perinatal outcomes data are reassuring. The incidence of chromosomal abnormalities in human embryos derived from cryopreserved oocytes is no different from that observed in control embryos derived from fresh oocytes (Gook DA, et al., 1994; Cobo A, et al., 2001). A study comparing outcomes in 200 infants derived from vitrified oocytes and in infants resulting from conventional fresh IVF found no differences in birth weight or in the incidence of birth defects (Chian RC, et al., 2008). A review of over 900 live births resulting from IVF of cryopreserved oocytes also observed no increase in the prevalence of congenital anomalies compared to that in the general population (Noyes N, et al., 2009). Oocyte cryopreservation is a viable fertility preservation strategy for women without partners seeking to preserve their fertility. Unfortunately few cancer patients have sufficient time to undergo ovarian stimulation before their treatment begins. The technology also holds enormous promise as a means to simplify oocyte donation, via egg banking, and is rapidly emerging as an elective fertility preservation strategy for women anticipating delayed childbearing and concerned about their future fertility. Currently, elective oocyte cryopreservation to defer reproductive aging is controversial, primarily because the great majority of outcomes data have come from experience with cryopreserved oocytes obtained from healthy young oocyte donors and cannot be extrapolated to older women who represent the majority of those expressing interest in elective oocyte cryopreservation (Rybak EA & Lieman HJ 2009; ASRM Practice Committee). However, when age-stratified outcomes data become available, allowing women to be accurately informed about their prognosis for success, elective oocyte cryopreservation may realistically offer women the means to set their "biological clock."

10.2.1 Ovarian tissue cryopreservation

At least in theory, ovarian tissue cryopreservation offers the means to freeze thousands of primordial follicles for later in vitro maturation or to store tissue for xenografting into an animal host or later auto transplantation (Jeruss JS, Woodruff TK., 2009). Currently, autologous transplantation of ovarian tissue seems the most practical and effective approach because the technique has successfully restored fertility to women with ovarian failure resulting from cancer chemotherapy (Andersen CY,, et al., 2008; Demeestere I, 2006,2010; et al; Silber SJ 2009). Ovarian tissue is removed surgically via laparoscopy or laparotomy and frozen using either a slow-cool or vitrification technique, before the insult expected to result in ovarian failure. Later, it can be thawed and transplanted back into the patient in or near its original location (orthotopic transplantation) or to another site, such as the forearm or abdominal wall (heterotopic transplantation). The advantage of orthotopic transplantation is that pregnancy might be achieved without assistance, whereas heterotopic transplantation requires IVF (Jeruss JS & Woodruff TK. 2009). Live births have been achieved after transplantation of frozen-thawed ovarian tissue in sheep, (Candy CJ et al., 2000) and the first live birth in a primate after a fresh heterotopic ovarian transplantation has been reported (Lee DM, et al). Human oocytes have been obtained from heterotopic transplants and fertilized in vitro to yield embryos for transfer, resulting in a biochemical pregnancy (Rosendahl M, et al., 2006). The only human pregnancy achieved after heterotopic transplantation was achieved without assistance, indicating that the oocyte from which it arose came from the patient's existing ovary rather than from the transplant. Orthotopic transplantation has been successfully achieved in humans.

A number of live births have been reported after autologous orthotopic transplantation of cryopreserved ovarian tissue. Frozen ovarian tissue also has been transplanted successfully between monozygotic twin sisters after the receiving twin developed premature ovarian failure (Silber SJ, & Gosden RG, 2007). A 2008 systematic review identified 25 reports describing a total of 46 cases of ovarian tissue transplantation for treatment of premature ovarian failure or infertility, although most involved transplantation of fresh rather than frozen ovarian tissue (Bedaiwy MA, et al., 2008). The mean time to return of ovarian function was 120 days (range 60–244 days) and data were insufficient to evaluate function beyond 1 year. Fresh grafts were more likely to succeed, and in 25 women who sought pregnancy, eight conceived nine pregnancies. At least one potential risk of ovarian tissue cryopreservation and auto-transplantation is reseeding of tumor cells in women with malignancies. Future research focusing on defining patient suitability, tissue collection methods, and cryopreservation protocols is certainly warranted, but until effective techniques and the possibility for success can be defined, ovarian tissue cryopreservation will remain investigational and cannot be justified solely for the purpose of future use in healthy women.

11. References

Aboulghar MA, Mansour RT, Serour GA, Amin YM, Sattar MA, Ramzy AM, In vitro fertilization in a spontaneous cycle: a successful simple protocol, J Obstet Gynaecol (Tokyo 1995) 21:337, 1995.

Adhikari D, Liu K, Molecular mechanisms underlying the activation of mammalian primordial follicles, Endocr Rev; 30:438, 2009.

Ahmed-Ebbiary NA, Lenton EA, Cooke ID: Hypothalamic-pituitary ageing: progressive increases in FSH and LH concentrations throughout the reproductive life in regularly menstruating women. Clin Endocrinol; 41:199-206. 1994.

Akman MA, Erden HF, Tosun SB, Bayazit N, Aksoy E, Bahceci M, Comparison of agonistic fl are-up-protocol and antagonistic multiple dose protocol in ovarian stimulation of poor responders: results of a prospective randomized trial, Hum Reprod 16:868, 2001.

Albano C, Felberbaum RE, Smitz J, Riethmuller-Winzen H, Engel J, Diedrich K, Devroey P, Ovarian stimulation with HMG: results of a prospective randomized phase III European study comparing the luteinizing hormone-releasing hormone (LHRH)-antagonist cetrorelix and the LHRH-agonist buserelin. European Cetrorelix Study Group, Hum Reprod 15:526, 2000.

Albano C, Smitz J, Camus M, Riethmuller-Winzen H, Van Steirteghem A, Devroey P, Comparison of different doses of gonadotropin-releasing hormone antagonist Cetrorelix during controlled ovarian hyperstimulation, Fertil Steril 67:917, 1997.

Al-Inany HG, Abou-Setta AM, Aboulghar M, Gonadotrophinreleasing hormone antagonists for assisted conception, Cochrane Database Syst Rev 3:CD001750, 2006.

Anasti JN: Premature ovarian failure: an update. Fertil Steril 70:1-15. 1998.

Andersen CY, Rosendahl M, Byskov AG, Loft A, Ottosen C, Dueholm M, Schmidt KL, Andersen AN, Ernst E, Two successful pregnancies following autotransplantation of frozen/thawed ovarian tissue, Hum Reprod 23:2266, 2008.

Arora KK, Cheng Z, Catt KJ: Mutations of the conserved DRS motif in the second intracellular loop of the gonadotropin-releasing hormone receptor affect expression, activation, and internalization. Mol Endocrinol; 11:1203-1212. 1997.

Bancsi LF, Broekmans FJ, Eijkemans MJ, de Jong FH, Habbema JD, te Velde ER, Predictors of poor ovarian response in in vitro fertilization: a prospective study comparing basal markers of ovarian reserve, Fertil Steril 77:328, 2002.

Battaglia DE, Goodwin P, Klein NA, Soules MR, Influence of maternal age on meiotic spindle assembly in oocytes from naturally cycling women, Hum Reprod 11:2217, 1996.

Bedaiwy MA, El-Nashar SA, El Saman AM, Evers JL, Sandadi S, Desai N, Falcone T, Reproductive outcome after transplantation of ovarian tissue: a systematic review, Hum Reprod 23:2709, 2008.

Belsey EM, Pinol APY, and Task Force on Long-Acting Systemic Agents for Fertility Regulation, Menstrual bleeding patterns in untreated women, Contraception 55:57, 1997.

Bertherat J: Gonadotropin-releasing hormone receptor gene mutation: a new cause of hereditary hypogonadism and another mutated G-protein-coupled receptor. Eur J Endocrinol; 138:621-622. 1998.

Bianchi V, Coticchio G, Distratis V, Di Giusto N, Flamigni C, Borini A, Differential sucrose concentration during dehydration (0.2mol/l) and rehydration (0.3 mol/l) increases the implantation rate of frozen human oocytes, Reprod Biomed Online 14:64, 2007.

Blomenrohr M, Heding A, Sellar R, et al: Pivotal role for the cytoplasmic carboxyl-terminal tail of a nonmammalian gonadotropin-releasing hormone receptor in cell surface expression, ligand binding, and receptor phosphorylation and internalization. Mol Pharmacol; 56:1229-1237. 1999.

Boiso I, Marti M, Santalo J, Ponsa M, Barri PN, Veiga A, A confocal microscopy analysis of the spindle and chromosome configurations of human oocytes cryopreserved at the germinal vesicle and metaphase II stage, Hum Reprod 17:1885, 2002.

Branigan EF, Estes MA, Minimal stimulation IVF using clomiphene citrate and oral contraceptive pill pre-treatment for LH suppression, Fertil Steril 73:587, 2000.

Braunstein GD, Sundwall DA, Katz M, et al: Safety and efficacy of a testosterone patch for the treatment of hypoactive sexual desire disorder in surgically menopausal women: a randomized, placebo-controlled trial. Arch Intern Med; 165:1582-1589. 2005.

Broekmans FJ, Kwee J, Hendriks DJ, Mol BW, Lambalk CB, A systematic review of tests predicting ovarian reserve and IVF outcome, Hum Reprod Update 12:685, 2006.

Bromberger JT, Matthews KA, Kuller LH, et al: Prospective study of the determinants of age at menopause. Am J Epidemiol; 145:124-133. 1997.

Buckler HM, Evans A, Mamlora H, Burger HG, Anderson DC, Gonadotropin, steroid and inhibin levels in women with incipient ovarian failure during anovulatory and ovulatory 'rebound' cycles, J Clin Endocrinol Metab 72:116, 1991.

Bukman A, Heineman MJ, Ovarian reserve testing and the use of prognostic models in patients with subfertility, Hum Reprod Update 7:581, 2001.

Burger HD, Dudley EC, Hooper JL, et al: The endocrinology of the menopausal transition: a cross-sectional study of a population-based sample. J Clin Endocrinol Metab ; 80:3537-3545. 1995.

Burger HG 1993 Editorial: Clinical utility of inhibin measurements. J Clin Endocrinol Metab 76:1391–1396.

Burger HG, Dudley E, Manners P, Groome N, Robertson DM, Early follicular phase serum FSH as a function of age: the roles of inhibin B, inhibin A and estradiol, Climacteric 3:17, 2000.

Burger HG, Dudley EC, Cui J, et al: A prospective longitudinal study of serum testosterone, dehydroepiandrosterone sulfate, and sex hormone-binding globulin levels through the menopause transition. J Clin Endocrinol Metab; 85:2832-2838. 2000.

Burger HG, Dudley EC, Robertson DM, et al: Hormonal changes in the menopause transition. Recent Prog Horm Res; 57:257-275. 2002.

Burger HG, Hale GE, Dennerstein L, Robertson DM, Cycle and hormone changes during perimenopause: the key role of ovarian function, Menopause 15:603, 2008.

Burger HG, Hale GE, Dennerstein L, Robertson DM, Cycle and hormone changes during perimenopause: the key role of ovarian function, Menopause 15:603, 2008.

Burger HG, Hale GE, Robertson DM, et al: A review of the hormonal changes during the menopausal transition: focus on findings from the Melbourne Women's Midlife Health Project. Hum Reprod Update; 13:559-565. 2007.

Buyalos RP, Daneshmand S, Brzechffa PR, Basal estradiol and follicle-stimulating hormone predict fecundity in women of advanced reproductive age undergoing ovulation induction therapy, Fertil Steril 68:272, 1997.

Candy CJ, Wood MJ, Whittingham DG, Restoration of a normal reproductive lifespan after grafting of cryopreserved mouse ovaries, Hum Reprod 15:1300, 2000.

Castelo-Branco A, Frydman N, Kadoch J, Le Du A, Fernandez H, Fanchin R, Frydman R, The role of the semi natural cycle as option of treatment of patients with a poor prognosis for successful in vitro fertilization, J Gynecol Obstet Biol Reprod (Paris) 33:518, 2004.

Cedrin-Durnerin I, Bulwa S, Herve F, Martin-Pont B, Uzan M, Hugues JN, The hormonal fl are-up following gonadotrophin-releasing hormone agonist administration is influenced by a progestogen pretreatment, Hum Reprod 11:1859, 1996.

Centers for Disease Control and Prevention, 2007 Assisted Reproductive Technology Success Rates. National Summary and Fertility Clinic Reports. Atlanta, GA, 2009.

Chian RC, Huang JY, Tan SL, Lucena E, Saa A, Rojas A, Ruvalcaba astellon LA, Garcia Amador MI, Montoya Sarmiento JE, Obstetric and perinatal outcome in 200 infants conceived from vitrified oocytes, Reprod Biomed Online 16:608, 2008.

Cobo A, Kuwayama M, Perez S, Ruiz A, Pellicer A, Remohi J, Comparison of concomitant outcome achieved with fresh and cryopreserved donor oocytes vitrifi ed by the Cryotop method, Fertil Steril 89:1657, 2008.

Cobo A, Rubio C, Gerli S, Ruiz A, Pellicer A, Remohi J, Use of fluorescence in situ hybridization to assess the chromosomal status of embryos obtained from cryopreserved oocytes, Fertil Steril 75:354, 2001.

Collett ME, Wertenberger GE, Fiske VM, The effect of age upon the pattern of the menstrual cycle, Fertil Steril 5:437, 1954.

Colombat de L'Isere M: Diseases of Women. American edition translated by Meigs CD. Cited by Ricci JV. One Hundred Years of Gynaecology 1800–1900 (1850) Philadelphia, Blakiston Co. p 532. 1945.

Corfman RS, Milad MP, Bellavance TL, Ory SJ, Erickson LD, Ball GD, A novel ovarian stimulation protocol for use with the assisted reproductive technologies, Fertil Steril 60:864, 1993.

Couzinet B, Meduri G, Lecce MG, et al: The postmenopausal ovary is not a major androgen-producing gland. J Clin Endocrinol Metab; 86:5060-5066. 2001.

Coxworth JE, Hawkes K, Ovarian follicle loss in humans and mice: lessons from statistical model comparison, Hum Reprod 25:1796, 2010.

Cramer DW, Xu H, Harlow BL: Does "incessant" ovulation increase risk for early menopause?. Am J Obstet Gynecol ; 172:568-573. 1995.

Da Silva-Buttkus P, Marcelli G, Franks S, Stark J, Hardy K, Inferring biological mechanisms from spatial analysis: prediction of a local inhibitor in the ovary, Proc Natl Acad Sci U S A 106:456, 2009.

Davidson JS, Wakefield IK, Millar RP: Absence of rapid desensitization of the mouse gonadotropin-releasing hormone receptor. Biochem J; 300:299-302. 1994.

Daya S, Gonadotropin releasing hormone agonist protocols for pituitary desensitization in in vitro fertilization and gamete intrafallopian transfer cycles, Cochrane Database Syst Rev: CD001299, 2000.

De Jong D, Macklon NS, Eijkemans MJ, Mannaerts BM, Coelingh Bennink HJ, Fauser BC, Dynamics of the development of multiple follicles during ovarian stimulation for in vitro fertilization using recombinant follicle-stimulating hormone (Puregon) and various doses of the gonadotropin-releasing hormone antagonist ganirelix (Orgalutran/Antagon), Fertil Steril 75:688, 2001.

De Koning CH, McDonnell J, Themmen AP, de Jong FH, Homburg R, Lambalk CB, The endocrine and follicular growth dynamics throughout the menstrual cycle in women with consistently or variably elevated early follicular phase FSH compared with controls, Hum Reprod 23:1416, 2008.

De Roux N, Young J, Brailly-Tabard S, et al: The same molecular defects of the gonadotropin-releasing hormone receptor determine a variable degree of hypogonadism in affected kindred. J Clin Endocrinol Metab; 84:567-572. 1999.

De Santis L, Cino I, Rabellotti E, Papaleo E, Calzi F, Fusi FM, Brigante C, Ferrari A, Oocyte cryopreservation: clinical outcome of slow-cooling protocols differing in sucrose concentration, Reprod Biomed Online 14:57, 2007.

De Ziegler D, Jaaskelainen AS, Brioschi PA, Fanchin R, Bulletti C, Synchronization of endogenous and exogenous FSH stimuli in controlled ovarian hyperstimulation (COH), Hum Reprod 13:561, 1998.

Demeestere I, Simon P, Buxant F, Robin V, Fernandez SA, Centner J, Delbaere A, Englert Y, Ovarian function and spontaneous pregnancy after combined heterotopic and orthotopic cryopreserved ovarian tissue transplantation in a patient previously treated with bone marrow transplantation: case report, Hum Reprod 21:2010, 2006.

Dhont M, Onghena A, Coetsier T, De Sutter P, Prospective randomized study of clomiphene citrate and gonadotrophins versus goserelin and gonadotrophins for follicular stimulation in assisted reproduction, Hum Reprod 10:791, 1995.

Dickey RP, Taylor SN, Rye PH, Lu PY, Future use of clomiphene in ovarian stimulation. A role for clomiphene in the 21st century?, Hum Reprod 13:2361, 1998.

Diedrich K, Diedrich C, Santos E, Zoll C, al-Hasani S, Reissmann T, Krebs D, Klingmuller D, Suppression of the endogenous luteinizing hormone surge by the gonadotrophin-releasing hormone antagonist Cetrorelix during ovarian stimulation, Hum Reprod 9:788, 1994.

Dor J, Ben-Shlomo I, Levran D, Rudak E, Yunish M, Mashiach S, The relative success of gonadotropin-releasing hormone analogue, clomiphene citrate, and gonadotropin in 1,099 cycles of in vitro fertilization, Fertil Steril 58:986, 1992.

Dumesic DA, Damario MA, Session DR, Famuyide A, Lesnick TG, Thornhill AR, McNeilly AS, Ovarian morphology and serum hormone markers as predictors of ovarian follicle recruitment by gonadotropins for in vitro fertilization, J Clin Endocrinol Metab 86:2538, 2001.

Eldar-Geva T, Ben-Chetrit A, Spitz IM, Rabinowitz R, Markowitz E, Mimoni T, Gal M, Zylber-Haran E, Margalioth EJ, Dynamic assays of inhibin B, anti-Mullerian hormone and estradiol followingFSH stimulation and ovarian ultrasonography as predictors of IVF outcome, Hum Reprod 20:3178, 2005.

El-Hage G, Eden JA, Manga RZ: A double-blind, randomized, placebo-controlled trial of the effect of testosterone cream on the sexual motivation of menopausal hysterectomized women with hypoactive sexual desire disorder. Climacteric; 10:335-343. 2007

Elizur SE, Aslan D, Shulman A, Weisz B, Bider D, Dor J, Modified natural cycle using GnRH antagonist can be an optional treatment in poor responders undergoing IVF, J Assist Reprod Genet 22:75, 2005.

Everest HM, Hislop JN, Harding T, et al: Signalling and anti-proliferative effects mediated by GnRH receptors after expression in breast cancer cells using recombinant adenovirus. Endocrinology; 142:4663-4672. 2001.

Evers JL, Slaats P, Land JA, Dumoulin JC, Dunselman GA, Elevated levels of basal estradiol-17beta predict poor response in patients with normal basal levels of follicle-stimulating hormone undergoing in vitro fertilization, Fertil Steril 69:1010, 1998.

Fabbri R, Porcu E, Marsella T, Rocchetta G, Venturoli S, Flamigni C, Human oocyte cryopreservation: new perspectives regarding oocyte survival, Hum Reprod 16:411, 2001.

Faddy MJ, Gosden RG, A model conforming the decline in follicle numbers to the age of menopause in women, Hum Reprod 11:1484, 1996.

Fanchin R, Cunha-Filho JS, Schonauer LM, Kadoch IJ, Cohen- Bacri P, Frydman R, Coordination of early antral follicles by luteal estradiol administration provides a basis for alternative controlled ovarian hyperstimulation regimens, Fertil Steril 79:316, 2003.

Fanchin R, Cunha-Filho JS, Schonauer LM, Righini C, de Ziegler D, Frydman R, Luteal estradiol administration strengthens the relationship between day 3 follicle-stimulating hormone and inhibin B levels and ovarian follicular status, Fertil Steril 79:585, 2003.

Fanchin R, Salomon L, Castelo-Branco A, Olivennes F, Frydman N, Frydman R, Luteal estradiol pre-treatment coordinates follicular growth during controlled ovarian hyperstimulation with GnRH antagonists, Hum Reprod 18:2698, 2003.

Fanchin R, Taieb J, Lozano DH, Ducot B, Frydman R, Bouyer J, High reproducibility of serum anti-Mullerian hormone measurements suggests a multi-staged follicular secretion and strengthens its role in the assessment of ovarian follicular status, Hum Reprod 20:923, 2005.

Fauser BC, de Jong D, Olivennes F, Wramsby H, Tay C, Itskovitz- Eldor J, van Hooren HG, Endocrine profiles after triggering of final oocyte maturation with GnRH agonist after co-treatment with the GnRH antagonist ganirelix during ovarian hyper-stimulation for in vitro fertilization, J Clin Endocrinol Metab 87:709, 2002.

Ferrell RJ, Simon JA, Pincus SM, Rodríguez G, O'Connor KA, Holman DJ, Weinstein M, The length of perimenopausal menstrual cycles increases later and to a greater degree than previously reported, Fertil Steril 86:619, 2006.

Fiedler K, Ludwig M, Use of clomiphene citrate in in vitro fertilization (IVF) and IVF/intracytoplasmic sperm injection cycles, Fertil Steril 80:1521, 2003.

Findlay JK, Xiao S, Shukovski L The role of inhibin-related peptides as intragonadal regulators. Reprod Fertil Dev 2:205–218. 1990.

Fluker M, Grifo J, Leader A, Levy M, Meldrum D, Muasher SJ, Rinehart J, Rosenwaks Z, Scott Jr RT, Schoolcraft W, Shapiro DB, Effi cacy and safety of ganirelix acetate versus leuprolide acetate in women undergoing controlled ovarian hyperstimulation, Fertil Steril 75:38, 2001.

Frattarelli JL, Lauria-Costab DF, Miller BT, Bergh PA, Scott RT, Basal antral follicle number and mean ovarian diameter predict cycle cancellation and ovarian responsiveness in assisted reproductive technology cycles, Fertil Steril 74:512, 2000.

Garcia JE, Padilla SL, Bayati J, Baramki TA, Follicular phase gonadotropin-releasing hormone agonist and human gonadotropins: a better alternative for ovulation induction in in vitro fertilization, Fertil Steril 53:302, 1990.

Gold EB, Bromberger J, Crawford S, et al: Factors associated with age at natural menopause in a multiethnic sample of midlife women. Am J Epidemiol; 153:865-874. 2001.

Gonen Y, Jacobson W, Casper RF, Gonadotropin suppression with oral contraceptives before in vitro fertilization, Fertil Steril 53:282, 1990.

Gook DA, Osborn SM, Bourne H, Johnston WI, Fertilization of human oocytes following cryopreservation; normal karyotypes and absence of stray chromosomes, Hum Reprod 9:684, 1994.

Gougeon A, Echochard R, Thalabard JC, Age-related changes of the population of human ovarian follicles: increase in the disappearance rate of non-growing and early-growing follicles in aging women, Biol Reprod 50:653, 1994.

Grifo JA, Noyes N, Delivery rate using cryopreserved oocytes is comparable to conventional in vitro fertilization using fresh oocytes: potential fertility preservation for female cancer patients, Fertil Steril 93:391, 2010.

Grifo JA, Noyes N, Delivery rate using cryopreserved oocytes is comparable to conventional in vitro fertilization using fresh oocytes: potential fertility preservation for female cancer patients, Fertil Steril 93:391, 2010.

Haisenleder DJ, Dalkin AC, Ortolano GA, et al: A pulsatile gonadotropin-releasing hormone stimulus is required to increase transcription of the gonadotropin subunit genes: evidence for differential regulation of transcription by pulse frequency in vivo. Endocrinology; 128:509-517. 1991.

Hale GE, Zhao X, Hughes CL, Burger HG, Robertson DM, Fraser IS, Endocrine features of menstrual cycles in middle and late reproductive age and the menopausal transition classifi ed according to the Staging of Reproductive Aging Workshop (STRAW) staging system, J Clin Endocrinol Metab 92:3060, 2007.

Hall JE, Lavoie HG, Marsh EE, et al: Decrease in gonadotropin-releasing hormone pulse frequency with aging in postmenopausal women. J Clin Endocrinol Metab; 85:1794-1800. 2000.

Harlow SD, Mitchell ES, Crawford S, Nan B, Little R, Taffe J, for the ReSTAGE Collaboration, The ReSTAGE Collaboration: defining optimal bleeding criteria for onset of early menopausal transition, Fertil Steril 89:129, 2008.

Hazout A, Bouchard P, Seifer DB, Aussage P, Junca AM, Cohen- Bacrie P, Serum anti-mullerian hormone/mullerian-inhibiting substance appears to be a more discriminatory marker of assisted reproductive technology outcome than follicle-stimulating hormone, inhibin B, or estradiol, Fertil Steril 82:1323, 2004.

Heding A, Vrecl M, Hanyaloglu AC, et al: The rat gonadotropin-releasing hormone receptor internalizes via a beta arrestin independent, but dynamin-dependent, pathway: addition of a carboxyl-terminal tail confers beta-arrestin dependency. Endocrinology; 141:299-306. 2000.

Hee J, MacNaughton J, Bangah M, Burger HG, Perimenopausal patterns of gonadotrophins, immunoreactive inhibin, oestradiol and progesterone, Maturitas 18:9, 1993.

Hehenkamp WJ, Looman CW, Themmen AP, de Jong FH, Te Velde ER, Broekmans FJ, Anti-Mullerian hormone levels in the spontaneous menstrual cycle do not show substantial fluctuation, J Clin Endocrinol Metab 91:4057, 2006.

Hernandez ER, Embryo implantation and GnRH antagonists: embryo implantation: the Rubicon for GnRH antagonists, Hum Reprod 15:1211, 2000.

Hill MJ, McWilliams GD, Miller KA, Scott Jr RT, Frattarelli JL, A luteal estradiol protocol for anticipated poor-responder patients may improve delivery rates, Fertil Steril 91:739, 2009.

Hreinsson JG, Scott JE, Rasmussen C, et al: Growth differentiation factor-9 promotes the growth, development, and survival of human ovarian follicles in organ culture. J Clin Endocrinol Metab; 87:316-321. 2002.

Hughes EG, Fedorkow DM, Daya S, Sagle MA, Van de Koppel P, Collins JA, The routine use of gonadotropin-releasing hormone agonists prior to in vitro fertilization and gamete intrafallopian transfer: a meta-analysis of randomized controlled trials, Fertil Steril 58:888, 1992.

Hughes EG, Robertson DM, Handelsman DJ, Hayward S, Healy DL, DeKrester DM Inhibin and estradiol responses to ovarian hyper stimulation: effects of age and predictive value for in vitro fertilization outcome. J Clin Endocrinol Metab, 70:358–364.,1990.

Illing N, Troskie BE, Nahorniak CS, et al: Two gonadotropin-releasing hormone receptor subtypes with distinct ligand selectivity and differential distribution in brain and pituitary in the goldfish (Carassius autatus). Proc Natl Acad Sci U S A; 96:2256-2531. 1999

Ingerslev HJ, Hojgaard A, Hindkjaer J, Kesmodel U, A randomized study comparing IVF in the unstimulated cycle with IVF following clomiphene citrate, Hum Reprod 16:696, 2001.

Ismael NN: A study of the menopause in Malaysia. Maturitas; 19:205-209. 1994.

Jeruss JS, Woodruff TK, Preservation of fertility in patients with cancer, New Engl J Med 360:902, 2009.

Kaiser UB, Jakubowiak A, Steinberger A, et al: Differential effects of gonadotropin-releasing hormone (GnRH) pulse frequency on gonadotropin subunit and GnRH receptor messenger ribonucleic acid levels in vitro. Endocrinology; 138:1224-1231. 1997.

Karacan M, Erkan H, Karabulut O, Sarikamis B, Camlibel T, Benhabib M, Clinical pregnancy rates in an IVF program. Use of the flare-up protocol after failure with long regimens of GnRH-a, J Reprod Med 46:485, 2001.

Karande V, Morris R, Rinehart J, Miller C, Rao R, Gleicher N, Limited success using the "fl are" protocol in poor responders in cycles with low basal follicle-stimulating hormone levels during in vitro fertilization, Fertil Steril 67:900, 1997.

King JA, Millar RP: Coordinated evolution of GnRHs and their receptors. In: Parhar, IS, Sakuma Y, ed. GnRH Neurones: Gene to Behavior, Toyko: Brain Shuppan;:51-77. 1997.

King JA, Millar RP: Structure of chicken hypothalamic luteinizing hormone-releasing hormone. II. Isolation and characterization. J Biol Chem; 257:10729-10732. 1982.

Klein NA, Battaglia DE, Miller PB, Branigan EF, Giudice LC, Soules MR, Ovarian follicular development and the follicular fluid hormones and growth factors in normal women of advanced reproductive age, J Clin Endocrinol Metab 81:1946, 1996.

Klein NA, Harper AJ, Houmard BS, Sluss PM, Soules MR, Is the short follicular phase in older women secondary to advanced or accelerated dominant follicle development?, J Clin Endocrinol Metab 87:5746, 2002.

Klein NA, Illingworth PJ, Groome NP, McNeilly AS, Battaglia AS, Soules MR Decreased inhibin B secretion is associated with the monotropic FSH rise in older, ovulatory women: a study of serum and follicular fluid levels of dimeric inhibin A and B in spontaneous menstrual cycles. J Clin Endocrinol Metab, , 81:7:2742–2745. 1996.

Klein NA, Soules MR: Endocrine changes of the perimenopause. Clin Obstet Gynecol;41:912-920.1998.

Knauff EA, Eijkemans MJ, Lambalk CB, ten Kate-Booij MJ, Hoek A, Beerendonk CC, Laven JS, Goverde AJ, Broekmans FJ, Themmen AP, de Jong FH, Fauser BC, Anti-Mullerian hormone, inhibin B, and antral follicle count in young women with ovarian failure, J Clin Endocrinol Metab 94:786, 2009.

Kolibianakis E, Bourgain C, Albano C, Osmanagaoglu K, Smitz J, Van Steirteghem A, Devroey P, Effect of ovarian stimulation with recombinant follicle-stimulating hormone, gonadotropin releasing hormone antagonists, and human chorionic gonadotropin on endometrial maturation on the day of oocyte pick-up, Fertil Steril 78:1025, 2002.

Kolibianakis E, Zikopoulos K, Albano C, Camus M, Tournaye H, Van Steirteghem A, Devroey P, Reproductive outcome of polycystic ovarian syndrome patients treated with GnRH antagonists and recombinant FSH for IVF/ICSI, Reprod Biomed Online 7:313, 2003.

Kolibianakis E, Zikopoulos K, Camus M, Tournaye H, Van Steirteghem A, Devroey P, Modified natural cycle for IVF does not offer a realistic chance of parenthood in poor responders with high day 3 FSH levels, as a last resort prior to oocyte donation, Hum Reprod 19:2545, 2004.

Kolibianakis EM, Albano C, Camus M, Tournaye H, Van Steirteghem AC, Devroey P, Relationship between LH and oestradiol in IVF cycles before GnRH antagonist initiation, Reprod Biomed Online 7:190, 2003.

Kolibianakis EM, Albano C, Kahn J, Camus M, Tournaye H, Van Steirteghem AC, Devroey P, Exposure to high levels of luteinizing hormone and estradiol in the early follicular phase of gonadotropinreleasing hormone antagonist cycles is associated with a reduced chance of pregnancy, Fertil Steril 79:873, 2003.

Kupesic S, Kurjak A, Bjelos D, Vujisic S, Three-dimensional ultrasonographic ovarian measurements and in vitro fertilization outcome are related to age, Fertil Steril 79:190, 2003.

Lasley BL, Santoro N, Randolph JF, Gold EB, Crawford S, Weiss G, McConnell DS, Sowers MF, The relationship of circulating dehydroepiandrosterone, testosterone, and estradiol to stages of the menopausal transition and ethnicity, J Clin Endocrinol Metab 87:3760, 2002.

Lass A, Skull J, McVeigh E, Margara R, Winston RM, Measurement of ovarian volume by transvaginal sonography before human menopausal gonadotrophin superovulation for in-vitro fertilization can predict poor response, Hum Reprod 12:294, 1997.

Lee DM, Yeoman RR, Battaglia DE, Stouffer RL, Zelinski- Wooten MB, Fanton JW, Wolf DP, Live birth after ovarian tissue transplant, Nature 428:137, 2004.

Lin YH, Hwang JL, Seow KM, Huang LW, Hsieh BC, Tzeng CR, Comparison of outcome of clomiphene citrate/human menopausal gonadotropin/cetrorelix protocol and buserelin long protocol—a randomized study, Gynecol Endocrinol 22:297, 2006.

Lobo RA: Treatment of the Postmenopausal Woman. Basic and Clinical Aspects. 2nd ed. Baltimore, Lippincott Williams & Wilkins, p 67. 1999.

Loffler KA, Zarkower D, Koopman P: Etiology of ovarian failure in blepharophimosis ptosis epicanthus inversus syndrome: FOXL2 is a conserved, early-acting gene in vertebrate ovarian development. Endocrinology; 144:3237-3243. 2003.

Longscope C, Franz C, Morello C, et al: Steroid and gonadotropin levels in women during the perimenopausal years. Maturitas ; 8:189-196. 1986.

Loumaye E, Vankrieken L, Depreester S, Psalti I, de Cooman S, Thomas K, Hormonal changes induced by short-term administration of gonadotropin-releasing hormone agonist during ovarian hyper-stimulation for in vitro fertilization and their consequences for embryo development, Fertil Steril 51:105, 1989.

Loutradi KE, Kolibianakis EM, Venetis CA, Papanikolaou EG, Pados G, Bontis I, Tarlatzis BC, Cryopreservation of human embryos by vitrifi cation or slow freezing: a systematic review and meta-analysis, Fertil Steril 90:186, 2008.

Ludwig M, Katalinic A, Banz C, Schroder AK, Loning M, Weiss JM, Diedrich K, Tailoring the GnRH antagonist cetrorelix acetate to individual patients' needs in ovarian stimulation for IVF: results of a prospective, randomized study, Hum Reprod 17:2842, 2002.

MacDougall MJ, Tan SL, Hall V, Balen A, Mason BA, Jacobs HS, Comparison of natural with clomiphene citrate-stimulated cycles in in vitro fertilization: a prospective, randomized trial, Fertil Steril 61:1052, 1994.

Macklon NS, Stouffer RL, Giudice LC, Fauser BC, The science behind 25 years of ovarian stimulation for in vitro fertilization, Endocr Rev 27:170, 2006.

MacNaughton J, Bangah M, McCloud P, Hee J, Burger HG, Age related changes in follicle stimulating hormone, luteinizing hormone, oestradiol and immunoreactive inhibin in women of reproductive age, Clin Endocrinol 36:339, 1992.

Mansour R, Aboulghar M, Serour GI, Al-Inany HG, Fahmy I, Amin Y, The use of clomiphene citrate/human menopausal gonadotropins in conjunction with GnRH antagonist in an IVF/ICSI program is not a cost effective protocol, Acta Obstet Gynecol Scand 82:48, 2003.

Marshall JC, Dalkin AC, Haisenleder DJ, et al: GnRH pulses-the regulators of human reproduction. Trans Am Clin Climatol Assoc; 104:31-46. 1993.

Matikainen T, Ding YQ, Vergara M, Huhtaniemi I, Couzinet B, Schaison G, Differing responses of plasma bioactive and immunoreactive follicle-stimulating hormone and luteinizing hormone to gonadotropin-releasing hormone antagonist and agonist treatments in postmenopausal women, J Clin Endocrinol Metab 75:820, 1992.

McIlveen M, Skull JD, Ledger WL, Evaluation of the utility of multiple endocrine and ultrasound measures of ovarian reserve in the prediction of cycle cancellation in a high-risk IVF population, Hum Reprod 22:778, 2007.

McKinlay SM, Brambilla DJ, Posner JG: The normal menopause transition. Am J Hum Biol.; 4:37-46. 1992.

McLachlan RI, Robertson DM, Healy DL, de Kretser DM, Burger HG Plasma inhibin levels during gonadotropin-induced ovarian hyper stimulation for IVF: a new index of follicular function? Lancet 1:1233–1234. 1986.

Messinis IE, Milingos SD, Future use of clomiphene in ovarian stimulation. Clomiphene in the 21st century, Hum Reprod 13:2362, 1998.

Meyer PM, Zeger SL, Harlow SD, Sowers M, Crawford S, Luborsky JL, Janssen I, McConnell DS, Randolph JF, Weiss G, Characterizing daily urinary hormone profi les for women at midlife using functional data analysis, Am J Epidemiol 165:936, 2007.

Millar R: Brain Peptides Section. In: Kastin AJ, ed. Handbook on Biologically Active Peptides, Burlington, MA: Elsevier;:635-644. 2005.

Millar RP, Lu Z-L, Pawson AJ, et al: Gonadotropin-releasing hormone receptors. Endocr Rev; 25(2):235-275. 2004.

Millar RP: Gonadotropin-releasing hormones and their receptors. In: Fauser BCJM, ed. Reproductive medicine: molecular cellular and genetic fundamentals, Lancaster: Parthenon Publishing; 2002:199-224.

Munster K, Schmidt L, Helm P, Length and variation in the menstrual cycle—a cross-sectional study from a Danish county, Br J Obstet Gynaecol 99:422, 1992.

Nagy ZP, Chang CC, Shapiro DB, Bernal DP, Elsner CW, Mitchell-Leef D, Toledo AA, Kort HI, Clinical evaluation of the efficiency of an oocyte donation program using egg cryo-banking, Fertil Steril 92:520, 2009.

Nargund G, Waterstone J, Bland J, Philips Z, Parsons J, Campbell S, Cumulative conception and live birth rates in natural (unstimulated) IVF cycles, Hum Reprod 16:259, 2001.

Nilsson E, Rogers N, Skinner MK, Actions of anti-Mullerian hormone on the ovarian transcriptome to inhibit primordial to primary follicle transition, Reproduction 134:209, 2007.

Noyes N, Porcu E, Borini A, Over 900 oocyte cryopreservation babies born with no apparent increase in congenital anomalies, Reprod Biomed Online 18:769, 2009.

Oktay K, Cil AP, Bang H, Effi ciency of oocyte cryopreservation: a meta-analysis, Fertil i R, Seracchioli R, Ciotti PM, Magrini O, Flamigni C, Birth of a healthy female after intracytoplasmic sperm injection of cryopreserved human oocytes, Fertil Steril 68:724, 1997.

Olivennes F, Alvarez S, Bouchard P, Fanchin R, Salat-Baroux J, Frydman R, The use of a GnRH antagonist (Cetrorelix) in a single dose protocol in IVF-embryo transfer: a dose fi nding study of 3 versus 2 mg, Hum Reprod 13:2411, 1998.

Olivennes F, Belaisch-Allart J, Emperaire JC, Dechaud H, Alvarez S, Moreau L, Nicollet B, Zorn JR, Bouchard P, Frydman R, Prospective, randomized, controlled study of in vitro fertilization-embryo transfer with a single dose of a luteinizing hormone-releasing hormone (LH-RH) antagonist (cetrorelix) or a depot formula of an LH-RH agonist (triptorelin), Fertil Steril 73:314, 2000.

Olivennes F, Cunha-Filho JS, Fanchin R, Bouchard P, Frydman R, The use of GnRH antagonists in ovarian stimulation, Hum Reprod Update 8:279, 2002.

Olivennes F, Diedrich K, Frydman R, Felberbaum RE, Howles CM, Safety and effi cacy of a 3 mg dose of the GnRH antagonist cetrorelix in preventing premature LH surges: report of two large multicentre, multinational, phase IIIb clinical experiences, Reprod Biomed Online 6:432, 2003.

Ortmann O, Weiss JM, Diedrich K, Embryo implantation and GnRH antagonists: ovarian actions of GnRH antagonists, Hum Reprod 16:608, 2001.

Padilla SL, Dugan K, Maruschak V, Shalika S, Smith RD, Use of the fl are-up protocol with high dose human follicle stimulating hormone and human menopausal gonadotropins for in vitro fertilization in poor responders, Fertil Steril 65:796, 1996.

Pandian Z, McTavish AR, Aucott L, Hamilton MP, Bhattacharya S, Interventions for 'poor responders' to controlled ovarian hyper-stimulation (COH) in in-vitro fertilization (IVF). Cochrane Database Syst Rev 20:CD004379, 2010.

Pawson AJ, Katz A, Sun YM, et al: Contrasting internalization kinetics of human and chicken gonadotropin-releasing hormone receptors mediated by C-terminal tail. J Endocrinol 1998; 156:R9-12.

Pearlstone AC, Fournet N, Gambone JC, Pang SC, Buyalos RP, Ovulation induction in women age 40 and older: the importance of basal follicle-stimulating hormone level and chronological age, Fertil Steril 58:674, 1992.

Pelinck MJ, Hoek A, Simons AH, Heineman MJ, Efficacy of natural cycle IVF: a review of the literature, Hum Reprod Update 8:129, 2002.

Pelinck MJ, Vogel NE, Hoek A, Simons AH, Arts EG, Mochtar MH, Beemsterboer S, Hondelink MN, Heineman MJ, Cumulative pregnancy rates after three cycles of minimal stimulation IVF and results according to subfertility diagnosis: a multicentre cohort study, Hum Reprod 21:2375, 2006.

Polak de Fried E, Notrica J, Rubinstein M, Marazzi A, Gomez Gonzalez M, Pregnancy after human donor oocyte cryopreservation and thawing in association with intracytoplasmic sperm injection in a patient with ovarian failure, Fertil Steril 69:555, 1998.

Practice Committee of the American Society for Reproductive Medicine, ASRM Practice Committee resonse to Rybak and Lieman: elective self-donation of oocytes, Fertil Steril 92:1513, 2009.

Quigley MM, Schmidt CL, Beauchamp PJ, Pace-Owens S, Berkowitz AS, Wolf DP, Enhanced follicular recruitment in an in vitro fertilization program: clomiphene alone versus a clomiphene/ human menopausal gonadotropin combination, Fertil Steril 42:25, 1984.

Rannevik G, Jeppsson S, Johnell O, et al: A longitudinal study of the perimenopausal transition: altered profiles of steroid and pituitary hormones, SHBG, and bone mineral density. Maturitas; 21:103-113. 1995.

Reissmann T, Felberbaum R, Diedrich K, Engel J, Comaru- Schally AM, Schally AV, Development and applications of luteinizing hormone-releasing hormone antagonists in the treatment of infertility: an overview, Hum Reprod 10:1974, 1995.

Reynaud K, Cortvrindt R, Smitz J, et al: Alterations in ovarian function of mice reduced amounts of KIT receptor. Reproduction; 121:229-237.2001.

Robertson DM, Burger HG: Reproductive hormones: ageing and the perimenopause. Acta Obstet Gynecol Scand; 81:612. 2002.

Rosendahl M, Loft A, Byskov AG, Ziebe S, Schmidt KT, Andersen AN, Ottosen C, Andersen CY, Biochemical pregnancy after fertilization of an oocyte aspirated from a heterotopic autotransplant of cryopreserved ovarian tissue: case report, Hum Reprod 21: 2006.

Rossmanith WG, Scherbaum WA, Lauritzen C: Gonadotropin secretion during aging in postmenopausal women. Neuroendocrinology 1991; 54:211-218.

Rybak EA, Lieman HJ, Egg freezing, procreative liberty, and ICSI: the double standards confronting elective self-donation of oocytes, Fertil Steril 92:1509, 2009.

San Roman GA, Surrey ES, Judd HL, Kerin JF, A prospective randomized comparison of luteal phase versus concurrent follicular phase initiation of gonadotropin-releasing hormone agonist for in vitro fertilization, Fertil Steril 58:744, 1992.

Santoro N, Banwell T, Tortoriello D, et al: Effects of aging and gonadal failure on the hypothalamic-pituitary axis in women. Am J Obstet Gynecol; 178:732-741. 1998.

Santoro N, Brown JR, Adel T, Skurnick JH, Characterization of reproductive hormonal dynamics in the perimenopause, J Clin Endocrinol Metab 81:1495, 1996.

Santoro N: The menopause transition: an update. Hum Reprod Update; 8:155-160. 2002.

Schwanzel-Fukuda M, Pfaff DW: Origin of luteinizing hormone-releasing hormone neurons. Nature; 338:161-164. 1989.

Schwingl PJ, Hulka BS, Harlow SD: Risk factors for menopausal hot flashes. Obstet Gynecol 1994; 64:29.

Scott Jr RT, Elkind-Hirsch KE, Styne-Gross A, Miller KA, Frattarelli JL, The predictive value for in vitro fertility delivery rates is greatly impacted by the method used to select the threshold between normal and elevated basal follicle-stimulating hormone, Fertil Steril 89:868, 2008.

Scott Jr RT, Hofmann GE, Prognostic assessment of ovarian reserve, Fertil Steril 63:1, 1995.

Scott RT, Navot D, Enhancement of ovarian responsiveness with microdoses of gonadotropin-releasing hormone agonist during ovulation induction of in vitro fertilization, Fertil Steril 61:880, 1994.

Seifer DB, Gardiner AC, Lambert-Messerlian G, Schneyer AL Differential secretion of dimeric inhibin in cultured luteinized granulosa cells as a function of ovarian reserve. J Clin Endocrinol Metab 81:7:736–739. 1996.

Shaw JM, Oranratnachai A, Trounson AO, Fundamental cryobiology of mammalian oocytes and ovarian tissue, Theriogenology 53:59, 2000.

Sherman BM, West JH, Korenman SG, The menopausal transition: analysis of LH, FSH, estradiol, and progesterone concentrations during menstrual cycles of older women, J Clin Endocrinol Metab 42:629, 1976.

Silber SJ, Fresh ovarian tissue and whole ovary transplantation, Seminars Reprod Med 27:479, 2009.

Silber SJ, Gosden RG, Ovarian transplantation in a series of monozygotic twins discordant for ovarian failure, New Engl J Med 356:1382, 2007.

Soules MR, Sherman S, Parrott E, et al: Executive summary: Stages of Reproductive Aging Workshop (STRAW). Fertil Steril; 76:874-878. 2001.

Sowers MR, Eyvazzadeh AD, McConnell D, Yosef M, Jannausch ML, Zhang D, Harlow SD, Randolph Jr. JF, Anti-müllerian hormone and inhibin B in the defi nition of ovarian aging and the menopause transition, J Clin Endocrinol Metab 93:3478, 2008.

Sowers MR, Eyvazzadeh AD, McConnell D, Yosef M, Jannausch ML, Zhang D, Harlow S, Randolph Jr JF, Anti-mullerian hormone and inhibin B in the defi nition of ovarian aging and the menopause transition, J Clin Endocrinol Metab 93:3478, 2008.

Sowers MR, Zheng H, McConnell D, Nan B, Harlow SD, Randolph Jr. JF, Estradiol rates of change in relation to the final menstrual period in a population-based cohort of women, J ClinEndocrinol Metab 93:3847, 2008.

Speroff L, Glass H, Kase NG: Clinical Gynecologic Endocrinology and Infertility. 6th ed. Baltimore, Lippincott Williams & Wilkins, p 116. 1999.

Stachecki JJ, Willadsen SM, Cryopreservation of mouse oocytes using a medium with low sodium content: effect of plunge temperature, Cryobiology 40:4, 2000.

Steptoe PC, Edwards RG, Birth after the reimplantation of a human embryo, Lancet 2:366, 1978.

Sun YM, Flanagan CA, Illing N, et al: A chicken gonadotropin-releasing hormone receptor that confers agonist activity to mammalian antagonists. Identification of D-Lys(6) in the ligand and extracellular loop two of the receptor as determinants. J Biol Chem ; 276:7754-7761. 2001.

Surrey ES, Bower J, Hill DM, Ramsey J, Surrey MW, Clinical and endocrine effects of a micro-dose GnRH agonist fl are regimen administered to poor responders who are undergoing in vitro fertilization, Fertil Steril 69:419, 1998.

Surrey ES, Schoolcraft WB, Evaluating strategies for improving ovarian response of the poor responder undergoing assisted reproductive techniques, Fertil Steril 73:667, 2000.

Tamada T, Iwasake H: Age at natural menopause in Japanese women. Nippon Sanka Fujinka Gakkai Zasshi; 47:947-952. 1995.

Tensen C, Okuzawa K, Blomenrohr M, et al: Distinct efficacies for two endogenous ligands on a single cognate gonadoliberin receptor. Eur J Biochem ; 243:134-140,1997.

The European Middle East Orgalutran Study Group, Comparable clinical outcome using the GnRH antagonist ganirelix or a long protocol of the GnRH agonist triptorelin for the prevention of premature LH surges in women undergoing ovarian stimulation, Hum Reprod 16:644, 2001.

Tibilette MG, Testa G, Vegetti W, et al: The idiopathic forms of premature menopause and early menopause show the same genetic pattern. Hum Reprod ; 14:2731-2734. 1999.

Trad FS, Toner M, Biggers JD, Effects of cryoprotectants and ice seeding temperature on intracellular freezing and survival of human oocytes, Hum Reprod 14:1569, 1999.

Treloar AE, Boynton RE, Borghild GB, Brown BW, Variation of the human menstrual cycle through reproductive life, Int J Fertil 12:77, 1967.

Treloar AE, Menstrual cyclicity and the pre-menopause, Maturitas 3:249, 1981.

Tsepelidis S, Devreker F, Demeestere I, Flahaut A, Gervy C, Englert Y, Stable serum levels of anti-Mullerian hormone during the menstrual cycle: a prospective study in normo-ovulatory women, Hum Reprod 22:1837, 2007.

Ulloa-Aguirre A, Stanislaus D, Arora V, et al: The third intracellular loop of the rat gonadotropin-releasing hormone receptor couples the receptor to Gs- and G(q/11)-mediated signal transduction pathways: evidence from loop fragment transfection in GGH3 cells. Endocrinology 1998; 139:2472-2478.

Utian WH: The International Menopause Society. Menopause-related terminology definitions. Climacteric; 2:284-286. 1999.

van Rooij IA, Broekmans FJ, Scheffer GJ, Looman CW, Habbema JD, de Jong FH, Fauser BJ, Themmen AP, te Velde ER, Serum antimullerian hormone levels best refl ect the reproductive decline with age in normal women with proven fertility: a longitudinal study, Fertil Steril 83:979, 2005.

van Rooij IA, Tonkelaar I, Broekmans FJ, Looman CW, Scheffer GJ, de Jong FH, Themmen AP, te Velde ER, Anti-mullerian hormone is a promising predictor for the occurrence of the menopausal transition, Menopause 11:601, 2004.

Verberg MF, Macklon NS, Nargund G, Frydman R, Devroey P, Broekmans FJ, Fauser BC, Mild ovarian stimulation for IVF, Hum Reprod Update 15:13, 2009.

Visser JA, De Jong FH, Laven JS, Themmen AP, Anti-müllerian hormone: a new marker for ovarian function, Reproduction 131:1, 2006.

Vrecl M, Anderson L, Hanyaloglu A, et al: Agonist-induced endocytosis and recycling of the gonadotropin-releasing hormone receptor: effect of beta-arrestin on internalization kinetics. Mol Endocrinol; 12:1818-1829. 1998.

Wang L, Bogerd J, Choi HS, et al: Three distinct types of gonadotropin-releasing hormone receptor characterized in the bullfrog. Proc Natl Acad Sci U S A 2001; 98:361-366.

Weel AE, Utterlinden AG, Westendorp IC, et al: Estrogen receptor polymorphism predicts the onset of natural and surgical menopause. J Clin Endocr Metab; 84:3146-3150. 1999.

Weghofer A, Margreiter M, Bassim S, Sevelda U, Beilhack E, Feichtinger W, Minimal stimulation using recombinant follicle stimulating hormone and a gonadotropin-releasing hormone antagonist in women of advanced age, Fertil Steril 81:1002, 2004.

Weigert M, Krischker U, Pohl M, Poschalko G, Kindermann C, Feichtinger W, Comparison of stimulation with clomiphene citrate in combination with recombinant follicle-stimulating hormone and recombinant luteinizing hormone to stimulation with a gonadotropin-releasing hormone agonist protocol: a prospective, randomized study, Fertil Steril 78:34, 2002.

Welt CK, McNicholl DJ, Taylor AE, Hall JE, Female reproductive aging is marked by decreased secretion of dimeric inhibin, J Clin Endocrinol Metab 84:105, 1999.

Whiteman MK, Staropoli CA, Benedict JC, et al: Risk factors for hot flashes in midlife women. J Women's Health; 12:459-472. 2003.

WHO Scientific Group: Research on Menopause in the 1990s. Report of a WHO Scientific Group. WHO Technical Report Series 866. Geneva, World Health Organization, 1996.

Williams SC, Gibbons WE, Muasher SJ, Oehninger S, Minimal ovarian hyperstimulation for in vitro fertilization using sequential clomiphene citrate and gonadotropin with or without the addition of a gonadotropin-releasing hormone antagonist, Fertil Steril 78:1068, 2002.

Yong PY, Baird DT, Thong KJ, McNeilly AS, Anderson RA, Prospective analysis of the relationships between the ovarian follicle cohort and basal FSH concentration, the inhibin response to exogenous FSH and ovarian follicle number at different stages of the normal menstrual cycle and after pituitary down-regulation, Hum Reprod 18:35, 2003.

Zapantis G, Santoro N: Ovarian ageing and the menopause transition. Best Pract Res Clin Obstet Gynaecol 2002; 16:263-276. Psychiatry; 60:29-36. 2003.

Zumoff B, Straw GW, Miller LK, et al: Twenty-four hour mean plasma testosterone concentration declines with age in normal premenopausal women. J Clin Endocrinol Metab; 80:1429-1430. 1995